Critical Care Pediatric Nephrology and Dialysis: A Practical Handbook

Sidharth Kumar Sethi • Rupesh Raina
Mignon McCulloch • Timothy E. Bunchman
Editors

Critical Care Pediatric Nephrology and Dialysis: A Practical Handbook

Springer

Editors
Sidharth Kumar Sethi
Kidney & Urology Institute
Medanta, The Medicity Kidney
& Urology Institute
Gurugram, Haryana
India

Mignon McCulloch
Red Cross War Memorial Children's Hospital
University of Cape Town
Cape Town
South Africa

Rupesh Raina
Department of Nephrology
Cleveland Clinic Akron General Medical
center and Akron Children's Hospital
Akron, OH
USA

Timothy E. Bunchman
Pediatric Nephrology
Children's Hospital of Richmond at the
Virginia Commonwealth University
Richmond, VA
USA

ISBN 978-981-13-2275-4 ISBN 978-981-13-2276-1 (eBook)
https://doi.org/10.1007/978-981-13-2276-1

Library of Congress Control Number: 2018966698

This Springer imprint is published by the registered company Springer Nature Singapore Pte Ltd.
The registered company address is: 152 Beach Road, #21-01/04 Gateway East, Singapore 189721, Singapore

Dedicated to our patients who are our teachers

Contents

Part V Outcomes

Part VI Advances

About the Editors

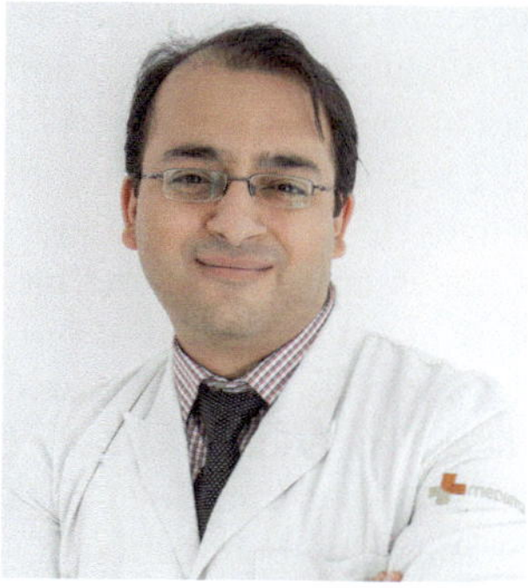

Sidharth Kumar Sethi is a Senior Consultant in Pediatric Nephrology and Pediatric Renal Transplant Medicine at the Kidney and Urology Institute, Medanta, India. He completed his fellowship (International Pediatric Nephrology Association Fellowship) and senior residency in Pediatric Nephrology at the All India Institute of Medical Sciences, New Delhi, and the Division of Pediatric Nephrology and Transplant Immunology at Cedars Sinai Medical Centre, Los Angeles, California. He has been involved in numerous national and international meetings on pediatric acute kidney injury and pediatric dialysis. His chief interests include acute kidney injury, dialysis, and pediatric renal transplantation. He has been actively involved in the care of children with all kinds of complex renal disorders, including acute kidney injury, nephrotic syndrome, tubular disorders, urinary tract infections, hypertension, and chronic kidney disease. He was honored by Case Western Reserve University for his outstanding contributions to the field in 2014. He was part of an eight-member committee responsible for writing the Indian guidelines on steroid-sensitive nephrotic syndrome and member of an expert committee involved in the formulation of guidelines on pediatric renal disorders, including steroid-resistant nephrotic syndrome and urinary tract infections. He has published several international papers on pediatric nephrology and chapters in nephrology textbooks. He is also Co-Convener of the Indian Society of Pediatric Nephrology-CKD Registry. He is currently Secretary of the Indian Society of Pediatric Nephrology and Editor of the *Journal of Clinical Pediatric Nephrology*.

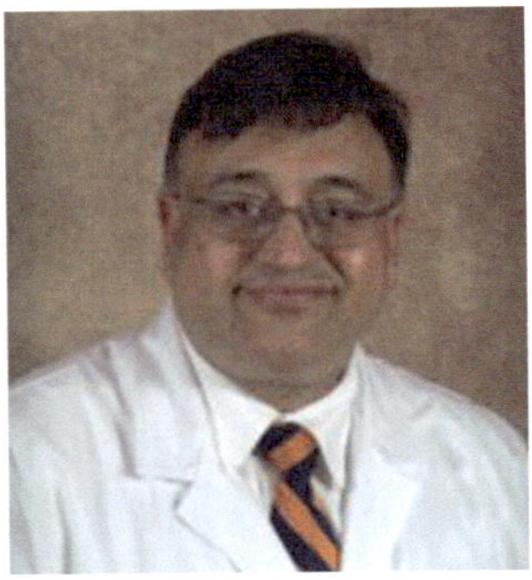

Rupesh Raina is an Associate Professor and currently a combined Adult and Pediatric Nephrologist and Director of Medical Research in Internal Medicine at the Cleveland Clinic Foundation's Akron General Medical Center and the Akron Children's Hospital. He is also a member of the faculty and research staff at Case Western Reserve University School of Medicine. Dr. Raina is a member of the University Council of Medicine at Northeast Ohio Medical University. His research interests include the pathophysiology and prevention of the progression of renal cystic disease, transition of nephrology care from pediatrics to adults, renal replacement therapy, and high-flow ultrafiltration for management of inborn errors of metabolism. He has a particular interest in developing medical curricula and case-based workshops to enhance medical students' and residents' clinical knowledge. He has trained numerous scientists and clinical researchers from the United States and abroad and has written several peer-reviewed articles, editorials, and book chapters related to biomedical research and clinical activities. He is currently a member of the National Kidney Foundation's Medical Advisory Board; fellow of the American College of Physicians, the American Association of Pediatrics, and the American Society of Nephrology; and fellow and board member of the National Kidney Foundation.

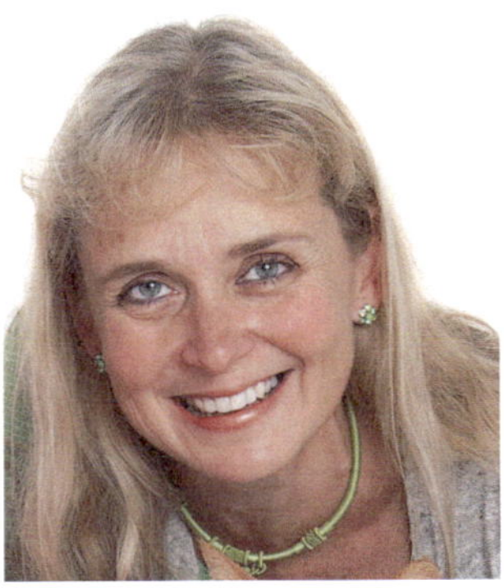

Mignon McCulloch is currently a Pediatric Nephrologist and Consultant at the Pediatric Intensive Care Unit at the Red Cross War Memorial Children's Hospital, Cape Town, as well as a Senior Lecturer at the University of Cape Town, South Africa. She is also an Honorary Consultant at Evelina London Children's Hospital, United Kingdom. Her interests include developing pediatric nephrology and care of critically ill children, specifically acute kidney injury (AKI), and all forms of dialysis in infants and children especially in poorly resourced regions, adolescent transition, and pediatric transplantation (renal, liver, and cardiac). She is the current President Elect of the International Pediatric Transplant Association (IPTA), Assistant Secretary of International Pediatric Nephrology Association (IPNA), and President of the African Pediatric Nephrology Association. She is actively involved in the "Saving Young Lives (SYL)" steering committee—providing hands-on training in pediatric dialysis to teams of doctors and nurses at residential courses, including bedside PD catheter insertion, vascular access training, basic resuscitation, and all forms of dialysis.

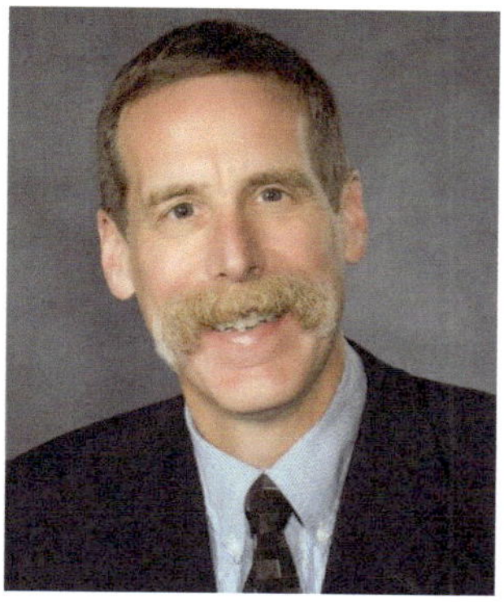

Timothy E. Bunchman is currently tenured Professor and Division Chief, Children's Hospital of Richmond at Virginia Commonwealth University (VCU), USA. His primary departmental program area is Pediatric Nephrology. He is trained in Pediatric Nephrology from the University of Minnesota, Minneapolis. His areas of expertise and interest are pediatric transplantation, acute kidney injury, renal replacement therapy, and vasculitis. He has published papers in international journals and contributed chapters in books on pediatric nephrology and pediatric critical care. He has multiple awards to his credit and has been nominated by the American Society of Pediatric Nephrology to the National Advisory Committee on Children and Disasters (NACCD). He is on the editorial board of many reputed international journals including *Pediatric Critical Care Medicine*, *Pediatric Nephrology*, and *Nephrology Dialysis Transplantation*. He has also been an Associate Editor for the *American Journal of Kidney Diseases*. He is the organizer and program director of the International Conference on Pediatric Continuous Renal Replacement Therapy (PCRRT) endorsed by the International Pediatric Nephrology Association (IPNA) as well as the critical care section of the American Academy of Pediatrics (AAP).

Part I

Acute Kidney Injury in a Sick Child

Acute Kidney Injury: Definitions and Epidemiology

1

Neziha Celebi and Ayse Akcan Arikan

Case 1

An 11-year-old female with history of acute myeloid leukemia who underwent bone marrow transplant 34 days ago developed fever to 104 °F; her blood pressure was 50/20 and heart rate was 180 beats/min. On physical exam she appeared lethargic, pale, and cold to touch. She was empirically started on broad-spectrum antibiotics and underwent emergency resuscitation with multiple fluid boluses ultimately requiring intubation and pressor support. Her urine output was previously reported as 1 ml/kg/day; however, she made only 30 ml of urine in 6 h after admission to the intensive care unit (ICU). Laboratory studies on ICU admission demonstrated that the electrolytes were normal, the blood urea nitrogen was 50 mg/dl, and creatinine was 0.9 mg/dl (creatinine was 0.6 mg/dl 2 days ago). The urinalysis was unremarkable.

N. Celebi
Department of Pediatrics, Renal Section, Baylor College of Medicine, Houston, TX, USA

Department of Pediatrics, Critical Care Section, Baylor College of Medicine, Houston, TX, USA

A. A. Arikan (✉)
Department of Pediatrics, Renal Section, Baylor College of Medicine, Houston, TX, USA

Department of Pediatrics, Critical Care Section, Baylor College of Medicine, Houston, TX, USA

Critical Care Nephrology, Texas Children's Hospital, Houston, TX, USA
e-mail: aysea@bcm.edu

S. K. Sethi et al. (eds.), *Critical Care Pediatric Nephrology and Dialysis: A Practical Handbook*, https://doi.org/10.1007/978-981-13-2276-1_1

Case 2
A 14-year-old previously healthy male presented to emergency department for complaints of lower back pain and malaise for which he reported taking ibuprofen in appropriate doses daily last week. Otherwise he did not have fever and reported unchanged amount of urine output. On physical examination the height and weight were normal, the blood pressure was 117/75, and he appeared pale. Laboratory studies demonstrated that the electrolytes were normal, the blood urea nitrogen was 57 mg/dl, and creatinine was 3.2 mg/dl. The urinalysis was unremarkable. Renal ultrasonography demonstrated normal sized kidneys with increased echogenicity and loss of corticomedullary differentiation.

1.1 Acute Kidney Injury: Definition

Acute kidney injury (AKI) is defined as a rapid decline in glomerular filtration rate (GFR) leading to accumulation of waste products. AKI is common, affecting one third of the children admitted to intensive care unit (ICU) and is associated with poor outcomes including increased mortality and morbidity among critically ill children [1]. Severity and progressions of AKI is directly associated with stepwise increase in mortality and other adverse outcomes. Therefore, a standardized definition of AKI is particularly important to diagnose AKI and stratify AKI severity, in order to manage these patients better. In the past, available literature included multiple definitions for renal failure based on different thresholds of serum creatinine or blood urea nitrogen, with or without contribution from urine output, or requirement of renal replacement therapy, which made detection, diagnosis, classification, and study of AKI rather difficult. In an effort to better define AKI, three standardized consensus classifications have been proposed: (1) RIFLE (Risk, Injury, Failure, Loss, End-stage kidney disease) criteria was developed by the Acute Dialysis Quality Initiative (ADQI) in 2004 for adult patients by using changes in serum creatinine levels from baseline and/or decrease in urine output (Table 1.1) [2]. RIFLE definition was adapted for children by using change in estimated creatinine clearance from baseline, which is referred to as pediatric RIFLE (pRIFLE) definition (Table 1.1) [3]. In an adult study, increase of serum creatinine 0.3 mg/dl was found to be associated with 70% increase in risk of death; those results were replicated later in a pediatric study where increase of serum creatinine of 0.3 mg/dl was associated with increased mortality risk in a population with decompensated heart failure [4, 5]. (2) Further refinement of RIFLE criteria was developed by acute kidney injury network (AKIN) in 2007 which included the additional criterion of 0.3 mg/dl increase in serum creatinine in less than 48 h (Table 1.2) [6]. (3) Finally, in 2012 several aspects of RIFLE, pRIFLE, and AKIN criteria were integrated into a single definition for pediatric and adult patients by the Kidney Disease Improving Global Outcomes (KDIGO) classification (Table 1.3) [7].

Table 1.1 RIFLE/pRIFLE criteria for acute kidney injury

	Cr/GFR criteria	Urine output criteria
Risk (R)	Increased Cr × 1.5 or decreased GFR by 25% eCCl decrease by 25%[a]	Urine output <0.5 ml/kg/h × 6 h Urine output <0.5 ml/kg/h × 8 h[a]
Injury (I)	Increased Cr × 2 or decreased GFR by 50% eCCl decrease by 50%[a]	Urine output <0.5 ml/kg/h × 12 h Urine output <0.5 ml/kg/h × 16 h[a]
Failure (F)	Increased Cr × 3 or decreased GFR by 75% or Cr >4 mg/dl (with acute rise of >0.5 mg/dl) eCCl decrease by 75% or Cl <35 ml/min/1.73 m^2[a]	Urine output <0.3 ml/kg/h × 24 h or Anuria × 12 h
Loss (L)	Persistent failure—complete loss of renal function for >4 weeks	
ESRD (E)	End-stage renal disease-persistent failure >3 months	

[a]pRIFLE criteria; *eCCL* estimated creatinine clearance, *Cr* creatinine

Table 1.2 AKIN criteria for acute kidney injury

	Cr/GFR criteria	Urine output criteria
Stage 1	Increased Cr × 1.5–1.9 from baseline or increase by ≥0.3 mg/dl	Urine output <0.5 ml/kg/h × 6 h
Stage 2	Increased Cr × 2–2.9 from baseline	Urine output <0.5 ml/kg/h × 12 h
Stage 3	Increased Cr × ≥3 or sCr ≥4 mg/dl with acute rise of ≥0.5 mg/dl	Urine output < 0.3 ml/kg/h × 24 h or Anuria × 12 h

Table 1.3 KDIGO criteria for acute kidney injury

	Cr/GFR criteria	Urine output criteria
Stage 1	Increased Cr × 1.5–1.9 from baseline or increase by ≥0.3 mg/dl	Urine output <0.5 ml/kg/h × 6–12 h
Stage 2	Increased Cr × 2–2.9 from baseline	Urine output <0.5 ml/kg/h × 12 h
Stage 3	Increased Cr × ≥3 or increase in sCr ≥4 mg/dl or initiation of renal replacement therapy or, in patients <18 years, decrease in GFR <35 ml/min/1.73 m^2	Urine output <0.3 ml/kg/h × 24 h or Anuria × 12 h

All three definitions have subtle differences and different advantages. Baseline creatinine interpretation differs among definitions; most notably, AKIN uses first creatinine available as the baseline creatinine, whereas pRIFLE requires height to calculate eCCL. Thus, pRIFLE, AKIN, and KDIGO result in different AKI epidemiology. pRIFLE is more sensitive to detect mild AKI. AKIN is less sensitive but more specific to diagnose severe AKI; whereas, pRIFLE and KDIGO detect severe AKI similarly. Since KDIGO is applicable to both pediatric and adult population it has come into wide use. Overall, all three definitions highly correlate with staging of AKI and outcomes [8, 9].

Table 1.4 Modified KDIGO criteria for neonatal acute kidney injury

	Cr/GFR criteria	Urine output criteria
Stage 0	No change in sCr or rise <0.3 mg/dl	Urine output >1 ml/kg/h
Stage 1	sCr rise ≥0.3 mg/dl within 48 h or sCr rise ≥1.5 to 1.9 × reference sCr[a] within 7 days	Urine output >0.5 ml/kg/h and ≤1 ml/kg/h
Stage 2	sCr rise ≥2 to 2.9 × reference sCr	Urine output >0.3 ml/kg/h and ≤0.5 ml/kg/h
Stage 3	sCr rise ≥3 × reference SCr or sCr ≥2.5 mg/dl or receipt of dialysis	Urine output ≤0.3 ml/kg/h

[a]Reference serum creatinine, defined as the lowest previous serum creatinine value available

The criteria for the diagnosis of AKI and staging of severity of AKI are based on changes in serum creatinine and urine output. The caveat here is that serum creatinine is a late marker of decreasing GFR. Additionally, serum creatinine concentrations can be influenced by malnutrition, liver dysfunction, decreased muscle mass, and volume overload, which all can cause underestimation of the degree of renal dysfunction. On the other hand, changes in urine output usually precede the changes in serum creatinine [10]. If only creatinine criteria are used, up to 70% of AKI are missed [1]. However, relying on urine output solely will obviously miss nonoliguric AKI, such as presented in Case 2 in the beginning of the chapter. Since urine output may not be measured routinely in non-intensive care settings, early AKI might easily be missed. The worry for catheter associated urinary tract infection has led to a tendency of not placing indwelling bladder catheters or early removal in the intensive care settings. Clinicians need to be aware of when closer monitoring is needed and order this simple intervention accordingly. All patients who get admitted in shock should receive an indwelling bladder catheter until shock is resolved.

Definition of AKI in critically ill neonates has lagged behind that in older populations. Serum creatinine is difficult to interpret in newborns since it may reflect maternal creatinine during first week of life in term neonates and may persist at maternal levels up to 2–3 weeks in preterm infants. Monitoring the trend of the serum creatinine may be more helpful. Progressive increase in serum creatinine or failure to decrease is consistent with decreased renal function. KDIGO AKI definition was adapted and used for study purposes in the neonatal population (Table 1.4). The overall incidence of AKI in neonates and infants is about 30% and is associated with poor outcomes including higher mortality, similar to other age groups [11].

1.2 Acute Kidney Injury: Epidemiology

Although precise incidence of pediatric AKI is not known, overall incidence of AKI is thought to be increasing and depends on the clinical setting and patient's clinical condition. An administrative dataset screening for physician coding revealed AKI rate of 3.9 per 1000 at-risk pediatric hospitalizations [11]. Twenty seven percent of the critically ill children at pediatric intensive care unit (PICU) developed AKI with 10% of them developing severe AKI (AKI stage 2 and stage 3), and 1% requiring renal replacement therapy. Twelve percent of severe AKI develops within 7 days after ICU admission [1].

Multiorgan dysfunction, need for mechanical ventilation, documented infection, extracorporeal membrane oxygenation, and nephrotoxic medication exposure are identified as risk factors for developing AKI in critically ill children, while nephrotoxic medication exposure has the greatest independent risk [12, 13]. Development of AKI is associated with higher mortality, PICU length of stay, and duration of mechanical ventilation [13, 14]. Severe AKI (stage II or III) has the highest association with mortality. Patients with resolved AKI or those who have improvement in their severity of AKI stage tend to have lower mortality; however, patients with any degree of AKI, even mild, despite complete resolution, still have higher rates of mortality than patients who do not develop AKI at all in the ICU setting [15]. Outside of the PICU, 25% of the non-critically ill children who are exposed to three or more nephrotoxic medications developed AKI [16, 17]. AKI rates of 30% have been reported in infants; whereas, 48% of extremely preterm infants (less than 28 weeks of gestation) develop AKI [18]. The incidence increases to 40–65% in the infants undergoing cardiac surgery depending on the definition used, the rate increasing with lower age at surgery, longer cardiopulmonary bypass, type of repair, and lower gestational age [19, 20] (Table 1.5).

Table 1.5 Risk factors associated with AKI [21]

Critical illness
  Sepsis
  Shock—hypotension, vasopressor requirement
  Mechanical ventilation
  Extracorporeal membrane oxygenation

Preexisting renal, hepatic, cardiac, neurologic, or respiratory disease
Oncologic disease

Neonates
  Low gestational age
  Low birth weight
  Perinatal asphyxia
  Congenital diaphragmatic hernia
  Bronchopulmonary dysplasia
  Maternal exposure to angiotensin-converting enzyme (ACE) inhibitors

Solid organ transplants
Bone marrow transplants
Intravascular volume depletion—diabetic ketoacidosis, nephrotic syndrome, diarrhea, vomiting
Venous congestion—congestive heart failure, right heart failure, pulmonary hypertension
Post cardiac surgery—prolonged cardiopulmonary bypass

Nephrotoxic medication exposure[a]
  Aminoglycosides
  Vancomycin
  Piperacillin/tazobactam
  Amphotericin B
  Chemotherapeutics
  Immune modulators
  Non-steroidal anti-inflammatory drugs
  ACE inhibitors
  Intravenous contrast media

[a]List in not exhaustive

1.3 Acute Kidney Injury: Pathophysiology

1.3.1 Functional AKI

Functional (prerenal) AKI is caused by decreased renal perfusion due to decrease in either absolute or effective circulating volume. Hypotension, decreased cardiac function, renovascular compromise, and volume depletion can all lead to functional AKI. The hallmark is the improvement of renal function with correction of underlying problem, hence the term functional. Systemic hypoperfusion triggers the activation of sympathetic nervous system, renin-angiotensin axis, and nonosmotic antidiuretic hormone secretion leading to compensatory mechanisms that raise blood pressure. GFR is initially preserved by several intrarenal autoregulatory mechanisms including generation of intrarenal vasodilatory prostaglandins and intrinsic myogenic mechanisms [22]. Prolonged duration and increased severity of the trigger lead to decrease in GFR, manifested as functional AKI. During this phase, subclinical intrinsic renal injury may be demonstrated by novel biomarkers, which typically are proteins expressed in cellular stress and repair. Longer duration of this phase can easily transition into intrinsic injury.

1.3.2 Intrinsic Renal Injury

Prolonged duration of processes leading to functional AKI, exposure to nephrotoxins, or sepsis, among other causes, can lead to intrinsic AKI, especially in the setting of critical illness. Though traditionally referred to as acute tubular necrosis (ATN), histological evidence of ATN is exceedingly rare in the critically ill patients suffering from AKI. Endothelial cell injury can promote the initiation and extension of intrinsic AKI via disrupting the microvascular blood flow. Straight segment (S3 segment) of proximal tubule and medullary thick ascending limb of Henle are particularly sensitive to ischemic changes given inherent high cellular energy needs and relative low oxygen tension in the adjoining renal medulla. Cellular injury leads to cell sloughing from disrupted adhesion molecules and cell necrosis which may further cause tubular obstruction with leakage of proteinaceous material (Tamm–Horsfall protein). Inflammatory processes also contribute to the sequence of events in intrinsic AKI [22].

1.3.3 Postrenal AKI/Obstructive Nephropathy

Anatomic abnormalities of the genitourinary system (for example, posterior urethral valves), functional problems (for example, neurogenic bladder, dysfunctional bladder, or other voiding dysfunction), obstruction at the bladder outlet or bilateral ureters, or blockage of tubules with protein and crystals can lead to urinary retention and AKI. Obstruction affecting bilateral collecting systems is the hallmark of obstructive AKI. Backward pressure from obstruction is transmitted up through the

Table 1.6 Determining type of the renal injury

	FeNa: ([U/P] Na)/([U/P]/Cr) × 100	FeUrea: ([U/P] Urea)/([U/P]/Cr) × 100
Functional AKI	FeNa <1%	FeUrea <35%
	Urine sodium: <20 mEq/l Urine osmolality: >400 mOsm/kg Urine specific gravity: >1020 Urine sediment: bland Urine protein: none to low	
Intrinsic AKI	FeNa >2%	FeUrea >50 to 65%
	Urine sodium: >30 mEq/l Urine osmolality: <350 mOsm/kg Urine specific gravity: <1012 Urine sediment: broad brownish granular cast Urine protein: none to low	

Sodium (Na), Creatinine (Cr), Urine (U), Plasma (P)

urinary system, which counteracts the hydrostatic pressure for filtration at the glomerulus. When it eventually overcomes the hydrostatic pressure in the glomerulus, glomerular filtration stops and AKI occurs [22].

1.4 Differentiation of Functional and Intrinsic AKI

Urinary indices are derived from the assumption that tubular integrity is maintained in the setting of functional AKI. In prerenal/functional AKI state, sodium-retaining mechanism is activated, reducing the urinary sodium; whereas tubular cell damage of ATN causes impaired resorptive capacity of proximal tubule leading to urinary sodium rise. Thus, urine sodium is used as an indicator of volume status and renal tubular integrity. Fractional excretion of sodium (FeNa) evaluates urinary sodium excretion. However, diuretic use limits sodium reabsorption and makes FeNa calculation unreliable in patients who have received diuretics. Fractional excretion of urea (FeUrea), based on the same principal, can be used in these instances (Table 1.6).

References

1. Kaddourah A, et al. Epidemiology of acute kidney injury in critically ill children and young adults. N Engl J Med. 2017;376(1):11–20.
2. Bellomo R, et al. Acute renal failure - definition, outcome measures, animal models, fluid therapy and information technology needs: the Second International Consensus Conference of the Acute Dialysis Quality Initiative (ADQI) Group. Crit Care. 2004;8(4):R204–12.
3. Akcan-Arikan A, et al. Modified RIFLE criteria in critically ill children with acute kidney injury. Kidney Int. 2007;71(10):1028–35.
4. Chertow GM, et al. Acute kidney injury, mortality, length of stay, and costs in hospitalized patients. J Am Soc Nephrol. 2005;16(11):3365–70.
5. Price JF, et al. Worsening renal function in children hospitalized with decompensated heart failure: evidence for a pediatric cardiorenal syndrome? Pediatr Crit Care Med. 2008;9(3):279–84.

6. Mehta RL, et al. Acute Kidney Injury Network: report of an initiative to improve outcomes in acute kidney injury. Crit Care. 2007;11(2):R31.
7. Khwaja A. KDIGO clinical practice guidelines for acute kidney injury. Nephron Clin Pract. 2012;120(4):c179–84.
8. Sutherland SM, et al. AKI in hospitalized children: comparing the pRIFLE, AKIN, and KDIGO definitions. Clin J Am Soc Nephrol. 2015;10(4):554–61.
9. Zappitelli M, et al. Ascertainment and epidemiology of acute kidney injury varies with definition interpretation. Clin J Am Soc Nephrol. 2008;3(4):948–54.
10. Bellomo R. Defining, quantifying, and classifying acute renal failure. Crit Care Clin. 2005;21(2):223–37.
11. Jetton JG, Askenazi DJ. Update on acute kidney injury in the neonate. Curr Opin Pediatr. 2012;24(2):191–6.
12. Slater MB, et al. Risk factors of acute kidney injury in critically ill children. Pediatr Crit Care Med. 2016;17(9):e391–8.
13. Alkandari O, et al. Acute kidney injury is an independent risk factor for pediatric intensive care unit mortality, longer length of stay and prolonged mechanical ventilation in critically ill children: a two-center retrospective cohort study. Crit Care. 2011;15(3):R146.
14. Wang HE, et al. Acute kidney injury and mortality in hospitalized patients. Am J Nephrol. 2012;35(4):349–55.
15. Sanchez-Pinto LN, et al. Association between progression and improvement of acute kidney injury and mortality in critically ill children. Pediatr Crit Care Med. 2015;16(8):703–10.
16. Moffett BS, Goldstein SL. Acute kidney injury and increasing nephrotoxic-medication exposure in noncritically-ill children. Clin J Am Soc Nephrol. 2011;6(4):856–63.
17. Goldstein SL, et al. Electronic health record identification of nephrotoxin exposure and associated acute kidney injury. Pediatrics. 2013;132(3):e756–67.
18. Jetton JG. Incidence and outcomes of neonatal acute kidney injury (AWAKEN): a multicenter, multinational, observational cohort study. Lancet Child Adolesc Health. 2017;1:184–94.
19. Morgan CJ, et al. Risk factors for and outcomes of acute kidney injury in neonates undergoing complex cardiac surgery. J Pediatr. 2013;162(1):120–7. e1
20. Skippen PW, Krahn GE. Acute renal failure in children undergoing cardiopulmonary bypass. Crit Care Resusc. 2005;7(4):286–91.
21. Joyce EL, et al. Drug-associated acute kidney injury: who's at risk? Pediatr Nephrol. 2017;32(1):59–69.
22. Kher KK, William Schnaper H, Greenbaum LA. Clinical pediatric nephrology. In: Prasad Devarajan SLG, editor. Acute kidney injury. 3rd ed. Boca Raton, FL: CRC Press; 2017.

Biomarkers in Pediatric Acute Kidney Injury

2

Eileen Ciccia and Prasad Devarajan

2.1 Clinical Case

NB is a 4-month-old male with hypoplastic left heart syndrome who underwent a cardiac repair procedure requiring cardiopulmonary bypass 3 days ago. He has made no urine postoperatively despite aggressive dosing of furosemide and bumetanide. His serum potassium has been trending 6.1–6.3 mEq/L and serum bicarbonate 15–18 mEq/L. He remains intubated and has not tolerated weaning of respiratory support or vasoactive drips. NB is currently 8% fluid overloaded and appears mildly edematous on exam. The team would like to provide full parenteral nutrition to this postoperative patient but they are concerned that he will not tolerate the volume needed.

Outcome 1 The team decides to initiate renal replacement therapy. Because of previous abdominal procedures, NB is not a candidate for peritoneal dialysis; therefore, a central line is placed and he receives three sessions of daily hemodialysis. Subsequent laboratory tests suggest renal recovery, and no further dialysis is performed.

Outcome 2 The team has been trending NGAL, a non-invasive, inexpensive laboratory test marker of structural acute kidney injury, which demonstrates that the kidney injury is improving, although other labs and urine output remain unchanged. Fluid restriction is maintained and electrolyte abnormalities are managed medically.

E. Ciccia · P. Devarajan (✉)
Nephrology and Hypertension, Cincinnati Children's Hospital Medical Center, Cincinnati, OH, USA
e-mail: prasad.devarajan@cchmc.org

S. K. Sethi et al. (eds.), *Critical Care Pediatric Nephrology and Dialysis: A Practical Handbook*, https://doi.org/10.1007/978-981-13-2276-1_2

The next day, NB begins producing small amounts of urine and within 48 h all fluid and electrolyte restrictions are discontinued. The increased cost and morbidity of renal replacement therapy are avoided.

Which outcome would you prefer for your patient?

2.2 The Unmet Need for Acute Kidney Injury Biomarkers

Acute kidney injury (AKI) is common in hospitalized children and is a significant cause of morbidity and mortality. Approximately one-third of all pediatric patients worldwide develop AKI during hospital admission [1]. Over 25% of critically ill children develop AKI and over 10% of these cases can be classified as severe, which is defined as Stage 2 or 3 AKI by the Kidney Disease Improving Global Outcomes Work Group staging system [2, 3]. Severe AKI has been shown to confer increased risk of mortality [2, 4], longer hospital stay [3], and heightened risk of developing chronic kidney disease [5, 6].

Traditionally, clinicians have utilized functional indicators to assess a patient's renal status. The most common of these functional markers, serum creatinine and urine output, have several significant limitations, particularly in children. Serum creatinine is a delayed marker of renal impairment, with levels only rising hours to days following kidney insult. Early recognition of structural kidney injury is limited given that a baseline healthy kidney's functional reserve requires a significant injury and functional loss prior to creatinine elevation. It also can be unreliable in several specific clinical contexts, such as variable muscle mass and fluid overload. A large prospective, multinational observational study of pediatric intensive care patients confirmed the inadequacy of serum creatinine for AKI diagnosis, since 67.2% of patients with oliguria-diagnosed AKI would not have been recognized using creatinine-based definitions alone [2]. Unfortunately, urine production is a difficult measure to obtain with high accuracy, particularly in young children without indwelling urinary catheters and patients in non-ICU settings. Furthermore, urine output can be confounded by the hydration status as well as the common use of diuretics in critically ill children.

In contrast to these functional indicators, the use of a structural AKI biomarker improves diagnostic and therapeutic patient care by allowing earlier detection of tissue injury at a time when inciting factors can still be modified and response to interventions trended in real-time [7]. A good biomarker is expected to be valid, reliable, and clinically useful, with biomarker results being both clearly actionable and promptly available to effectively drive clinical care. Non-invasive technique, cost-effectiveness, and the ability to process the biomarker ubiquitously in hospital clinical laboratories or even at the bedside are additional features that render a biomarker more generalizable across a spectrum of patient populations.

Table 2.1 Urinary biomarkers in AKI

Biomarker	Source	Physiologic role	Clinical utility
NGAL	Distal tubule and collecting duct	Regulates iron trafficking, promotes tubule cell survival	• Confirmed early marker of AKI severity, renal replacement need, mortality, and renal recovery • Standard clinical platforms widely available • Results in 15–30 min
KIM-1	Proximal tubule	Promotes epithelial regeneration, regulates apoptosis	• Delayed marker of AKI compared with NGAL • Awaits confirmatory studies • No clinical assays available
IL-18	Proximal tubule	Promotes tubule cell apoptosis and necrosis	• Predicts AKI in post-CPB • No clinical assays available
L-FABP	Proximal tubule	Antioxidant, suppresses tubulo-interstitial damage	• Awaits confirmatory studies • No clinical assays available
TIMP-2, IGFBP7	Proximal tubule	Limits proliferation of damaged tubule cells	• Delayed marker of AKI compared with NGAL • AUC comparable to NGAL for predicting AKI • Requires specialized testing platform

Abbreviations: *AKI* acute kidney injury, *NGAL* neutrophil gelatinase-associated lipocalin, *KIM-1* kidney injury molecule-1, *IL-18* interleukin-18, *CPB* cardiopulmonary bypass, *L-FABP* liver-type fatty acid-binding protein, *TIMP-2* tissue inhibitor of metalloproteinases-2, *IGFBP7* insulin-like growth factor-binding protein 7, *AUC* area under the curve

A number of promising structural biomarkers have been investigated in AKI research with varying degrees of clinical applicability ([8], Table 2.1). Of these, neutrophil gelatinase-associated lipocalin (NGAL) is the most well-established, validated in many patient populations, and is already being employed effectively in the clinical setting using widely available standardized clinical platforms [9, 10]; thus, NGAL will be primarily discussed further here.

2.3 Neutrophil Gelatinase-Associated Lipocalin (NGAL)

Neutrophil gelatinase-associated lipocalin (NGAL), also known as lipocalin-2, is a 25 kDa glycoprotein released by epithelial tissues and as such can be increased in the systemic circulation in a number of human disease processes apart from AKI (Table 2.2). In the majority of these conditions, urinary NGAL remains low unless there is concomitant renal tubular injury that prevents any filtered NGAL from being efficiently reabsorbed. It is one of the most upregulated genes in the kidney following conditions of ischemic or toxic stress and is released directly into the

Table 2.2 Clinical settings in which NGAL can be elevated independent of AKI

Urinary tract infection
Sepsis
Chronic kidney disease
Malignancy
Pancreatitis

Abbreviations: *NGAL* neutrophil gelatinase-associated lipocalin, *AKI* acute kidney injury

urine by kidney tubule cells, where its role in the iron-chelation process assists in renal protection and tubule cell recovery and proliferation [11]. Following AKI, the released NGAL is also partially reabsorbed into the circulation, thus contributing to the systemic NGAL pool.

NGAL remains stable when stored at 4 °C for up to 24 h in urine and up to 48 h in plasma/serum [12, 13]. While both urine and plasma NGAL levels have been shown to increase within 2–4 h of intrinsic structural AKI, data utilizing urine NGAL is overall more prevalent in the available pediatric clinical and research AKI literature. There are currently three clinical platforms available for testing NGAL levels, one of which is easily adaptable to most standard clinical laboratory platforms and is already in routine clinical use in several institutions worldwide.

Clinically, NGAL has been extensively validated to predict and differentiate intrinsic structural AKI from functional AKI (previously referred to as a prerenal state) and to predict the adverse outcomes of AKI. Several groups have completed systemic analyses of the extensive published literature to date looking at the accuracy of NGAL in predicting AKI diagnosis and prognosis across a variety of clinical settings.

A meta-analysis published by Haase et al. in 2009 looked at 19 prospective, observational, single-center cohort studies investigating the diagnostic and prognostic accuracy of NGAL to predict creatinine-based AKI, dialysis initiation, and in-hospital mortality [14]. These studies represent data from a total of 2538 patients (of which 663 were children) from 8 different countries. It was found that NGAL level accuracy improved with more severe AKI definitions and that an NGAL cut-off of >150 ng/mL using a standardized clinical platform provided optimal sensitivity and specificity to predict AKI with an area under the curve for the receiver-operating characteristic (AUC-ROC) of 0.83 (95% CI 0.741–0.918). Overall, the AKI predictive value of NGAL in children was shown to be substantially high than in adults, with the diagnostic odds ratio (DOR) in children at 25.4 (AUC-ROC 0.93) versus 10.6 (AUC-ROC 0.782) in adults. The predictive values of urine and plasma NGAL were similar (DOR 17.9, AUC-ROC 0.775 and DOR 18.6, AUC-ROC 0.837, respectively). When used to prognosticate adverse outcomes of AKI in all-age pooled data

Table 2.3 AKI risk categories based on urinary NGAL level

AKI risk category	Urinary NGAL level (ng/mL)	Interpretation
Low	<50	Intrinsic structural AKI unlikely
Equivocal	50–149	Gray zone; clinical risk factors and repeat NGAL measurements needed to clarify
Moderate	150–300	Predicts intrinsic structural AKI
High	>300	Predicts severe AKI and adverse outcomes

Abbreviations: *AKI* acute kidney injury, *NGAL* neutrophil gelatinase-associated lipocalin

evaluation, NGAL was shown to be useful, with DOR 12.9, AUC-ROC 0.782 for initiation of renal replacement therapy and DOR 8.8, AUC 0.706 for in-hospital mortality.

In a 2017 meta-analysis, Filho et al. looked at 13 studies (6 which overlapped with the Haase analysis) with a total of 1629 pediatric patients [15]. Through this analysis it was determined that NGAL was able to predict AKI development in children with a sensitivity of 0.76 (95% CI 0.62–0.86) in urine, 0.80 (95% CI 0.64–0.90) in plasma and specificity of 0.93 (95% CI 0.88–0.96) in urine, 0.87 (95% CI 0.74–0.94) in plasma. Overall, the DOR for AKI detection was 26 (95% CI 8–82) and AUC 0.90 (95% CI 0.87–0.94), substantiating previous analyses demonstrating NGAL to have good predictive value and discriminative power in predicting AKI in children. In particular, the negative predictive value of NGAL is especially high, such that a normal NGAL result effectively rules out true structural AKI (irrespective of the serum creatinine or the urine output).

Summative assessment of the NGAL literature to date has demonstrated that AKI risk, severity stratification, and prognosis are dose-dependent. As such, NGAL level thresholds (Table 2.3) have been established for the standardized clinical laboratory platforms, with cut-off levels derived during previous meta-analyses, and their effective application in pediatric clinical care has already been reported in the literature [9, 10]. One example of a clinical algorithm for use of NGAL in the hospital setting is detailed in Fig. 2.1.

It is important to note that, as with every test ordered in patient care, the proper clinical application and interpretation of NGAL levels is only optimized when a patient's clinical status, individual medical history, and AKI risk factors are taken into account. As such, it can be helpful to use a clinical risk stratification method to assist in deciding who should have NGAL testing done and how to act on the results. One example is the renal angina index, a scoring tool developed to identify patients at risk of AKI within the first 24 h of pediatric intensive care admission [16, 17] based on admission characteristics.

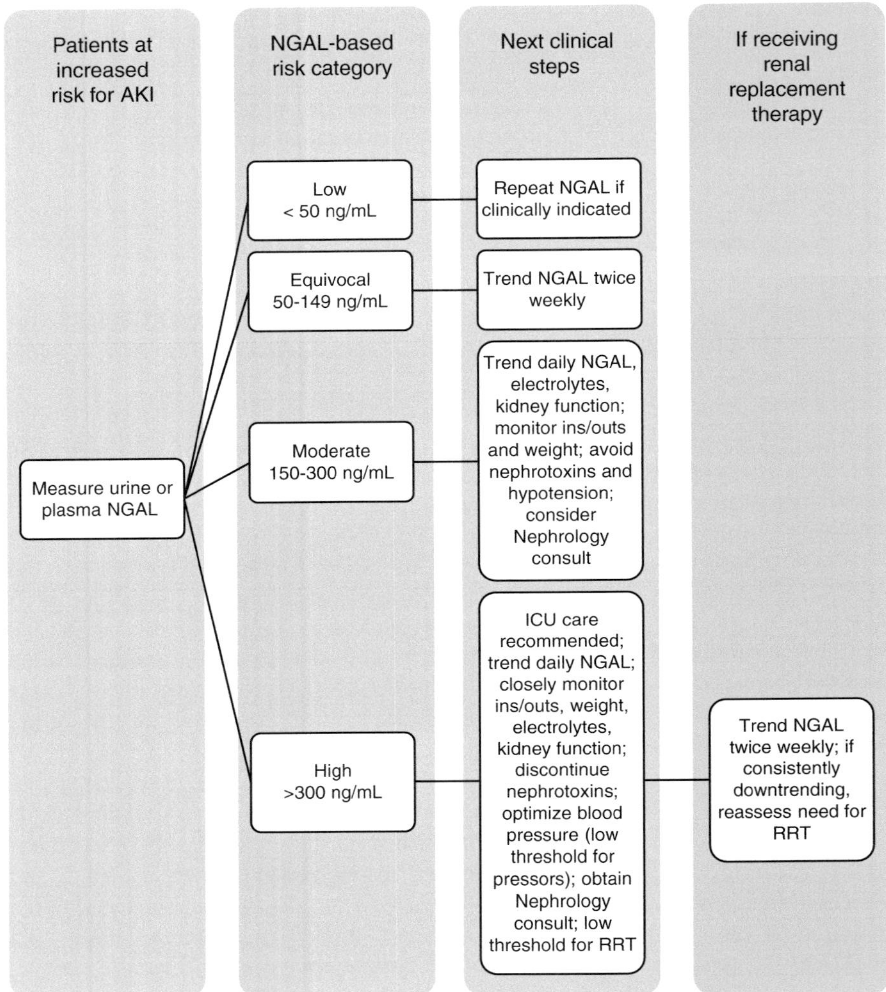

Fig. 2.1 Clinical algorithm for NGAL in AKI

2.4 Conclusion: Key "Take Home" Points

1. Current functional markers of AKI (serum creatinine and urine output) are delayed and inadequate to allow for early detection or to trend intervention effects in real-time.
2. Neutrophil gelatinase-associated lipocalin (NGAL) is a protein biomarker upregulated in and released into urine and plasma from injured kidney tubule cells.

3. Use of NGAL as a non-invasive AKI biomarker is well-established, validated across many patient care settings, and already effectively being used clinically to assist in modifying fluid balance, ameliorating renal stress exposures, and optimizing the timing and duration of renal replacement therapy.
4. AKI risk, severity stratification, and prognosis are dose-dependent and can be trended in real-time using categories based on NGAL levels: low risk <50 ng/mL, equivocal 50–150 ng/mL, moderate risk 150–300 ng/mL, and high risk >300 ng/mL.
5. Increasing NGAL-based AKI risk indicates a correlating escalation in monitoring, intervention, and nephrology specialty involvement.

References

1. Susantitaphong P, Cruz DN, Cerda J, Abulfaraj M, Algahtani F, Koulouridis I, Jaber BL, Acute Kidney Injury Advisory Group of the American Society of Nephrology. World incidence of AKI: a meta-analysis. Clin J Am Soc Nephrol. 2013;8(9):1482–93. Erratum in: Clin J Am Soc Nephrol. 2014; 9(6):1148.
2. Kaddourah A, Basu RK, Bagshaw SM, Goldstein SL. Epidemiology of acute kidney injury in critically ill children and young adults. N Engl J Med. 2017;376:11–20.
3. Kellum JA, Lameire N, Aspelin P, et al. Kidney disease: improving global outcomes (KDIGO) acute kidney injury working group. KDIGO clinical practice guideline for acute kidney injury. Kidney Int Suppl. 2012;2(1):1–138.
4. Sutherland SM, Byrnes JJ, Kothari M, et al. AKI in hospitalized children: comparing the pRIFLE, AKIN, and KDIGO definitions. Clin J Am Soc Nephrol. 2015;10(4):554–61.
5. Cooper DS, Claes D, Goldstein SL, Bennett MR, Ma Q, Devarajan P, Krawczeski CD. Follow-up renal assessment of injury long-term after acute kidney injury (FRAIL-AKI). Clin J Am Soc Nephrol. 2016;11(1):21–9.
6. Madsen NL, Goldstein SL, Froslev T, Christiansen CF, Olsen M. Cardiac surgery in patients with congenital heart disease is associated with acute kidney injury and the risk of chronic kidney disease. Kidney Int. 2017;92(3):751–6.
7. Devarajan P. Neutrophil gelatinase-associated lipocalin: a promising biomarker for human acute kidney injury. Biomark Med. 2010;4:265–80.
8. Ciccia E, Devarajan P. Pediatric acute kidney injury: prevalence, impact and management challenges. Int J Nephrol Renov Dis. 2017;10:77–84.
9. Varnell CD Jr, Goldstein SL, Devarajan P, Basu RK. Impact of near real-time urine neutrophil gelatinase-associated lipocalin assessment on clinical practice. Kidney Int Rep. 2017;2:1243–9.
10. Devarajan P. Kidney attack: is NGAL set to take the stage with troponins? In: Rangaswami J, Lerma EV, Ronco C, editors. Cardio-nephrology: confluence of the heart and kidney in clinical practice. 1st ed. Cham: Springer; 2017.
11. Ostermann M, Phillips BJ, Forni LG. Clinical review: biomarkers of acute kidney injury: where are we now? Crit Care. 2012;16(5):233.
12. Schuh MP, Nehus E, Ma Q, Haffner C, Bennett M, Drawczeski CD, Devarajan P. Long-term stability of urinary biomarkers of acute kidney injury in children. Am J Kidney Dis. 2016;67(1):56–61.
13. Pedersen KR, Ravn HB, Hjortdal VE, Nørregaard R, Povlsen JV. Neutrophil gelatinase-associated lipocalin (NGAL): validation of commercially available ELISA. Scand J Clin Lab Invest. 2010;70(5):374–82.
14. Haase M, Bellomo R, Devarajn P, Schlattmann P, Haase-Fielitz A, NGAL Meta-analysis Investigator Group. Accuracy of neutrophil gelatinase-associated lipocalin (NGAL) in diagno-

sis and prognosis in acute kidney injury: a systemic review and meta-analysis. Am J Kidney Dis. 2009;54(6):1012–24.
15. Filho LT, Grande AJ, Colonetti T, Possamai Della ES, da Rosa MI. Accuracy of neutrophil gelatinase-associated lipocalin for acute kidney injury diagnosis in children: systematic review and meta-analysis. Pediatr Nephrol. 2017;32(10):1979–88.
16. Basu RK, Wang Y, Wong HR, Chawla LS, Wheeler DS, Goldstein SL. Incorporation of biomarkers with the renal angina index for prediction of severe AKI in critically ill children. Clin J Am Soc Nephrol. 2014;9(4):654–62.
17. Goldstein SL. The renal angina index to predict acute kidney injury: are adults just large children? Kidney Int Rep. 2018;3(3):516–8.

Part II

Managing a Sick Child with AKI

Acute Kidney Injury: Principles of Management

3

Jitendra Meena and Arvind Bagga

Acute kidney injury (AKI) is characterized by rapid decline in renal function with accumulation of nitrogenous waste and inability of kidney to maintain fluid and electrolyte homeostasis. The term acute renal failure had been replaced by AKI since it represents renal dysfunction as a continuum rather than a discrete finding of failed function. The manifestations of AKI are wide, ranging from minimal elevation of serum creatinine to anuric renal failure. AKI can occur in variety of clinical settings and is associated with several short- and long-term morbidities and increased mortality [1].

3.1 Definition and Staging

While previous studies on the epidemiology of renal failure have used various definitions, attempts have been made to standardize the definition of AKI in order to better estimate disease burden and outcomes. Standardization of the definition of AKI began in 2004 when the acute dialysis quality initiative (ADQI) proposed the RIFLE criteria [2], later modified for use in children (pRIFLE) [3]. The latter used urine output and estimated glomerular filtration rate (eGFR) instead of absolute change in serum creatinine to account for expected change with somatic growth (Table 3.1). Since even small changes in serum creatinine are associated with adverse outcomes, the criteria were revised by the acute kidney injury network (AKIN 2007), to include minor change of serum creatinine (>0.3 mg/dl) in AKI stage 1 and those receiving renal replacement therapy in stage III [4].

In an attempt to harmonize definitions, the Kidney Disease: Improving Global Outcome (KDIGO) Conference in 2012 proposed a standard definition, where AKI

J. Meena · A. Bagga (✉)
Division of Nephrology, Department of Pediatrics, ICMR Center for Advanced Research in Nephrology, All India Institute of Medical Sciences, New Delhi, India

S. K. Sethi et al. (eds.), *Critical Care Pediatric Nephrology and Dialysis: A Practical Handbook*, https://doi.org/10.1007/978-981-13-2276-1_3

Table 3.1 Acute kidney injury definitions

pRIFLE			KDIGO		
Class	Estimated CCI	Urine output	Stage	Serum creatinine	Urine output
R	eCCI decreased by ≥25%	<0.5 ml/kg/h for ≥8 h	1	Rise in SCr 1.5 to <2 times from baseline within 7 days, *or* increase in SCr >0.3 mg/dl from baseline within 48 h period	<0.5 ml/kg/h for 6–12 h
I	eCCI decreased by ≥50%	<0.5 ml/kg/h for ≥16 h	2	Rise in SCr 2–3 times from baseline	<0.5 ml/kg/h for >12 h
F	eCCI decreased by 75%, *or* eCCI <35 ml/min/1.73 m^2	<0.3 ml/kg/h for 24 h or anuria for 12 h	3	Rise in SCr ≥3 times from baseline, *or* increase in SCr >4 mg/dl from baseline, *or* initiation of renal replacement therapy, *or* decrease in eGFR <35 ml/min/1.73 m^2	<0.3 ml/kg/h for 24 h or anuria for >12 h
L	Persistent failure (F) >4 weeks				
E	Persistent failure >3 months				

eCCI estimated creatinine clearance, *SCr* serum creatinine, *R* risk, *I* injury, *F* failure, *L* loss, *E* end stage, *KDIGO* Kidney Disease: Improving Global Outcome

is defined by increase in serum creatinine >0.3 mg/dl within 48 h or ≥1.5-fold increase in the prior 7 days, or decrease in urine output <0.5 ml/kg/h for 6–12 h (Table 3.1) [5]. The KDIGO definition is currently used for defining and staging AKI in children. Few modifications have been proposed for defining neonatal AKI. First, the lowest serum creatinine is consider as the reference value; second, the rise in serum creatinine of >2.5 mg/dl is used to define stage 3 AKI, instead of >4 mg/dl for children and adults.

The above definition has some limitations. While the etiology of AKI in adults is rather homogeneous, children have varied causes that are not distinguished in this classification. Rise in serum creatinine is affected by multiple factors, including muscle mass, age, volume status, and metabolic state. Measurement of urine output helps in early diagnosis, but is cumbersome to assess in children. Despite limitations, estimation of blood levels of creatinine and urine output provides the most pragmatic definition of AKI.

3.2 Epidemiology

AKI is common in hospitalized children, with incidence depending on the patient population. In the multicenter AWARE study, 26% and 11.6% critically ill children showed AKI and severe AKI, respectively [6]. Patients with severe AKI showed increased risk of mortality. Similarly the incidence of AKI in the retrospective

AWAKEN study in neonatal intensive care units was 30% [7]. Young children undergoing cardiac surgery are also at risk for AKI, with estimates ranging between 30 and 65%, and associated with increased mortality and duration of hospital stay. The incidence of AKI in non-critically ill hospitalized patients ranges from 4 to 6%.

While AKI in the developed world predominately occurs in hospital settings and is associated with multiple risk factors (e.g., sepsis, hypotension, surgery, nephrotoxic agents), the illness in developing countries is chiefly community acquired and often due to a single cause, e.g., acute gastroenteritis, malaria, snake bite, or poisonings [8, 9]. Incident AKI in tertiary care hospitals in developing countries often shows a spectrum of illness that is similar to the developed world.

3.3 Etiology

The etiology of AKI is traditionally classified, according to the anatomical location of the insult, into three categories: prerenal, renal (intrinsic), and postrenal causes (Table 3.2). AKI is a heterogeneous syndrome that involves multiple pathophysiological pathways for tissue injury (inflammatory, immunological, autoregulatory, and adaptive process); the primary mechanism for renal injury is thus not the same. Prerenal cause includes dehydration, where serum creatinine rises due to functional adaptive drop in GFR and it is fluid responsive while in other prerenal etiology like congestive cardiac failure or nephrotic syndrome, structure damage to kidney may be present and administration of fluid in such setting may be detrimental to the final

Table 3.2 Important causes of acute kidney injury in children

Prerenal	*Hypovolemia*: Gastroenteritis, vomiting, hemorrhage, bleeding, nasogastric drainage, diuretic use *Third space loss*: Nephrotic syndrome, sepsis, burns Congestive heart failure; hepatorenal syndrome *Medications:* Non-steroidal anti-inflammatory drugs, angiotensin converting enzyme inhibitors, angiotensin receptor blockers, calcineurin inhibitors
Intrinsic renal	*Vascular:* Renal vein or renal artery thrombosis; renal artery stenosis Hemolytic uremic syndrome, thrombotic thrombocytopenic purpura; malignant hypertension; disseminated intravascular coagulation *Glomerular:* Rapidly progressive GN (ANCA associated vasculitides, immune mediated disease, anti-glomerular basement membrane disease) Immune mediated GN (postinfectious, IgA nephropathy, lupus nephritis, membranoproliferative) *Acute tubular necrosis*: Hypoxic/ischemic injury; medications (aminoglycosides, amphotericin, acyclovir, cisplatin, radiocontrast); exogenous toxins (ethylene glycol, methanol, heavy metals); intrinsic toxins (myoglobin, hemoglobin, tumor lysis syndrome); any prolonged prerenal cause *Interstitial nephritis:* Drug induced, idiopathic *Infection* : Pyelonephritis, malaria, leptospirosis
Postrenal	Posterior urethral valves, urethral stricture; bilateral pelviuretric junction obstruction Ureteral obstruction: stenosis, stone, ureterocele

ANCA antineutrophil cytoplasmic antibodies, *GN* glomerulonephritis outcome. Differentiation between fluid responsive and other prerenal causes of structural AKI damage is of importance since it helps mitigate further renal injury. The conventional approach of classification does not provide insight into the nature of injury and is not used for initial management.

Chief causes of AKI in the developing world are systemic sepsis, diarrhea, infections such as malaria, leptospirosis, and dengue, and the use of nephrotoxic agents [8]. Appropriate use of antibiotics and change in patterns of epidemiology have resulted in significant decline in the occurrence of poststreptococcal glomerulonephritis and shigatoxin-associated hemolytic uremic syndrome (HUS), respectively. Systemic sepsis and atypical HUS are the chief causes of severe AKI, requiring renal replacement therapy.

3.3.1 Neonatal AKI

Prerenal causes including hypoxemia, hypovolemia, and hypotension account for ~85% of neonatal AKI; intrinsic and postrenal causes are uncommon. Perinatal hypoxemia secondary to birth asphyxia or respiratory distress syndrome is a leading cause; 50–60% babies with severe birth asphyxia have AKI. Hypovolemia, secondary to dehydration, intraventricular hemorrhage, twin-to-twin transfusion syndrome, placental hemorrhage, and increased insensible losses (radiant warmer, phototherapy) are important causes [10]. Congenital malformations of the kidney and urinary tract can present with AKI in babies. Neonates are highly sensitive to inhibition of angiotensin converting enzyme (ACE); there is thus high risk for AKI when exposed to ACE inhibitors. Renal vein thrombosis, in patients with history of maternal diabetes, perinatal asphyxia, polycythemia, umbilical vein catheterization, dehydration, and sepsis, is an uncommon but important cause. Such patients also require screening for protein C and S deficiency, homocystinuria, and rare inherited prothrombotic disorders [11].

3.4 Diagnostic Evaluation

3.4.1 Renal Angina Index

Early identification of AKI is essential as no proven curative therapy is available and early institution of preventive measures can help mitigate renal injury. Analogous to concept of cardiac angina, where myocardial infarction is identified by precordial pain, the concept of renal angina has been proposed for AKI. This is a collection of multiple clinical risk factors and evidence of kidney injury used for stratification of patients at risk of AKI (Table 3.3) [12].

Renal angina index = Risk of AKI × Sign of kidney injury

Renal angina score ranges from 1 to 40; the negative predictive value of a score <8 for occurrence of AKI is 92%. The tool can be utilized for identification of high risk patients, who can then be screened for standard and novel biomarker(s).

Table 3.3 Renal angina index[a]

Risk of AKI		Sign of kidney injury		
Risk factor	Score	Reduced creatinine clearance	Fluid overload (%)	Score
Sepsis, ICU admission	1	No change	≤5	1
Stem-cell, solid organ transplant	3	0–24.99%	5–9.99	2
Mechanical ventilation and inotropic support	5	25–49.99%	10–14.99	4
		>50%	≥15	8

$$\text{Fluid over load} \equiv \text{Fluid In} - \text{Fluid Out} \times 100 \div \text{Admission body weight}$$

[a]Renal angina index is the product of risk and severity of kidney injury within 24 h of admission

3.4.2 Novel Biomarkers

The diagnosis of AKI depends on serial monitoring of serum creatinine and urine output, both functional biomarkers that rise late in the pathophysiology of AKI and when large part of renal parenchyma is damaged. Efforts have been made to discover biomarkers that identify structural renal injury, including neutrophil gelatinase associated lipocalin (NGAL), kidney injury molecule 1 (KIM-1), interleukin-18 (IL18), and liver-type fatty acid binding protein (L-FABP). Studies show increase of these biomarkers, 2–12 h after the insult, enabling an early diagnosis of AKI that precedes the rise in serum creatinine at 48 h. These markers need validation before they can be used as point of care test for children, especially in those undergoing cardiac surgery, or with multiorgan failure and sepsis. Two biomarkers, insulin-like growth factor binding protein 7 (IGFBP7) and tissue inhibitor of metalloproteinase-2 (TIMP-2) are approved by the US FDA for clinical use [13].

3.4.3 Clinical Evaluation

A careful history provides clues to underlying etiology of AKI. In a child with history of reduced urine output, patients should be screened for features of prerenal cause: vomiting, diarrhea, blood and volume loss, and history of fluid intake in last 24 h. Acute tubular necrosis is most common cause of AKI in hospitalized children and can occur in multiple settings, i.e., sepsis with capillary leak, burns, cardiac dysfunction, and inadequate fluid replacement. Attention should be paid to the overall fluid balance; negative balance suggests dehydration and hypovolemia while progressive increase in weight suggests excessive fluid accumulation and severe form of AKI.

History is obtained for additional features: edema, hematuria, and hypertension (acute glomerulonephritis); dysentery, pallor, and petechiae (HUS); sudden onset pallor, jaundice, and cola colored urine (intravascular hemolysis); rash and arthritis (systemic lupus, vasculitis). History of colic with hematuria and dysuria suggests nephrolithiasis, while history of interrupted urinary stream and palpable urinary bladder suggests obstruction in lower urinary tract. Urine output is usually normal in patients with AKI secondary to nephrotoxic medications (aminoglycosides, amphotericin B, calcineurin inhibitors, and angiotensin converting enzyme inhibitors) and radiocontrast agents. Anuria is present in patient with urinary tract obstruction, acute cortical necrosis, bilateral vascular occlusion, and severe glomerulonephritis. Polyuria may be seen in patients with partial ureteral obstruction, pre-existing tubular disorders such as diabetes insipidus, or hyperglycemia.

AKI may occasionally occur in patient with chronic kidney disease, suggested by the presence of failure to thrive, bony deformities, hypocalcemia, hyperphosphatemia, and small contracted kidneys. AKI may be precipitated by hypotension, urinary tract infection, and nephrotoxic drug intake. Patients with AKI may present with altered sensorium and seizures secondary to severe hypertension or uremia. They may show features of fluid overload (pulmonary edema, heart failure); metabolic acidosis manifests with rapid and deep breathing.

3.4.4 Laboratory Evaluation

Investigations help confirm the underlying etiology and assess severity of AKI. Differentiating prerenal from intrinsic causes is important. Acute tubular necrosis in the setting of hypoperfusion results in reduced tubular function with high urinary sodium (>40 mEq/L) and dilute urine (osmolality <300 mOsm/kg). In prerenal state, the GFR is reduced but tubular reabsorption is normal; urine sodium (<20 mEq/L) and its fractional excretion are low (<1%), and there is high ratio of blood urea to creatinine (>20 mg/mg). These indices have limited role in non-oliguric failure.

Investigations performed in patients with AKI are shown in Table 3.4. Peripheral smear is examined for evidence of microangiopathic hemolytic anemia and

Table 3.4 Laboratory investigations in acute kidney injury (AKI)

Urinalysis	Protein, red blood cells (RBC) and morphology, RBC and leukocyte casts, granular casts culture[a]
Blood	Complete blood count, peripheral smear for microangiopathy, and malarial parasite Creatinine, urea Potassium, sodium, calcium, phosphate, albumin[a] pH, bicarbonate, base deficit Coagulation profile[a] Autoimmune profile: Antinuclear antibody, antineutrophil cytoplasmic antibody[a] Complement C3 and C4[a] Serology: leptospirosis, rickettsial, dengue
Imaging	Abdominal ultrasonography Chest X-ray, electrocardiogram Doppler study[a] Micturating cystourethrogram[a]
Biopsy[a]	Diagnosis of glomerulonephritis, interstitial nephritis, allograft rejection Unexplained cause for AKI

[a]Required if suggested by history and physical examination to determine underlying cause of AKI

thrombocytopenia. Urinalysis helps evaluate for glomerulonephritis, indicated by proteinuria, hematuria, and red cell casts. The presence of renal epithelial cells and muddy brown tubular casts supports the diagnosis of acute tubular necrosis. Serum C3 and titer of ASO other streptococcal antibodies is done in patients suspected to have poststreptococcal glomerulonephritis.

Ultrasonography is an important investigation for evaluating AKI, since it allows delineation of kidney anatomy, congenital anomalies, obstruction in urinary tract, and renal vascular thrombosis. Renal biopsy is indicated in the following patients with AKI: unclear etiology; prolonged unremitting course lasting beyond 2–3 weeks; suspected rapidly progressive GN, vasculitis, or interstitial nephritis; and AKI in renal allograft. In all these cases, histological diagnosis is likely to have clinical implications for management. Patients with severe azotemia should receive 2–3 sessions of dialysis to reduce severity of azotemia and the risk of bleeding.

3.5 Management

In a suspected case of prerenal AKI, the first step is *assessment of intravascular volume status*. If depleted, correction of hypovolemia leads to improved renal perfusion and subsequent urine output. Hypovolemia is corrected by administration of 20–30 ml/kg of isotonic solution over 45–60 min. During fluid administration vital signs and central venous pressure are monitored to determine adequacy of fluid replacement and avoid overhydration, which can be detrimental. If urine output is less than 1 ml/kg/h after 2 h and there are no signs of intravascular volume deficit, furosemide is given (1–2 mg/kg IV); if this fails to improve urine output, then an intrinsic cause for AKI is suspected.

The principles of management in established AKI comprise management of life-threatening complications, specific therapy of the underlying disorder, and supportive care in form of dialysis and nutrition. *Lower urinary tract obstruction should be ruled out in all cases by ultrasonography*. Patients with lower urinary tract obstruction require early intervention, although definitive surgery is usually performed after AKI has resolved.

3.5.1 Therapy for Complications

In patients with AKI and oligoanuria, attention is directed to detect life-threatening complications, including hyperkalemia, hyponatremia, pulmonary edema, severe hypertension, metabolic acidosis, and anemia. Appropriate clinical evaluation is necessary. Urgent laboratory investigations include blood electrolytes, urea, creatinine, pH, bicarbonate, and hemoglobin. Patients should undergo an electrocardiogram to screen for hyperkalemia, and chest-X-ray for pulmonary edema.

Hyperkalemia is the most dangerous life-threatening complication of AKI, and can result in cardiac arrhythmias and sudden death. Urgent treatment instituted

Table 3.5 Therapies for complications of acute kidney injury (AKI)

Fluid overload	Restrict fluid to 400 ml/m^2 plus urine output and losses; 5–10% dextrose for insensible loss and N/2 for urine output; prefer oral to intravenous fluids		
Pulmonary edema	Oxygen, IV furosemide 2–4 mg/kg, fluid restriction, dialysis		
Hypertensive emergency	Infusion of sodium nitroprusside 0.5–8 μg/kg/min or labetalol 0.25–3 mg/kg/h; furosemide if fluid overload 25% of desired blood pressure reduction is done within 8 h; remainder over next 12–24 h		
Metabolic acidosis	Sodium bicarbonate oral or IV (for bicarbonate levels <18 mEq/L); monitor for fluid overload and hypernatremia		
Hyponatremia	Restrict fluid intake If altered sensorium or seizures: 3% saline 6–12 ml/kg over 30–90 min		
Hyperkalemia			
	Dose	Onset	Remarks
Calcium gluconate, 10%	1 ml/kg IV over 3–5 min; repeat after 10 min	5 min	Stabilize cell membrane; prevent arrhythmias; give under cardiac monitoring
Sodium bicarbonate, 7.5%	1–2 ml/kg IV over 5–10 min	15–60 min	Shifts potassium into cells; do not give with calcium gluconate
Insulin-dextrose	0.1 U/kg insulin with 0.5 g/kg glucose IV over 30 min	20 min	Shifts potassium into cells; monitor for hypoglycemia
Salbutamol	5–10 mg by nebulization over 10 min	30 min	Shift potassium into cells
Calcium or sodium resonium	1 g/kg/d orally or per rectally	2 h	Slow action with variable efficacy

Patients with complications related to AKI should also be considered for early initiation of renal replacement therapy

depending on blood level of potassium level and changes on electrocardiograph. Hyponatremia is chiefly related to excessive hypotonic fluid administration and it best treated by restriction of fluid. Mostly patients with serum sodium >125 mEq/L are asymptomatic; those with symptomatic hyponatremia require treatment with 3% saline (Table 3.5). If complications are severe or refractory to medical measures, patients require urgent renal replacement therapy.

3.5.2 Specific Therapy

Immunosuppressive therapy with intravenous methylprednisolone and cyclophosphamide is instituted in patients with crescentic GN and severe lupus nephritis. Intensive plasmapheresis is additionally recommended for most patients with pauci-immune crescentic GN [14]. Patients with interstitial nephritis show satisfactory response to short-term therapy with prednisolone. While HUS secondary to shigatoxin infection is chiefly managed with supportive care, patients with atypical HUS require intensive plasma therapy and/or treatment with complement inhibitors. A subset of patients with anti-factor H associated HUS is effectively managed

Table 3.6 Specific treatment for common causes of acute kidney injury (AKI)

Atypical hemolytic uremic syndrome (HUS)	Plasma exchange; plasma infusions Eculizumab; novel complement inhibitors Immunosuppressive agents (corticosteroids, cyclophosphamide, azathioprine) for autoimmune HUS
Glomerulonephritis (GN)	IV methylprednisolone 3–6 pulses; *and either* IV cyclophosphamide q 3–4 weekly for 5–6 doses *or* rituximab infusions initially, q 4–6 months Plasma exchanges (pauci-immune crescentic GN; severe GN; anti GBM disease) Follow-up: Azathioprine or mycophenolate mofetil; taper prednisolone Antibiotics; removal of infected prosthesis
Interstitial nephritis	Discontinue offending agent; oral prednisolone 2–3 weeks
Urinary tract obstruction	Bladder catheterization; nephrostomy; radiological and surgically guided drainage

with intensive plasmapheresis, combined with immunosuppression; therapy with eculizumab may be indicated in specific instances (Table 3.6).

3.5.3 Fluid and Electrolytes

Careful fluid management is advised in patients with AKI to avoid complications of volume overload, which is associated with an adverse outcome. Daily fluid intake should be restricted to insensible losses (400 ml/m^2 body surface area) and ongoing losses. Insensible losses should be replaced with 10% dextrose, and urinary and extrarenal losses with 0.45% saline. The oral route is preferred for fluid administration. Patients with fluid overload should receive less than their daily requirement, in order to promote negative balance. Daily fluid prescription should be guided by strict input–output monitoring, physical examination, and estimation of daily weight and serum sodium. Judicious fluid administration with appropriate composition often results in 0.5–1% weight loss/day. Hyponatremia, hypertension, and failure to lose weight suggest excessive fluid intake, whereas excessive weight loss and hypernatremia suggest inadequate free water replacement.

Patients with AKI are at risk of electrolyte disturbances and need frequent monitoring. Potassium and sodium containing fluids should be restricted, especially in cases with oligoanuria. On the other hand, excessive fluid and electrolyte loss in non-oliguric AKI often requires supplements of potassium and sodium. Patients with AKI may show hyperphosphatemia that is managed by restriction of dietary phosphate and use of phosphate binders.

3.5.4 Pharmacological Therapy

There is currently no evidence-based pharmacological therapy for prevention or treatment of AKI. Dopamine in renal dose (0.5 μg/kg/min) improves renal blood flow and sodium excretion; the effect is short lasting and variable. Randomized trials in adults fail to show any utility of dopamine or fenoldopam for prevention and treatment of AKI [15]. Intravenous furosemide may result in improved urine output, but systematic reviews show no evidence of immediate renal recovery or long-term prognosis. KDIGO guidelines, however, state that therapy with IV frusemide be considered in patients with volume overload [5]. Such therapy may be useful in critically sick patients, awaiting initiation of dialysis. Systematic reviews suggest that single dose theophylline (5–8 mg/kg/day) is effective in reducing the incidence of renal dysfunction in term neonates with severe perinatal asphyxia. Agents like nesiritide, growth factors, and antioxidants require more evidence for use in clinical care.

3.5.5 Nutrition

Patients with AKI have increased metabolic requirements and are usually catabolic. Nutritional supplementation is a crucial component of the management plan for every patient. Most children with AKI are critically ill with increased protein catabolism, and should receive a minimum protein intake of 0.8–1.2 g/kg/day, that is increased to 1.5–1.8 g/kg/day in patients undergoing hemo- or peritoneal dialysis. The target energy intake should be close to the recommended dietary allowance. While on dialysis, these children require supplements of water soluble vitamins and micronutrients. Patients, who do not achieve desired intake with enteral feeding, are considered for parenteral alimentation [16, 17].

3.5.6 Renal Replacement Therapy

Advancement and innovation over the last decades have ensured that acute dialysis is currently the most effective therapy for management of AKI and can be provided safely to children of all age groups. Acute dialysis is used early to avoid severe complications related to AKI and facilitate renal recovery rather than as last resort for management. Indications for renal replacement therapy (RRT) include: hyperkalemia (>7 mEq/L); symptomatic hyponatremia and hypernatremia; severe metabolic acidosis (TCO_2 <10–12 mEq/L); neurological complications (seizures, altered sensorium); and fluid overload. *Fluid overload (exceeding 10–15%) is an independent predictor for mortality and prolonged hospital stay, and one of the chief indications for dialysis.* Fluid overload is calculated as follows:

$$\text{Fluid over load} \equiv \text{Fluid In} - \text{Fluid Out} \times 100 \div \text{Admission body weight}$$

Dialysis should also be considered early in patients in whom adequate nutrition intake is not achieved due to fluid restriction [18, 19].

Modalities for RRT in children include peritoneal dialysis, intermittent hemodialysis, and continuous renal replacement therapy (CRRT). Hemodialysis and peritoneal dialysis are equally effective for overall management of AKI. The choice of modality depends on patient size, clinical status, indication for RRT, and center specific expertise. In patients with hemodynamic instability, CRRT and peritoneal dialysis are preferred; in stable patients hemodialysis is as effective as CRRT. Removal of metabolic toxins and drugs is rapid and better achieved with hemodialysis and CRRT. In centers that lack expertise, peritoneal dialysis is the preferred modality since it is easy to perform, inexpensive, and needs minimal infrastructure; sick children and infants also tolerate the gradual removal of fluid better. Peritoneal dialysis should be avoided if the peritoneal membrane is damaged.

Several forms of CRRT are available, which include continuous venovenous hemodialysis, continuous venovenous hemofiltration, or continuous venovenous hemodiafiltration. CRRT requires expensive equipment and expertise, but is the preferred modality for AKI with heart failure, septic shock, and pulmonary edema. Patients with tumor lysis syndrome, hyperammonemia, and hypercatabolic state are also better managed with CRRT.

3.5.7 Use of Medications

Medication that worsen renal injury or delay recovery, e.g., aminoglycosides, nonsteroidal anti-inflammatory drugs (NSAIDs), amphotericin B should be avoided. The use of radiocontrast agents should be minimized. Drugs that impair renal perfusion (angiotensin converting enzyme inhibitors, NSAIDs) should not be used. Drug dosing should be adjusted as per residual renal function to avoid toxicity and prevent further renal injury. Agents excreted through the kidneys require dose modification once glomerular filtration rate decreases <50% of normal. Many medications are cleared during dialysis; standard charts should be used to determine whether additional dosing is required while receiving RRT. Monitoring of medication levels is applicable for few agents.

3.6 Outcome

Despite advancements in RRT, the mortality related to AKI has not improved significantly in children. The outcome is significantly determined by underlying etiology. While dehydration, diarrhea, intravascular hemolysis, and nephrotoxic drug related AKI have favorable prognosis, outcomes in crescentic GN, sepsis, and multiorgan failure are less satisfactory. Overall mortality rates of 30–40% are reported in low middle income countries with unsatisfactory survival among critically ill children. A recent 0by25 global snapshot study reported 7-day mortality of ~10% in hospitalized children in resource limited settings [20]. In a recent prospective study, the 28-day mortality rate of 13% was observed among the critically sick children and young adults with AKI [6].

Long-term studies also underscore the fact that AKI is not a one-time insult, and patients might be at risk of long-term adverse outcome. A meta-analysis in adult patients with AKI showed 9-times higher risk of developing chronic kidney disease

(CKD). A recent systematic review of morbidity following an episode of AKI in children showed proteinuria in 13.2%, hypertension in 6.6%, and CKD in 28%. Every patient should have long-term follow-up plan after an episode of AKI, with focus on detection of proteinuria, hypertension, and decline in GFR [21, 22]. The initial assessment should be made at 2–3 months and then every 3–6 months, depending upon risk factors and degree of recovery from AKI [23].

References

1. Lameire NH, Bagga A, Cruz D, De Maeseneer J, Endre Z, Kellum JA, et al. Acute kidney injury: an increasing global concern. Lancet. 2013;382:170–9.
2. Bellomo R, Ronco C, Kellum JA, Mehta RL, Palevsky P, Acute Dialysis Quality Initiative Workgroup. Acute renal failure - definition, outcome measures, animal models, fluid therapy and information technology needs: the Second International Consensus Conference of the Acute Dialysis Quality Initiative (ADQI) Group. Crit Care. 2004;8(4):R204–12.
3. Akcan-Arikan A, Zappitelli M, Loftis LL, Wasburn KK, Jefferson LS, Goldstein SL. Modified RIFLE criteria in critically ill children with acute kidney injury. Kidney Int. 2007;71:1028–35.
4. Mehta RL, Kellum JA, Shah SV, Molitoris BA, Ronco C, Warnock DG, et al. Acute Kidney Injury Network: report of an initiative to improve outcomes in acute kidney injury. Crit Care. 2007;11:R31.
5. Kellum JA, et al. Kidney disease: improving global outcome (KDIGO) acute kidney injury work group. KDIGO clinical practice guideline for acute kidney injury. Kidney Int Suppl. 2012;2:124–38.
6. Kaddourah A, Basu RK, Bagshaw SM, Goldstein SL, AWARE Investigators. Epidemiology of acute kidney injury in critically ill children and young adults. N Engl J Med. 2017;376(1):11–20.
7. Jetton JG, Boohaker LJ, Sethi SK, Wazir S, Rohatgi S, Soranno DE, et al. Incidence and outcomes of neonatal acute kidney injury (AWAKEN): a multicentre, multinational, observational cohort study. Lancet Child Adolesc Health. 2017;1(3):184–94.
8. Cerdá J, Bagga A, Kher V, Chakravarthi RM. The contrasting characteristics of acute kidney injury in developed and developing countries. Nat Clin Pract Nephrol. 2008;4(3):138–53.
9. Feehally J. The ISN 0by25 global snapshot study. Ann Nutr Metab. 2016;68(Suppl 2):29–31.
10. Jetton JG, Askenazi DJ. Update on acute kidney injury in the neonate. Curr Opin Pediatr. 2012;24(2):191–6.
11. Mian AN, Askenazi DJ, Mhanna MJ. Therapeutic options for neonatal acute kidney injury (AKI). Curr Treat Options Pediatr. 2016;2(2):69–81.
12. Goldstein SL, Chawla LS. Renal angina. Clin J Am Soc Nephrol. 2010;5(5):943–9.
13. Ciccia E, Devarajan P. Pediatric acute kidney injury: prevalence, impact and management challenges. Int J Nephrol Renovasc Dis. 2017;10:77–84.
14. Walters G. Role of therapeutic plasmapheresis in ANCA-associated vasculitis. Pediatr Nephrol. 2016;31:217.
15. Friedrich JO, Adhikari N, Herridge MS, Beyene J. Metaanalysis: low-dose dopamine increases urine output but does not prevent renal dysfunction or death. Ann Intern Med. 2005;142:510–24.
16. Li Y, Tang X, Zhang J, Wu T. Nutritional support for acute kidney injury. Cochrane Database Sys Rev. 2012;8:CD005426.
17. Sethi SK, Maxvold N, Bunchman T, Jha P, Kher V, Raina R. Nutritional management in the critically ill child with acute kidney injury: a review. Pediatr Nephrol. 2017;32(4):589–601.
18. Walters S, Porter C, Brophy PD. Dialysis and pediatric acute kidney injury: choice of renal support modality. Pediatr Nephrol. 2009;24:37–48.
19. Sutherland SM, Zappitelli M, Alexander SR, Chua AN, Brophy PD, Bunchman TE, et al. Fluid overload and mortality in children receiving continuous renal replacement therapy: the prospective pediatric continuous renal replacement therapy registry. Am J Kidney Dis. 2010;55:316–25.

20. Macedo E, Cerdá J, Hingorani S, Hou J, Bagga A, Burdmann EA, et al. Recognition and management of acute kidney injury in children: The ISN 0by25 Global Snapshot study. PLoS One. 2018;13(5):e0196586.
21. Greenberg JH, Coca S, Parikh CR. Long-term risk of chronic kidney disease and mortality in children after acute kidney injury: a systematic review. BMC Nephrol. 2014;15:184.
22. Sigurjonsdottir VK, Chaturvedi S, Mammen C, Sutherland SM. Pediatric acute kidney injury and the subsequent risk for chronic kidney disease: is there cause for alarm? Pediatr Nephrol. 2018;33(11):2047–55.
23. Mehta R, Bagga A, Patibandla R, Chakravarthi R. Detection and management of AKI in the Developing World: The 18th Acute Disease Quality Initiative (ADQI) International Consensus Conference. Kidney Int Rep. 2017;2(4):515–51.

Fluid Overload and Management

4

Leyat Tal, Manpreet Kaur Virk, and Ayse Akcan Arikan

Case 1: Oliguric AKI

A 19-year-old female with acute myeloid leukemia and neutropenia admitted to the PICU with 1 day history of fever, chills, malaise, decreased oral intake, and decreased urine output. Vital signs were temp 103 °F, heart rate 170, respiratory rate 28, blood pressure 90/50, oxygen saturation of 96%; admission weight was 75 kg. Her exam was significant for ill appearance and pallor with tachycardia, cool extremities, and a capillary refill of 4–5 seconds. She was otherwise euvolemic with the rest of her exam being unremarkable. Upon arrival to the PICU patient was intubated for impending respiratory failure and received 2.5 L of fluid resuscitation before being started on inotropic support for septic shock. Chemistry on admission to PICU showed Na 145 mEq/L, K 5.4 mEq/L, Cl 114 mmol/L, CO_2 17 mmol/L, BUN 45 mg/dL, Cr 2.82 mg/dL, Ca 8.1 mg/dL, Mg 1.7 mmol/L, and P 5.1 mmol/L. Baseline serum creatinine

L. Tal
Department of Pediatrics, Renal Section, Baylor College of Medicine, Houston, TX, USA

Critical Care Nephrology, Texas Children's Hospital, Houston, TX, USA

M. K. Virk
Department of Pediatrics, Critical Care Section, Baylor College of Medicine, Houston, TX, USA

A. A. Arikan (✉)
Department of Pediatrics, Renal Section, Baylor College of Medicine, Houston, TX, USA

Department of Pediatrics, Critical Care Section, Baylor College of Medicine, Houston, TX, USA

Critical Care Nephrology, Texas Children's Hospital, Houston, TX, USA
e-mail: aysea@bcm.edu

S. K. Sethi et al. (eds.), *Critical Care Pediatric Nephrology and Dialysis: A Practical Handbook*, https://doi.org/10.1007/978-981-13-2276-1_4

was 0.6–0.7 mg/dL. Within 24 h patient developed oliguria (<0.5 mL/kg/h) and fluid overload with net fluid balance of positive 6 L. Her physical exam was significant for anasarca with periorbital, sacral, and lower extremity pitting edema with 3+ ascites. Patient was started on continuous renal replacement therapy for fluid overload of 13% and oliguric acute kidney injury (AKI) Stage 3 from septic AKI.

Case 2: Non-oliguric AKI

A 12-year-old previously healthy male who presented to the emergency center with a 2 day history of fever, right leg pain, and inability to bear weight. Vital signs were temp 100.7 °F, heart rate 105, respiratory rate 22, blood pressure 115/70, oxygen saturation 99%; admission weight was 52 kg. His exam was significant for tenderness over lateral aspect of the right leg and inability to bear weight without signs of compartment syndrome. Serum chemistry showed Na 141 mEq/L, K 4.2 mEq/L, Cl 100 mmol/L, CO_2 24 mmol/L, BUN 15 mg/dL, Cr 0.6 mg/dL, Ca 9 mg/dL, Mg 1.8 mmol/L, and P 4.6 mmol/L. His CBC was remarkable for WBC 15 × 10^3/μL with 80% neutrophils, erythrocyte sedimentation rate 80 mm/h, and C-reactive protein 3.5 mg/L. Computed tomography scan with intravenous (IV) contrast was concerning for tibial osteomyelitis so a surgical bone biopsy was performed. He was admitted to the general pediatrics service and started on IV vancomycin every 8 h. Repeat chemistry 48 h after starting IV vancomycin showed Na 142 mEq/L, K 3.6 mEq/L, Cl 102 mmol/L, CO_2 25 mmol/L, BUN 20 mg/dL, Cr 4.3 mg/dL, Ca 8.8 mg/dL, and Phos 5 mmol/L. The vancomycin trough level prior to the fourth dose was elevated at 35. A fractional excretion of sodium (FeNa) was 3%. He was started on D5 1/2NS at 110 ml/h. His fluid intake/output balance since admission showed him at positive fluid balance of 1.5 L with urine output of 2 ml/kg/h. Repeat weight was 55 kg with physical exam significant for 2+ lower extremity edema, 1+ periorbital edema, and ascites. Patient was diagnosed with non-oliguric acute kidney injury Stage 3 from presumed acute tubular necrosis secondary to nephrotoxic medication and IV contrast exposure with 5% fluid overload. He was started on IV Lasix 30 mg every 12 h and was able to achieve negative fluid balance and he returned back to his baseline weight. IV vancomycin was discontinued once bone culture results returned and within 72 h serum creatinine had returned to baseline 0.65 mg/dL.

4.1 Fluid Overload: Pathophysiology

Fluid administration remains the cornerstone of medical therapy in order to restore effective circulatory volume and maintain end organ perfusion in critically ill patients. Fluid resuscitation is often carried out in critically ill patients in order to maintain organ perfusion and to correct hemodynamic instability. Ongoing massive volume resuscitation can commonly lead to fluid overload and contribute to organ dysfunction [1]. In addition, critically ill patients frequently have high obligate fluid intake due to requirement for continuous infusions and multiple medications used in supportive care. In this chapter we will focus on the assessment and management of fluid overload in the context of oliguric and non-oliguric AKI.

Critically ill patients have a multitude of reasons contributing to fluid overload:

1. Positive pressure ventilation: Increased intrathoracic pressure associated with invasive mechanical ventilation leads to activation of feedback mechanisms to restore intravascular volume. These mechanisms along with capillary leak, increasing extravascular lung water, and defective alveolar fluid clearance [2] all lead to worsening gaseous exchange.
2. Activation of renin-angiotensin-aldosterone system (RAAS) pathway: In states of true hypovolemia or decrease in effective circulating volume (advanced end stage liver disease with portal hypertension and ascites, congestive heart failure), neurohumoral compensatory mechanisms get triggered. Aldosterone stimulates sodium reabsorption by the principal cells of the late distal tubule and collecting duct resulting in salt and water retention to maintain effective arterial blood volume. Unfortunately, in certain cases, especially with low effective circulating volume in the setting of increased total body water, these compensatory mechanisms become maladaptive and contribute to excess fluid retention. In certain cases, RAAS activation could be partially responsible for "diuretic resistance" observed where despite increasing doses of loop diuretics, urine output response is not maintained or even decreased.
3. Non-osmotic control of antidiuretic hormone (ADH) release: Sympathetic stimulation particularly alpha and beta adrenergic stimulation alters renal water excretion by controlling ADH release via baroreceptor pathways. Various stimuli such as hypovolemia, nausea, vomiting, hypoglycemia, and elevated IL-6 concentrations lead to inappropriate ADH secretion leading to fluid retention. Similar to the mechanism described above, adaptive responses might become maladaptive, contributing further to fluid accumulation.
4. Syndrome of inappropriate ADH secretion (SIADH): Commonly seen in conditions such as CNS tumors, pulmonary disease (viral infections), spinal surgery, and medications (especially chemotherapeutic agents such as vincristine and etoposide). SIADH is characterized by a euvolemic hyponatremia resulting in retention of free water and expansion of intravascular space. SIADH is very common in the critically ill patients and contributes to oliguria and fluid retention.

5. Oliguric acute kidney injury: Widespread inflammation, microvascular congestion, and thrombosis along with decreased end organ perfusion cause AKI and oliguria further contributing to fluid imbalance. Furthermore, creatinine commonly used as a marker of kidney function may be falsely low given increased total body water in fluid overloaded patients and hence mislead practitioners. Some adult data have suggested that creatinine production decreases in the critically ill patients. In liver failure, musculoskeletal diseases with decreased muscle mass, or malnutrition, serum creatinine levels, and estimated creatinine clearance significantly overestimate true glomerular filtration rate. Some authors have proposed that serum creatinine levels be corrected for degree of fluid overload for more accurate diagnosis of AKI in the critically ill.
6. Obligate fluid intake and relative oliguria—Limited data exists on obligatory maintenance fluids in the critically ill. In the early phase of illness, fluid administration is required to establish therapy and reach hemodynamic stability, but might lead to fluid accumulation. Awareness of total fluid exposure including fluid administered with medications would be beneficial once resuscitation phase is completed. Oliguria (absolute or relative) in the setting of acute kidney injury needs to be assessed to avoid missed diagnoses, where increases in creatinine could be masked due to the dilutional effect of total body fluid overload on serum creatinine.
7. Congestive heart failure/pulmonary hypertension/right heart dysfunction: Altered angiogenesis, dysmorphic pulmonary circulation, and alveolar simplification in premature infants result in bronchopulmonary dysplasia and associated pulmonary hypertension. Elevated pulmonary vascular resistance with underlying abnormal vasoconstrictor response to hypoxia and decreased cross-sectional vascular surface area for gas exchange in these patients all contribute to pulmonary artery hypertension and right ventricular dysfunction [3] leading to elevated right sided pressures resulting in poor venous return. Positive pressure ventilation with increased intrathoracic pressure leads to increased resistance to venous return, which, along with compression of lymph vessels, results in poor lymphatic flow further worsening pulmonary edema. Premature infants with BPD also have LV dysfunction, which along with elevated left atrial pressure, pulmonary venous congestion, and poor pulmonary compliance result in pulmonary edema resistant to diuretics [4, 5].
8. Prolonged immobilization/deep sedation/neuromuscular blockade. Critically ill patients under neuromuscular blockade have abnormal vasomotor tone adversely affecting the venous pump further limiting venous return to the heart. Prolonged immobilization and lack of muscular activity and muscular contractions impair the so-called venous pump, leading to venous stasis and edema formation. Hypoalbuminemia and endothelial leak of critical illness also contribute to this phenomenon. Additionally, catabolism of critical illness, combined with muscle wasting due to disuse atrophy, leads to weight loss, potentially masking fluid accumulation, as weight seems stable.

Given multiple of the conditions above coexisting in the typical critically ill patient, it is easy to see how positive fluid balance could quickly lead to fluid overload. It is important to recognize and manage fluid overload early on in the clinical course, as reversal of fluid overload and restitution of euvolemia has not been shown to alter outcomes, although data is limited. Both adult and pediatric studies have signaled an association with increased morbidity and mortality after significant FO, somewhere between 10 and 20% [6–8].

4.1.1 Impact on Organ Function With Special Pediatric Considerations

Respiratory Failure Recent data [9, 10] has shown that daily positive fluid balance has adverse effect with increased morbidity and longer duration of mechanical ventilation in critically ill patients. Specifically in patients with respiratory failure requiring invasive mechanical ventilation, fluid imbalance, commonly seen in critically ill patients, has many deleterious consequences including worsening gas exchange and pulmonary compliance from increased extravascular lung water and defective alveolar fluid clearance. Cumulative fluid balance has been associated with longer duration of mechanical ventilation and higher mortality in pediatric patients with acute lung injury as well as worse oxygenation [9, 11, 12].

Intra-Abdominal Hypertension and Abdominal Compartment Syndrome Due to underlying inflammatory state and capillary leak, fluid imbalance also leads to increased intra-abdominal pressure and abdominal compartment syndrome further decreasing end organ perfusion. This could have profound consequences for intestinal, renal, and, hepatic function, among others.

Delayed Wound Healing Fluid overload in post-surgical patient leads to poor wound healing and tissue necrosis. In the general ICU population, it creates a predisposition to pressure ulceration further exacerbating a healthcare associated condition.

Pharmacokinetics/Pharmacodynamics Additionally, these patients can have altered volume of distribution (V_d) secondary to increased total body volume coupled with renal failure. Increased V_d can result in lower than required plasma concentrations of various medications importantly antibiotics further resulting in suboptimal therapeutic targets leading to under treatment. Hence, readjusting doses corresponding to the V_d is of paramount importance especially in the early phase of the illness.

Acute Kidney Injury It is unclear if fluid overload is a cause, a consequence, or a confounder of AKI in the ICU. It follows severe oliguric AKI and inability to appropriately restrict fluids due to obligate intake, however, not all patients who develop fluid overload are oliguric. No direct causative relationship between fluid overload and adverse outcomes has been demonstrated. Confounding by indication profoundly impacts this relationship: sicker kids receive a significantly higher number of obligate medications translating to a cumulative higher fluid intake. Decreased excretion as in covert acute kidney injury with accompanying absolute or relative oliguria has not been consistently demonstrated as the single unifying cause of fluid overload. Underlying confounders, such as the severity of illness, likely play a key role in the rate and volume of fluid exposure, but the content of intravenous fluid might also have unforeseen circumstances. For instance, 0.9% saline could exacerbate fluid overload due to its sodium content and lead to renal vasoconstriction exacerbating oliguria due to its high chloride content. Recent data has shown that hyperchloremia is independently associated with increased mortality in patients requiring CRRT [13]. On the other hand, synthetic starches could be directly nephrotoxic and contribute to AKI [14].

4.2 Assessment of Fluid Overload

Despite the increasing awareness of association between fluid overload and adverse outcomes, there is no consensus on how best to define fluid overload in the pediatric literature. A commonly used method of assessement of fluid overload is through measurement of changes in body weight. However, absolute changes in weight are not always available due to unit practices or critical nature of patients. In certain population, such as sick premature babies or neonates, increased insensible losses make the serial assessment of weights a must for accurate assessment of fluid balance. In the older critically ill population, severe catabolism can lead to weight loss masking fluid accumulation. There are different methods in defining the degree of fluid overload in a patient. This can be done either by measuring fluid intake and output (Method 1; [15]) or using weight-based formulas (Methods 2,3; [16])

Method 1 FO% = [(Sum of daily fluid in-out)/ICU admission weight] × 100

Method 2 FO% = [(calculation date weight−ICU admission weight)/ICU admission weight] × 100

Method 3 FO% = [(calculation date weight−hospital admission weight)/hospital admission weight] × 100

All three methods are generally comparable to one another thus there is no gold standard to calculating fluid overload [16]. However, in the neonatal intensive care unit, serial weights may be more desirable as insensible losses are higher than other pediatric populations and newborns are expected to lose weight in the first few days of life. Therefore, failure to lose weight might be an indication for positive fluid balance (Table 4.1 and 4.2).

Table 4.1 Clinical findings in fluid overload

• Physical exam findings	• Hypertension (if patient has capillary leak, they may still be fluid overloaded but normotensive or even hypotensive) • Cardiovascular: Tachycardia, tachypnea, gallop, jugular venous distention • Respiratory: Rales, tachypnea, decreased breath sounds • Abdomen: Hepatosplenomegaly, ascites • Extremities: Edema (lower extremity, sacral, chest wall, scalp, genitals)
• Laboratory findings	• Hyponatremia • Elevated BNP • Low BUN • Low creatinine • Dilutional anemia • Hypoalbuminemia (due to redistribution or decreased production)
Other findings	
• CXR	• Kerley lines, venous congestion, prominent pulmonary vasculature, pulmonary edema, pleural effusions
• Echo	• Dilated chambers, elevated end diastolic volume and pressure
• Hemodynamic monitoring	• Elevated CVP • Elevated PAP, pulmonary capillary wedge pressure (PCWP)
• Pulmonary mechanics	• Worsening pulmonary compliance • Worsening oxygenation (decrease in PaO_2, increasing P/F ratio, OI, OSI)
• Bioimpedance	• Evidence of increase in extracellular water, low resistance to include increased fat free mass)
• Lung US	• Increased extravascular lung water • B-lines (hyperechoic artifacts radiating from pleura–lung interface, perpendicular to probe)

Table 4.2 Available techniques to assess fluid overload

Technique	Measurement of interest	Studied in AKI	Studied in children	Limitation
Lung US	Extravascular lung water through B-line artifacts	Yes	Limited	Technologically limited in subcutaneous emphysema, post-surgical patients with dressings
Echo to assess IVC diameter	Respiratory variation in IVC diameter	No	Limited	Unreliable in spontaneously ventilating children
Serum biomarkers	BNP NT-proBNP	Yes	Limited	Unreliable in patients with heart failure and acute kidney injury
Bioimpedance vector analysis (BIVA)	Total body fluid content	Yes	Yes	Impacted by obesity

4.3 Management of Fluid Overload Under Medications Tab

The goal of managing a patient with fluid overload is to maintain a daily negative fluid balance. Depending on the patient, this can be done with either conservative management or renal replacement therapy. When considering the approach to treating fluid overload in a patient with AKI, the first step is to determine whether or not the patient is oliguric or non-oliguric.

Oliguric AKI—UOP of <0.5 ml/kg/h (KDIGO). This can also be assessed by evaluating the patient's intake/output status to see if they are in positive fluid balance.

Non-oliguric AKI—patients can have normal urine output or can even be polyuric.

FO in non-oliguric AKI

- Determine the negative balance fluid goal for the day
- Total output—fluid intake = goal negative fluid balance/day
- The negative fluid balance goal is determined based on size of patient, hemodynamic stability, degree of FO, and respiratory status. It should not exceed 5% of total body weight/24 h although safe rate remains unknown and might be lower than this threshold
- Monitor fluid intake/output (I/O) closely and adjust fluid intake as needed
- Monitor electrolytes closely as replacement may be needed

FO in oliguric AKI

- Fluid restriction
  - This will help avoid progressive fluid overload
  - Often leads to inadequate nutrition
  - Insensible fluid loss + ongoing losses (urinary, GI, respiratory) will maintain even fluid balance (starting point for fluid intake)
  - Insensible fluid loss calculation/day: 400 ml/m^2
- Medications

Loop diuretics are usually the first choice in the critically ill child. Furosemide is the most commonly used agent. Bumetanide and torsemide are other options. They can be used as intermittent bolus or continuous infusion. A meta-analysis has suggested continuous infusion to be more effective in achieving higher total urine output. Higher doses may be required to see adequate response [17]. Diuretics have not been shown to worsen AKI, but they cannot protect from it either. A "furosemide stress test" where the renal reserve tested in oliguria by assessing urine output has been proposed in adults to determine progression to severe AKI. Although not tested in an official manner, this is a clinical maneuver that has been carried out for decades in pediatric nephrology. Classical teaching entails that outcomes of oliguric AKI are worse with or without fluid overload. Conservative treatment of renal failure is often successful in the non-oliguric patient without requirement for renal replacement therapy (RRT). Alternatively, diuretic responsive FO can easily be treated with careful adjustment of diuretics and a stacked approach when necessary. Serum albumin is required to transport furosemide to the proximal tubule for secretion into the urinary space for ultimate action at the loop. Hence, patients who are hypoalbuminemic do not respond well to diuretics. Particularly in hypoalbuminemic patients with acute lung injury, loop diuretic and albumin combination infusions have led to improvement in oxygenation and ventilator parameters.

- Electrolyte management
  - In the presence of AKI, potassium should initially be removed from all fluids and TPN, also removal of phosphorus should be considered. However, in diuretic responsive FO, or FO without AKI, extra potassium supplementation will be needed to offset the urinary losses caused by loop diuretics. As intravenous potassium infusions are large volume, best approach is to start patients on enteral potassium supplementation at 2 meq/kg/day and titrate as needed. Frequent electrolyte monitoring, not only for hypokalemia but also for hyponatremia, hypomagnesemia, and hypercalcemia.
  - In hypoalbuminemic patients, careful albumin assisted diuresis with concentrated albumin infusion might augment urine output and facilitate fluid mobilization, partly due to improved medication delivery by the carrier protein albumin to the proximal tubule organic anion transporters and from there to the tubular lumen.

4.4 Renal Replacement Therapy (RRT)

RRT for pure FO should be considered in patients with FO >10% if they have failed conservative management especially if they are experiencing morbidity from fluid accumulation, such as impaired oxygenation. Additionally, the clinical picture of the patient must be assessed as a whole. In a patient with excessive obligate fluid intake due to high volume of medications or blood products, is relatively oliguric—ending each day with a positive fluid balance—and has suboptimal response to diuretics, RRT might need to be considered much sooner, even at lower FO% levels. Patients suffering from severe hypoxic respiratory failure with inadequate diuretic response will also need RRT sooner. Certain patient populations, such as stem cell transplant recipients or heart transplant recipients, are particularly sensitive to positive fluid balance, likely due to high obligate intake in the former and poor tolerance of the graft to stretching in that latter. A retrospective study has shown improvement in oxygenation and FO with CRRT in mechanically ventilated hematopoietic stem cell recipients [18]. Additionally, postoperative cardiac surgery patients frequently are started on RRT to assist with fluid balance, sternal closure, wound healing, and avoidance of overstretching of noncompliant chambers. In a small randomized controlled trial protocolized use of early PD led to higher negative fluid balance compared to diuretics alone [19]. Many centers will routinely place PD catheters for neonates/infants undergoing complex repairs with expected prolonged cardiopulmonary bypass times and initiate PD to assist with fluid removal immediately after surgery.

4.4.1 Modalities of RRT

- Continuous renal replacement therapy (CRRT) is the modality of choice for critically ill patients. It allows for gentle fluid removal in patients with hemodynamic instability, control of electrolyte and metabolic derangements, and delivery of adequate nutrition. Surgeon or pediatric intensivist with expertise in vascular access is needed. Dialysis catheter should be placed in the internal jugular vein or femoral vein. Younger patients will require a blood prime due to large extracorporeal volume. Dilutional coagulopathy could be a concern with small patients and large extracorporeal volume.
- Peritoneal dialysis (PD) is a very acceptable alternative to CRRT in pediatrics. Fluid removal is facilitated by the high dextrose concentration in the dialysate and fluid removal could be adjusted to a certain extent by increasing and decreasing the dextrose concentration. Previous abdominal surgery, significant ascites, or anasarca will limit the practical application. In patients with colostomies, especially freshly created stomas, PD is controversial and frequently not offered due to concern for infection. A typical wait time of 2 weeks is recommended before PD catheter is put to use to promote healing of the exit site and prevent leaks, which increase infection risk. However, low volume manual systems with continuous short cycles are safely instituted post-cardiopulmonary surgery in many institutions and rarely lead to infectious complications, as PD use is typically limited to 2–3 days in most patients. PD is a good alternative if the institution does not provide CRRT. It is not suitable for conditions that require high clearance, such as hyperammonemia or organic acidemias. In critically ill patients who are on high mean airway pressures for supporting oxygenation, PD often is not tolerated due to the restrictive physiology created and impact on venous return and thus cardiac output with each dwell. If significant fluid removal is required, high dextrose concentration in the dialysate could lead to hyperglycemia in the patient and requires close monitoring. It is also important to remember that automated machines currently available for children do not allow documentation of hourly fluid removal. In addition, it is difficult to tightly control the ultrafiltration.
- Intermittent hemodialysis: While not ideal for critically ill patients with hemodynamic instability, who have ongoing blood product requirement, or who are unable to fluid restrict, it can still be applicable in select patients, especially when renal recovery does not occur, as a transition to chronic dialysis. Additionally, it is contraindicated in patients who have elevated intracranial pressure, cerebral edema, or hepatic encephalopathy, as well as severe hypernatremia, due to rapid fluid shifts created with rapid solute removal. It is superior to all other modalities for efficiency of solute clearance, but has limited applicabil-

ity in the patient with fluid overload and ongoing critical illness due to poor tolerance of rapid fluid removal.

4.5 Take Home Points

- It is important to recognize fluid overload early.
- Management of FO in AKI may differ whether or not patient is oliguric or non-oliguric.
- Depending on the degree of fluid overload, conservative management may not be appropriate and patient may need to be started on CRRT.
- Fluid overload of ≥10% is associated with increased mortality.
- Fluid overload is a symptom and a biomarker rather than a stand-alone condition and requires multisystem assessment and intervention.

References

1. Claure-Del Granado R, Mehta RL. Fluid overload in the ICU: evaluation and management. BMC Nephrol. 2016;17(1):109.
2. Ware LB, Matthay MA. Alveolar fluid clearance is impaired in the majority of patients with acute lung injury and the acute respiratory distress syndrome. Am J Respir Crit Care Med. 2001;163(6):1376–83.
3. Khemani E, McElhinney DB, Rhein L, Andrade O, Lacro RV, Thomas KC, et al. Pulmonary artery hypertension in formerly premature infants with bronchopulmonary dysplasia: clinical features and outcomes in the surfactant era. Pediatrics. 2007;120(6):1260–9.
4. Malnick G, Pickoff AS, Ferrer PL, Peyser J, Bancalari E, Gelband H. Normal pulmonary vascular resistance and left ventricular hypertrophy in young infants with bronchopulmonary dysplasia: an echocardiographic and pathologic study. Pediatrics. 1980;66(4):589–96.
5. Mourani PM, Sontag MK, Younoszai A, Ivy DD, Abman SH. Clinical utility of echocardiography for the diagnosis and management of pulmonary vascular disease in young children with chronic lung disease. Pediatrics. 2008;121(2):317–25.
6. Soler YA, Nieves-Plaza M, Prieto M, García-De Jesús R, Suárez-Rivera M. Pediatric Risk, Injury, Failure, Loss, End-Stage renal disease score identifies acute kidney injury and predicts mortality in critically ill children: a prospective study. Pediatr Crit Care Med. 2013;14(4):e189–95.
7. Alobaidi R, Morgan C, Basu RK, Stenson E, Featherstone R, Majumdar SR, et al. Associations between fluid balance and outcomes in critically ill children: a protocol for a systematic review and meta-analysis. Can J Kidney Health Dis. 2017;4(8):2054358117692560.
8. Selewski DT, Askenazi DJ, Bridges BC, Cooper DS, Fleming GM, Paden ML, et al. The impact of fluid overload on outcomes in children treated with extracorporeal membrane oxygenation: a multicenter retrospective cohort study. Pediatr Crit Care Med. 2017;18(12):1126–35.
9. Arikan AA, Zappitelli M, Goldstein SL, Naipaul A, Jefferson LS, Loftis LL. Fluid overload is associated with impaired oxygenation and morbidity in critically ill children. Pediatr Crit Care Med. 2012;13(3):253–8.
10. Valentine SL, Sapru A, Higgerson RA, Spinella PC, Flori HR, Graham DA, et al. Fluid balance in critically ill children with acute lung injury. Crit Care Med. 2012;40(10):2883–9.
11. Flori HR, Church G, Liu KD, Gildengorin G, Matthay MA. Positive fluid balance is associated with higher mortality and prolonged mechanical ventilation in pediatric patients with acute lung injury. Crit Care Res Pract. 2011;2011(4):854142–5.

12. Sinitsky L, Walls D, Nadel S, Inwald DP. Fluid overload at 48 hours is associated with respiratory morbidity but not mortality in a general PICU: retrospective cohort study. Pediatr Crit Care Med. 2015;16(3):205–9.
13. Barhight MF, Lusk J, Brinton J, Stidham T, Soranno DE, Faubel S, et al. Hyperchloremia is independently associated with mortality in critically ill children who ultimately require continuous renal replacement therapy. Pediatr Nephrol. 2018;30(2):300.
14. Myburgh JA, Finfer S, Bellomo R, Billot L, Cass A, Gattas D, et al. Hydroxyethyl starch or saline for fluid resuscitation in intensive care. N Engl J Med. 2012;367(20):1901–11.
15. Goldstein SL, Currier H, Cd G, Cosio CC, Brewer ED, Sachdeva R. Outcome in children receiving continuous venovenous hemofiltration. Pediatrics. 2001;107(6):1309–12.
16. Selewski DT, Cornell TT, Lombel RM, Blatt NB, Han YY, Mottes T, et al. Weight-based determination of fluid overload status and mortality in pediatric intensive care unit patients requiring continuous renal replacement therapy. Intensive Care Med. 2011;37(7):1166–73.
17. Ng KT, Velayit A, Khoo DKY, Mohd Ismail A, Mansor M. Continuous infusion versus intermittent bolus injection of furosemide in critically ill patients: a systematic review and meta-analysis. J Cardiothorac Vasc Anesth. 2018;32(5):2303–10.
18. Elbahlawan L, West NK, Avent Y, Cheng C, Liu W, Barfield RC, et al. Impact of continuous renal replacement therapy on oxygenation in children with acute lung injury after allogeneic hematopoietic stem cell transplantation. Pediatr Blood Cancer. 2010;55(3):540–5.
19. Kwiatkowski DM, Goldstein SL, Cooper DS, Nelson DP, Morales DLS, Krawczeski CD. Peritoneal dialysis vs furosemide for prevention of fluid overload in infants after cardiac surgery: a randomized clinical trial. JAMA Pediatr. 2017;171(4):357–64.

Nutrition in Pediatric AKI and Critical Illness

5

Norma J. Maxvold and Timothy E. Bunchman

5.1 Introduction

Risk of AKI in the PICU is common. The primary disease process often effects hemodynamics that in turn redistributes the vascular volume to higher priority organs for immediate survival. This by itself sets the stage for renal insufficiency to some degree. The AWARE study found the overall incidence AKI in the PICU population to be 26.9% [1].

Literature supports higher AKI incidence in subsets of the PICU population; with congenital cardiac postop patients of 20–64% [2, 3], and in patients with acute respiratory failure requiring mechanical ventilation reports of AKI 53–82% [4, 5]. In addition, often the pediatric critically ill population require vasoactive medications during their support, these agents further alter the neuroendocrine influence on their metabolic state. Additive to this is the degree of malnutrition at the time of admission to the PICU. Pediatric studies to identify admission malnutrition have found moderate/severe (≤ 2 *Z* scores) malnutrition ranging from 17 to >50% of PICU children. Malnutrition being defined on *Z* scores of weight for age <2 years or BMI for children >2 years [6, 7].

This group of patients represent a wide heterogeneous base of primary disease processes with concurrent nutritional deficits preexisting from the base disease/disorder. Superimposed upon these deficits goes the catabolism associated with critical

N. J. Maxvold
Pediatric Intensive Care, Children's Hospital of Richmond at the Virginia Commonwealth University, Richmond, VA, USA

T. E. Bunchman (✉)
Pediatric Nephrology, Children's Hospital of Richmond at the Virginia Commonwealth University, Richmond, VA, USA
e-mail: timothy.bunchman@vcuhealth.org

S. K. Sethi et al. (eds.), *Critical Care Pediatric Nephrology and Dialysis: A Practical Handbook*, https://doi.org/10.1007/978-981-13-2276-1_5

Table 5.1 Physiologic response to critical illness

Immediate (0–72 h)	Acute (3–10 days)	Subacute: (>10 days)
Immediate fight or flight: Supply energy and APP: ↑Catecholamines, cortisol, glucagon ↓Insulin, androgens, leptin NEA-immediate stress: ↑GH (but also ↓GH receptors in tissue) ↑Lipolytic and insulin antagonism: ↑FFA and ↑ hyperglycemia ↓T3 and ↑rT3 (due to altered peripheral conversion of T4) ↑ACTH, ↓CBG, loss of diurnal variation	Catabolic phase: ↑Catecholamines, cortisol, glucagon Recovery of ↓insulin, androgens, leptin NEA response: GH resistance (↓GH receptors) ↓IGF-1, ↓ALS, ↓IGFBP-3 ↑ then ↔ TSH and T4 Normalizing ACTH yet ↑ Cortisol ↑Prolactin	Recovery phase: Diuresis, tissue repair, improved nitrogen balance weight gain begins NEA response: Normalizing cortisol
Physiologic response: ↓VO_2, ↓CO, ↓temperature Negative nitrogen balance Insulin resistance ↑ Substrate turnover	Physiologic response: ↑VO_2, ↑CO, ↑temperature Worsening negative nitrogen balance, continued substrate turnover and insulin resistance	Physiologic response: Normalize VO_2, CO, temperature Stabilizing substrate turnover, recovery of insulin sensitivity

illness and the nitrogen drain from the body's muscle mass to support the shift from anabolic growth to catabolic "fight or flight" survival of the individual throughout the ongoing illness (Table 5.1) [8]. Nutritional support for these children requires reassessments throughout their care with adjustment made of the components found to be lacking or in excess.

There is limited data on nutritional status in children admitted in pediatric intensive care with acute kidney injury. Studies (one on patients not on renal replacement therapy; other on children on continuous renal replacement therapy) showed a high prevalence of acute and chronic malnutrition among this population [9, 10]. It is important to note that fluid overload, which is quite common in this population, might underestimate the situation.

Kyle et al. in the retrospective analysis of 167 critically ill children, showed that underfeeding was accentuated in the children with AKI, and protein underfeeding was greater than the energy underfeeding in the first 5 days of ICU stay.

Using the median 5 day energy and protein intake expressed as percentile of prescribed daily energy–protein recommendation, PICU children with AKI received only 35.4% of energy prescribed and 0% or protein prescribed. Children without AKI received 58.2% of their prescribed energy and 22.5% of their prescribed protein. They noted the common practice that AKI children are often fasted or parts of the nutritional support avoided to delay need for renal replacement therapies.

The study confirmed the nutritional under support common in PICUs, regardless of the presence or absence of AKI, <68% of energy needs and <35% of protein needs were covered by the current nutrition practices of this study [9].

5.2 Approach to the Critically Ill Child with AKI

On admission to a PICU an intake assessment of the nutrition present is necessary. This will help define patients entering with malnutrition as well as existing deficits from their primary disease. Anthropometric measurements if available (mid arm circumference, Triceps skinfold) can be done with recognition of the effect that edema/fluid retention has on these measurements. Indirect calorimetry may be helpful in individual patients by measuring the basal energy expenditure and calculating the daily energy requirements, but for the young child often the measurements are limited due to the tidal volumes being lower than many instruments validation level (~150 mL). Recently a simplified version of IC using just volumetric CO_2 has been developed and trialed in intubated children with encouraging results [11, 12]. For now, estimated energy expenditures remain the mainstay for nutrition prescriptions, with evidence supporting use of Schofield/WHO equations as best fit for critically ill children [13].

Additional nutritional assessment on admission should include basic laboratory chemistries to help define the starting metabolic state of the child with AKI. This includes electrolytes, acid–base status, minerals: calcium/phosphorus/magnesium, and BUN and creatinine. Uric acid (metabolic by-product), triglyceride, and cholesterol (lipid metabolism) may also help define the state of AKI stress. Prealbumin (transthyretin) with a 24–48 h half-life additionally can be monitored intermittently as a surrogate for visceral protein pool [14]. This measurement though can be falsely elevated in AKI.

It has been suggested that caloric intake 20–30% above the estimated requirement will provide adequate calories in most children with AKI, without causing significant risk of overfeeding and associated complications. Recent 2017 ASPEN recommendations for the critically ill child suggest when not able to directly measure by indirect calorimetry, using the Schofield or the WHO predictive equations to estimate the basal energy requirements and not to add stress factors onto the calculation, so as to not risk the development of overfeeding [13]. This nutritional approach as demonstrated in the Kyle study significantly under-supported nutrition for these children, especially the AKI child. Until further studies can provide evidence that we as practitioners will routinely adhere to providing the estimated caloric intake, it may be best to continue with a starting caloric intake ~20 above estimate by Schofield/WHO equations.

At this time clinical practice frequently does not adhere to nutritional support based on basal estimates or IC in the early phase of the critical illness. Often no or at best limited nutrition is given during the first days of admission, growing the debt of energy and more so the nitrogen loss significantly before adequate support occurs. Ongoing debates/discussions/opinions on how much and when to supply the nutritional energy to the critically ill patient will continue but recent focus has helped us begin to address the nitrogen/protein debt.

5.2.1 Protein

Multiple hormonal and metabolic changes during critical illness contribute to the lean muscle mass loss (including increased hepatic gluconeogenesis, relative insulin resistance, elevated stress hormones, inflammatory mediator/cytokines) resulting in a catabolic state. Additive to this is AKI changes which occur (metabolic acidosis, reduce renal interconversion of amino acids, altered ammoniagenesis, impaired renal metabolism of proteins and hormones (rT3, RBP, triglyceride lipase, erythropoietin). Protein turnover is higher the younger the child is and is associated with increased energy expenditure [15, 16]. High protein turnover involves redistribution of amino acids from the skeletal muscle to the liver and other tissues involved in the inflammatory response. This hyper-catabolic state leads to a high rate of urea nitrogen appearance (180–250 mg/kg/day), and a net negative nitrogen balance in children with AKI [17].

It is known that even critically ill children who do not have AKI commonly have a negative nitrogen balance, despite the provision of protein as high as 2.5 g/kg/day [18]. The provision of dietary protein sufficient to improve nitrogen balance and optimize protein synthesis and preserve skeletal muscle mass is a most important nutritional intervention for critically ill children with AKI. It is difficult to maintain positive nitrogen balance in these children, especially in the presence of renal replacement therapy. Recent work by Kyle et al. has shown no negative effects in children with AKI while on high protein support recommended by the 2009 ASPEN guidelines [19].

5.2.2 Fat

Critically ill patients have increased lipid oxidation and FFAs provide a significant energy source during the altered early substrate metabolism with limited glucose oxidation rate [20]. Thus, due to increased lipid demands, and limited stores, critically ill children are susceptible to deficiency of essential fatty acids. Lipid support up to 40–50% of total energy needs can help reach the energy goals without risk of worsening hyperglycemia or visceral fat from lipogenesis of excess carbohydrate that cannot be fully oxidized.

5.2.3 Carbohydrates

Excess carbohydrate loads may induce lipogenesis. Providing an adequate energy supply to help maximize nitrogen balance has been investigated both in critically ill adults and children. Recent studies in critically ill children that were mechanically ventilated thus allowing IC measurements for energy expenditure found ~58 kcal/kg/day to support protein balance when given minimum intake of 1.5 g/kg/day of protein [21, 22]. How to best proportion the energy between carbohydrate (CHO)/fat/protein components is yet unknown. The common proportion of 50–60% CHO, 10–25% lipid, and 25–35% protein which supports the healthy child is likely not the same ratios needed by the acutely ill child. Indeed discussion continues whether protein should be used in calculating energy support during critical illness. Adhering to the 2017 ASPEN recommendation for supporting the critically ill child and bearing in mind the maximal oxidation rate of glucose at ~4–5 mg/kg/min then a proportional ratio of 35% CHO/45% lipid/20% protein would deliver the Schofield estimate of energy needs and the protein needs. Monitoring and preventing (by supplemental insulin) the hyperglycemia as a result of insulin resistance common in critical illness is also warranted from strong evidence linking hyperglycemia with poor clinical outcomes [23].

5.3 Changes in Nutrition When on Renal Replacement Therapy

When AKI worsens, intervention for control of the disturbed metabolic balance requires a renal support modality. Renal replacement therapy (RRT) allows for "room" to give sufficient nutrition. Modalities of RRT have unique impact upon losses of nutrition.

Hemodialysis (high flux or standard) or sustained low efficiency dialysis (SLED) will have impact upon trace mineral losses as well as impact upon water-soluble vitamins but less impact upon other components of nutrition.

Peritoneal dialysis (PD) will effect losses of amino acids and proteins with larger protein losses including albumin. Literature has demonstrated that these children (especially infants) will have significant protein losses and frequently result in immunoglobulin deficiency. Whereas it is difficult to understand how much additional protein is needed to be delivered in order to make these children "nitrogen neutral," it is estimated that protein delivery in the range of 3–4 g/kg/day may be needed [24, 25]. One can assess this by looking at a nitrogen balance measuring protein losses in the PD effluent and replacing it proportionally.

Continuous renal replacement therapy (CRRT) delivered by CVVHD was found to remove 10–20% of the amino acid daily intake [26]. Clearance of amino acids in children on CRRT was in the range of 20–40 ml/min/1.73 m^2. In this pediatric study, glutamine losses during CRRT accounted for 25% of all amino acid losses. Glutamine functions as a major nitrogen transporter for the body. It is known for its cell protective effects during insulin resistance of acute stress, it aids in induction of heat shock proteins (chaperone proteins) and as an energy source in rapid replicating cell lines (enterocytes, leukocytes). Glutamine additionally helps attenuate the oxidative stress in renal tubular cells. Due to the significant component glutamine represents of the total amino acid loss on CRRT consideration of supplementation may be prudent if available.

Recommendations issued by the American Society of Parenteral and Enteral Nutrition (2009 ASPEN) suggest the following age-adjusted intakes of protein for critically ill children in PICU: 0–2 years, 2–3 g/kg/day; 2–13 years, 1.5–2 g/kg/day; and 13–18 years, 1.5 g/kg/day. Studies are needed to validate these recommendations in critically ill children with AKI, either on renal replacement therapy or not. During CRRT, to account for losses in the ultrafiltrate/dialysate, additional 10–20% of amino acid intake should be supplemented to the diet.

5.3.1 Vitamins and Trace Elements

Literature on vitamin and trace element metabolism in critically ill patients with AKI is limited, with recent studies analyzing clearance of these by CRRT. Adult studies have found deficiencies in fat-soluble vitamins but that of vitamin K [27]. For children managed by CRRT, losses of water-soluble vitamins are likely over time. Thus, when supported on CRRT over prolonged periods >10 days, serum levels should be monitored, and additional supplementation may be required. Concern regarding supplementing vitamin C, which may contribute to the risk of oxalosis in renal failure, needs thoughtful discretion. Current research in high dose vitamin C in adults with sepsis has not identified this problem [28]. Current recommendations caution not to exceed 100 mg/day in patients not requiring CRRT, with supplementation up to 200 mg/day (adults) for patients requiring CRRT is allowed.

In a pediatric study (15 patients receiving CVVHD) evaluating the clearance of five trace elements (manganese, copper, selenium, chromium, and zinc) extraordinary losses during CRRT were not observed. This study only evaluated out to the 5th day of CRRT support, and the children were supported with standard parenteral vitamins and trace elements daily [26]. Adult studies have likewise shown that although losses do occur, replaced with a standard multiple trace element preparation and with additional 100 mcg/day of selenium (in adults) are capable to offset cumulative losses from CRRT.

Folate, being water soluble, was likewise found to be cleared readily on CRRT and it is possible that additional folate supplementation is needed in children who are receiving CRRT for prolonged periods. When beginning CRRT, recommended daily allowances should be provided with intermittent monitoring of water-soluble substances including vitamins, trace elements, and folate levels in children receiving prolonged renal replacement therapy.

5.4 Electrolytes

Dialytic modalities readily remove small molecular weight substances, this includes phosphorus and magnesium. Patients undergoing extended periods of intermittent or continuous dialysis are at increased risk of hypophosphatemia and depletion of magnesium. These assays should be monitored routinely and supplemented when indicated.

Peritoneal dialysis with high ultrafiltration requirements can result in sodium depletion and subsequent difficulties with perfusion/hypotension, sodium monitoring and supplementation should be done in these children.

5.5 Route and Timing of Nutritional Support

Institution of feeding and the speed of advancement remains in discussion in critically ill patients, both adults and children. For children, who represent active somatic and organ development, delay in beginning feeds will only compound the energy and protein debt of the critically ill state. Current 2017 ASPEN recommendations include beginning within the first 24–48 h of PICU admission. Amassed literature, both pediatric and adult, supports enteral nutrition as the primary route unless clear contra-indications are present. Feeding by an enteral route has been shown to reduce the risk of nosocomial infection and is cost-effective. A goal of providing at least 2/3 of the daily energy expenditure by day 5–7 of the PICU stay should be sought. There is insufficient evidence and potential harm in withholding supplemental parenteral nutrition to critically ill children who cannot meet their caloric needs by the enteral route, as has become common in the adult ICUs. Recent studies have confirmed the benefits of using enteral and parenteral nutrition in a complementary manner if energy intake targets are not met after 5 days, especially for children with acute kidney injury patients receiving renal replacement therapy. Supporting this combination approach are studies using intradialytic parenteral nutrition (IDPN) to augment protein delivery to chronic HD patients [29, 30].

To date insufficient data is present to provide a clear recommendation as to the site of feeding, gastric vs post-pyloric. Evidences suggest that post-pyloric is reasonably tolerated, but it bears remembering that intermittent bolus feeds give a more pulsatile amino acid flux which stimulates skeletal muscle protein synthesis [31]. One should consider this option in patients who do not tolerate gastric feeding or are at a greater risk of aspiration.

5.6 Conclusions

Children with acute kidney injury are at high risk of protein energy wasting, a significant negative prognostic factor. Studies support this accumulative protein/energy debt in critically ill children. To address this, early implementation of feeding within the first 24–48 h, starting with enteral nutrition is recommended. Goals of nutritional support in children with AKI are similar to critically ill children with normal renal function. Critically ill children with AKI present additional challenges by restricted urine output and solute clearances. When beginning renal supportive therapies, the additional nutrient losses from the renal replacement therapies should be factored into the nutritional prescription. Nutritional assessments including *Z* scores and laboratory analysis of solutes/nutrients should be done admission with scheduled reassessments. Nutritional goals should be frequently reassessed on a regular basis to ensure actual intake corresponds to the goals set and with special attention through individualization of the goals to avoid under/overfeeding.

Table 5.2 shows suggestions by these authors on consideration of components of nutrition needed during these times of critical illness.

Table 5.2 Nutrition prescription in AKI children

	Component prescription
Energy	Npkcal 40–65 kcal/kg/day 20–25% as carbohydrates (insulin as needed) ~ 5–6 mg/kg/min 30–40% lipid formulations (20% lipid emulsions) 40–50% protein
Protein	2–3 g/kg/day with AKI (increase intake if on high flow CRRT (by 20%)
Vitamins	Daily recommended intake (± replacement) Monitor serum folate, water-soluble vitamin levels
Trace elements	Daily recommended intake
Monitoring	MEE, nitrogen balance, electrolytes, vitamins, trace elements
Consider	– Pharmaconutrients: Glutamine, thiamine, L-carnitine

References

1. Kaddourah A, Basu RK, Bagshaw SM, AWARE Investigators. Epidemiology of acute kidney injury in critically ill children and young adults. N Engl J Med. 2017;376:11–20.
2. Gil-Ruiz Gil-Esparza MA, Alcaraz Romero AJ, Romero Otero A, Gil Villanueva N, Sanavia Moran E, Rodriguez Sanchez de la Blanca A, Lorente Romero J, Bellon Cano JM. Prognostic relevance of early AKI according to pRIFLE criteria in children undergoing cardiac surgery. Pediatr Nephrol. 2014;29:1265–72.
3. Sugimoto K, Toda Y, Iwasaki T, Shimizu K, Kanazawa T, Muto N, Kawase H, Morimatsu H, Morita K, Maeshima Y, Mori K, Sano S. Urinary albumin levels predict development of acute kidney injury after pediatric cardiac surgery: a prospective observational study. J Cardiothorac Vasc Anesth. 2016;30:64–8.
4. Villacres SM, Medar SS, Aydin SI. Acute kidney injury in children with acute respiratory failure. Clin Pediatr. 2018;57(11):1340–8. https://doi.org/10.1177/0009922818779222.
5. Akcan-Arikan A, Zappitelli M, Loftis LL, Washburn KK, Jefferson LS, Goldstein SL. Modified RIFLE criteria in critically ill children with acute kidney injury. Kidney Int. 2007;71:1028–35.
6. Delgado AF, Okay TS, Leone C, et al. Hospital malnutrition and inflammatory response in critically ill children and adolescents admitted to a tertiary intensive care unit. Clinics (San Paulo). 2008;63:357–62.
7. Mehta NM, Bechard LJ, Cahilll N, et al. Nutritional practices and their relationship to clinical outcomes in critically ill children—an international multicenter cohort study. Crit Care Med. 2012;40:2204–21.
8. Sethi SK, Maxvold N, Bunchman T, et al. Nutritional management in the critically ill child with acute kidney injury: a review. Pediatr Nephrol. 2017;32(4):589–601.
9. Kyle UG, Akcan-Arikan A, Orellana RA, Coss-Bu J. Nutritional support among critically ill children with AKI. Clin J Am Soc Nephrol. 2013;8:568–74.
10. Castillo A, Santiago MJ, López-Herce J, et al. Nutritional status and clinical outcome of children on continuous renal replacement therapy: a prospective observational study. BMC Nephrol. 2012;13:125.
11. Mehta NM, Smallwood CD, Joosten KF, et al. Accuracy of a simplified equation for energy expenditure based on bedside volumetric carbon dioxide elimination measurement-a-two-center study. Clin Nutr. 2015;34:151–5.
12. Kerklaan D, Augustus ME, Hulst JM, et al. Validation of ventilator derived VCO2 measurement to determine energy expenditure in ventilated critically ill children. Clin Nutr. 2017;36:452–7.
13. Mehta NM, Skillman HE, Irving SY, et al. Guidelines for the provision and assessment of nutrition support therapy in the pediatric critically ill patient: Society of Critical Care Medicine and American Society for Parenteral and Enteral Nutrition. J Parenter Enter Nutr. 2017;41(5):706–42.

14. Robison MK, Trujillo EB, Mogensen KM, Rounds J, McManus K, Jacobs DO. Improving nutritional screening of hospitalized patients: the role of prealbumin. J Parenter Enter Nutr. 2003;27:389–95.
15. Nissim I, Yudkoff M, Pereira G, Segal S. Effect of conceptual age and dietary intake on protein metabolism in premature infants. J Ped Gastrol Nutr. 1983;2:507–16.
16. Institute of Medicine. Dietary reference intakes for energy, carbohydrate, fiber, fat, fatty acids, cholesterol, protein, and amino acids (macronutrients). Washington, DC: The National Academies Press; 2005.
17. Maxvold NJ, Smoyer WE, Custer JR, et al. Amino acid loss and nitrogen balance in critically ill children with acute renal failure: a prospective comparison between classic hemofiltration and hemofiltration with dialysis. Crit Care Med. 2000;28(4):1161–5.
18. Coss-Bu JA, Jefferson LS, Walding D, David Y, O'Brian Smith E, Klish WJ. Resting energy expenditure and nitrogen balance in critically ill pediatric patients on mechanical ventilation. Nutrition. 1998;14:649–52.
19. Kyle UG, Akcan-Arikan A, Silva JC, Goldsworthy M, Shekerdemian LS, Coss-Bu JA. Protein feeding in pediatric acute kidney injury is not associated with a delay in renal recovery. J Ren Nutr. 2017;27:8–15.
20. Tappy L, Schwarz JM, Schneiter P, Cayeux C, Revelly JP, Fagerquist CK, Jéquier E, Chioléro R. Effects of isoenergetic glucose-based or lipid-based parenteral nutrition on glucose metabolism, de novo lipogenesis, and respiratory gas exchanges in critically ill patients. Crit Care Med. 1998;26:860–7.
21. Chaparro CJ, Depeyre JL, Longchamp D, Perez MH, Taffe P, Cotting J. How much protein and energy are needed to equilibrate nitrogen and energy balances in ventilated critically ill children? Clin Nutr. 2016;335:460–7.
22. Bechard LJ, Parott S, Mehta NM. Systematic review of the influence of energy and protein intake on protein balance in critically ill children. J Peds. 2012;161:333–9.
23. Faustino DV, Apkon M. Persistent hyperglycemia in critically ill children. J Peds. 2005;146:30–4.
24. Quan A, Baum M. Protein losses in children on continuous cycler peritoneal dialysis. Pediatr Nephrol. 1996;10:728–31.
25. Edefonti A, Picca M, Damiani B, Loi S, Ghio L, Giani M, Consalvo G, Grassi G. Dietary prescription based on estimated nitrogen balance during peritoneal dialysis. Pediatr Nephrol. 1999;13:253–8.
26. Zappitelli M, Juarez M, Castillo L, et al. Continuous renal replacement therapy amino acid, trace metal and folate clearance in critically ill children. Intensive Care Med. 2009;35:698–706.
27. Druml W, Schwarzenhofer M, Aspner R, Horl WH. Fat-soluble vitamins in patients with acute renal failure. Miner Electrolyte Metab. 1998;24:220–2.
28. Tenj J, Pourmand A, Maxer-Amirshahi M. Vitamin C: the next step in sepsis management? J Crit Care. 2018;43:230–4.
29. Goldstein SL, Baronette S, Gambrell TV, Currier H, Brewer ED. nPCR assessment and IDPN treatment of malnourishment in pediatric hemodialysis patients. Pediatr Nephrol. 2002;17:531–4.
30. Smolle KH, Kaufmann P, Holzer H, Druml W. Intradialytic parenteral nutrition in malnourished patients on chronic hemodialysis therapy. Nephrol Dial Transplant. 1995;10:1441–16.
31. El-Kadi SW, Suryawan A, Gazzaneo MC, et al. Anabolic signaling and protein deposition are enhanced by intermittent compared with continuous feeding in skeletal muscle of neonates. Am J Physiol Endocrinol Metab. 2012;302:E674–86.

6 Pharmacology of a Critically Ill Child and Drug Dosing

Joshua Zaritsky and Carl Gerdine

6.1 Introduction

We will be focusing on CRRT, a difficult topic due to the following:

- *PICU patients on CRRT represent an overlap of*:
  - Disturbed pharmacokinetics induced by critical illness
  - Extracorporeal drug removal
  - Often a rapidly changing clinical situation
- *Current drug dosing during CRRT*:
  - Are based on a wider variation of CRRT techniques
  - Use a very heterogeneous (often ADULT) population
  - Often lack data to back them up

6.2 Pharmacokinetics (General)

Pharmacokinetics describes the way drugs are absorbed, distributed, metabolized, and eliminated. Each drug has unique physicochemical properties that influence how it is processed by the body. Is it a small or large molecule? Hydrophilic or lipophilic? Highly protein bound or not? Metabolized by liver enzymes or excreted by the kidney as unchanged drug?

J. Zaritsky (✉)
Pediatric Nephrology, Nemours/A.I. duPont Hospital for Children, Wilmington, DE, USA
e-mail: Joshua.Zaritsky@nemours.org

C. Gerdine
Pediatric Cardiac Intensive Care, Nemours/A.I. duPont Hospital for Children, Wilmington, DE, USA
e-mail: Carl.Gerdine@nemours.org

S. K. Sethi et al. (eds.), *Critical Care Pediatric Nephrology and Dialysis: A Practical Handbook*, https://doi.org/10.1007/978-981-13-2276-1_6

Pharmacokinetic studies determine such parameters as bioavailability, volume of distribution, and half-life. These help inform dosing regimens and administration frequency that maintain effective and safe drug levels.

What is effective and safe for a healthy patient may not be for one who is critically ill, where pharmacokinetic alterations are prevalent. Shock states, volume status variations, fluid shifts, and plasma protein disturbances can impact pharmacokinetic parameters. CRRT is sometimes indicated in these patients, and the impact on drug excretion depends on these variables.

This section will provide a practical review of pharmacokinetics as well as highlight certain alterations often seen in the critically ill. It will also be helpful for understanding the drug dosing methods in CRRT discussed later in the chapter.

6.3 Absorption

Absorption occurs when a drug crosses into the circulatory system from a different site of administration. The bioavailability of a drug is the fraction that makes it to the systemic circulation, dependent on the extent of absorption as well as, in some cases, the hepatic extraction ratio if the drug undergoes first pass metabolism (following enteral administration).

Enteral absorption of drugs can be diminished by splanchnic hypoperfusion. Vasopressors commonly used in the intensive care setting can further impact this. Subcutaneously administered medications can be similarly impacted when peripheral tissue perfusion is decreased by such drugs as well.

Intravenous administration, especially in the initial phases of ICU care, is recommended to avoid issues with absorption.

6.4 Volume of Distribution

Volume of distribution (V_d) describes the extent to which a drug distributes from the bloodstream into tissues. Said another way, V_d relates a drug dose to the resulting serum concentration. For example, if a patient receives a large intravenous dose of a drug, and the serum concentration is very small compared to the total blood volume, the V_d would be considered relatively high ($V_d > 1$). These are typically also lipophilic drugs. On the other hand, more hydrophilic drugs, such as most beta-lactams and aminoglycosides, have a low V_d (<0.7 l/kg) and generally stay in the intravascular compartment. They are affected to a greater extent by the pharmacokinetic changes seen in critically ill patients. These variables can change with a patient's condition, and vigilant monitoring is ultimately necessary.

Drugs with lower V_d are more prone to changes in blood volume and fluid shifts, which can occur in shock states. Fluid resuscitation increases intravascular volume, which can decrease drug concentration. Also, capillary leaks and third spacing can result in an increased apparent V_d for such drugs that would normally be confined to the intravascular space, but that under this condition, leak out.

The optimal way to monitor and adjust drug dosing is to use therapeutic drug monitoring by obtaining drug levels, such as with aminoglycosides and vancomycin. Because assays that determine drug levels are not available for all drugs, other methods to determine optimal dosing exist and will be discussed later in this chapter.

Also, plasma protein changes occur in critically ill patients. In the setting of hypoalbuminemia, a typically highly protein bound drug will instead have a higher free fraction. Only free (unbound) drug is capable of exerting its pharmacological effect. Logically, if free drug concentration rises, there is an increased risk for the patient to experience adverse drug effects. Note also that only unbound drug is prone to being dialyzed.

6.5 Metabolism

The primary site for drug metabolism is in the liver, though it can occur in a number of other sites including the gastrointestinal tract, kidney, and lung. Liver enzymes are responsible for metabolizing many drugs. Often lipophilic drugs (with a large V_d) are metabolized this way. The result of hepatic metabolism is usually that of a more polar, or hydrophilic, molecule that can then more readily be excreted by the kidney. The cytochrome P450 enzyme family is a prominent pathway in the liver, often responsible as the site for many drug–drug interactions among all patients, both healthy and ill. Metabolic enzyme activity, however, can change with the degree of critical illness. In general, the extent of hepatic metabolism depends on hepatic blood flow and the hepatic extraction ratio of a drug. Drugs can be classified by extraction ratio.

1. High (>0.7). These depend more on hepatic drug flow and are less sensitive to hepatic (intrinsic) function.
2. Intermediate (0.3–0.7).
3. Low (<0.3). These depend more on hepatic function and are less sensitive to hepatic blood flow.

6.6 Excretion

Renal clearance is the primary excretory pathway for most drugs or their metabolites. Generally the rate of renal clearance is proportional to the glomerular filtration rate. In the setting of acute kidney injury, glomerular filtration decreases substantially. Then drug clearance depends on non-renal mechanisms.

Renally excreted drugs need to be dose adjusted to account for reduced renal clearance to avoid toxic drug levels and adverse drug effects. Note that the initial dose of these drugs should usually not be changed, but the subsequent maintenance doses usually require a dose or frequency decrease. The decision to either decrease the dose, decrease the dosing interval, or both should be determined based on the pharmacodynamics of the drug. For example, it would be important to determine whether an affected antibiotic is time-dependent or concentration-dependent in terms of how it exerts its therapeutic effect.

Another option in this situation is to use medications that are cleared via non-renal mechanisms. Drugs with a large V_d that extensively distribute into tissues are usually less impacted by acute changes in kidney function and do not require a dose adjustment [1].

6.7 Antibiotics as an Example of Pharmacodynamics

(a) *Good news: Most data available for CRRT dosing*
(b) *Bad news: Must consider pharmacodynamics as well*
(c) *Beta-lactams and glycopeptides*:
- These are "time dependent" antibiotics
- Therefore the percentage that the plasma concentration remains above the MIC is the major determinant of efficacy
- In theory a continuous infusion would maximize pharmacodynamic exposure

(d) *Fluoroquinolones and aminoglycosides*:
- These are "concentration dependent" antibiotics with a post-antibiotic effect
- Aminoglycoside efficacy: ratio of the peak concentration to the MIC
- Fluoroquinolones efficacy: ratio of the AUC to MIC
- In both cases you want a high dosing with prolonged dosing interval

6.8 Extracorporeal Drug Removal During Renal Replacement Therapy

Another aspect of pharmacology in critically ill children is adjusting drug dosing during renal replacement therapy. Given the practical nature of this chapter the focus will be on factors affecting drug removal during continuous renal replacement therapy (CRRT) followed by a practical approach to drug delivery during CRRT.

Extracorporeal removal depends largely on both the physicochemical and pharmacokinetic properties of the drug in question. One of the most important characteristics of a drug is its volume of distribution (V_d). In very simplistic terms the dialyzer can only remove what it is present in the vascular compartment. The dialyzer access to the portion of drug present in deeper compartments (tissues) is related to the rate of extracorporeal removal and rate of transfer between compartments. This can lead to very complex models of drug removal and can also lead to post-treatment rebound of certain drugs as there is a re-equilibration between the central and peripheral compartments. Fortunately given the continuous nature of CRRT the impact of V_d is lessened as there is an ongoing equilibration between the various compartments.

Clearly another aspect of drug removal via CRRT is the treatment characteristics. CRRT can employ both diffusive and convective clearances. Convective clearance, provided via hemofiltration, describes the movement of solutes along with water across the dialysis membrane. It is the simplest to model as the solute's movement is simply driven by a pressure gradient and is independent of its molecular weight with an absolute upper limit cutoff being the pore size of the membrane. The ability of a drug to move via convection is it sieving coefficient (SC) which can be expressed as a ratio between its effluent and plasma concentration, $C_{effluent}$ and C_{plasma}, respectively. Mathematically $SC = C_{effluent}/C_{plasma}$ and for most cases, since SC is driven by the drug's protein binding (PB), SC can be simplified to 1-PB. One caveat is that available values for PB may not reflect, that is, can vary between health and critical illness states.

For purely convective clearance delivered via post-dilution hemofiltration, the clearance (Cl) can be mathematically expressed as: CL = SC × effluent flow ($Q_{effluent}$) and thus in cases of drugs with molecular weights below the membrane cut off that are not significantly protein bound (SC = 1); the clearance is simply equal to effluent flow. In the case of predilution hemofiltration the blood entering the filter is diluted reducing the efficiency by the ratio of blood flow (Q_b) to blood flow + predilution flow (Q_{pre}). Mathematically then $CL = S\,C\times Q_{effluent} \times (Q_b/[Q_b + Q_{pre}])$

With dialysis modalities two additional concepts need to be introduced. First and unlike convective clearance, a drug's diffusive removal is proportional to its molecular weight. In order to account for this a drugs relative (to that of creatinine) diffusive mass transfer coefficient (Kdrel) is often used [2]. It can be calculated using the equation: $K_{drel} = (MW_{drug}/113)^{-0.42}$.

Additionally the degree of dialysate saturation (DS) must be considered and can lead to very complex modeling with the high dialysate flow (Q_d) rates in hemodialysis. However, the slow flow rates of dialysate used during CRRT generally result in complete dialysate saturation (dialysate concentration = plasma concentration) for those drugs with a very low protein binding. So once again clearance is largely proportional to 1-PB and DS, similar to how SC in convective clearance can be approximated by 1-PB. Combining this with Kdrel leads to the following equation describing clearance via CRRT dialysis: $CL = DS \times Q_d \times Kdrel$.

In the case of hemodiafiltration CRRT, for simplicity's sake, convective and diffusive clearances can be combined and thus for small drugs with little PB, CL can be approximated by $Q_{effluent}$.

6.9 A Practical Approach to Drug Dosing During CRRT

What follows is a practical approach to drug delivery during renal replacement therapy. The following considerations need to be made for each drug.

1. Is the drug highly protein bound or hepatically cleared?
   In essence the answer to this question will determine how much clearance of the drug will occur through the CRRT circuit. Given the typical pore size of the membranes used in dialysis (20–30,000 Daltons), any drug that is bound to plasma proteins will not be removed via diffusion or filtration [2]. Thus assuming high protein binding (>75%) there will be very limited clearance of the drug via CRRT and no dose adjustment (when compared to an anuric patient) would

be necessary. Conversely, if a drug is only partially protein bound, its free fraction (1-protein bound fraction) can be used to estimate clearance.

Similar considerations should be made when it comes to drugs eliminated via non-renal pathways. In anuric non-dialysis patients, most non-renal clearance is via the hepatic route. Thus, to estimate whether dose adjustment is needed in CRRT, it becomes important to know hepatic clearance at least qualitatively. Drugs that are almost exclusively hepatically cleared, such as acetaminophen, will not need any adjustments even with very high CRRT clearances.

2. Is the drug's fractional extracorporeal clearance < or >25%?

In order to know if CRRT clearance is clinically relevant and a drug dosing will need to be altered during CRRT, it can be helpful to calculate a fractional extracorporeal clearance [3, 4]. Essentially this represents the relative clearance of a drug via CRRT versus other metabolic or clearance pathways and can be expressed mathematically as: $Fr_{EC} = Cl_{EC}/(Cl_{EC} + Cl_{NR} + Cl_{R})$. Cl_{EC} represents CRRT or extracorporeal clearance, ClNR represents any non-renal clearance, and Cl_R is residual renal clearance. Using the FrEC allows for a practical rule that if extracorporeal clearance is less than 25%, drug dosing can remain unchanged. While this equation may appear complicated in most clinical situations, it allows for drug dosing adjustments to be made at least qualitatively. For example, as considered above, if the hepatic clearance is dominant, i.e., Cl_{NR} is very high, the Fr will be correspondingly low and extracorporeal clearance will not be clinically relevant. Similarly if the drug is highly protein bound, Fr_{EC} will be low as Cl_{EC} will be low. A specific example would be dosing levofloxacin vs. moxifloxacin during CRRT. Levofloxacin, due to its low protein binding and low hepatic elimination, has a high Fr_{EC} and would require dosing adjustments while moxifloxacin, given its high protein binding and high hepatic elimination (Cl_{NR}), has a low Fr_{EC} and does not require dosing adjustments. Finally, in most clinical situations where CRRT is employed, Cl_R will not be clinically relevant.

Methods for drug dosage adjustments: Below several methods are presented to help estimate drug dosing in the setting of CRRT. It is important to note that these methods have, in general, not been prospectively tested to see how closely they can attain therapeutic target concentrations, and there is no data to see if their use can improve patient outcomes. Additionally, the methods below can result in significantly different dosing than in popular dosage guidelines [5]. Importantly, with a single drug there can be significant differences in dosing between the methods below [6].

6.9.1 Method 1: Use a General Table or Literature Values for Specific Medications

This method relies on previously published dosing guidelines (for example, see [7–9]) to make dosing adjustments during CRRT. While convenient and straightforward, there are several shortfalls associated with this method. Actual pharmacokinetic studies of drugs conducted in critically ill patients receiving CRRT are extremely rare. More importantly, even when data is available its validity often is questionable given heterogeneous patient populations and the use of different CRRT techniques and setting. A common problem is that newer machines and the ability to deliver much higher CRRT doses can lead to a situation where critically important drugs, such as antibiotics, will end up being under dosed since the data was derived using much older technology and lower CRRT dosing.

6.9.2 Method 2a: Dose as If the "Total Creatinine Clearance (Cl_{cr})" Is Approximately 20–50 ml/min

This method assumes that the combination of CRRT clearance (using current dosing guidelines) along with the patient's residual renal and non-renal clearance falls in the range of 20–50 ml/min. This allows the drug to be dosed using widely available dosing guidelines for patients who have a native GFR in the 20–50 ml/min range. This method is simple and easily employed; however, it relies heavily on the underlying assumption that the total Cl_{cr} is 20–50 ml/min which might not be the case. A simple example would be drugs that are cleared via renal tubular secretion would end up being overdosed as CRRT, unlike native renal function, does not clear drug via an active secretion mechanism. Conversely, drugs that undergo renal tubular re-absorption, such as fluconazole, have the possibility of being underdosed since CRRT clearance may be actually higher than in patients with normal renal function.

6.9.3 Method 2b: Divide Hourly CRRT Effluent Rate by 60 to Get Estimated "Total Creatinine Clearance (Cl_{cr})"

This method drops any consideration of renal and non-renal clearance and takes advantage of the ease of estimating CRRT clearance via the CRRT effluent rate. Similar to method 2a, once a total Cl_{cr} is estimated, widely available dosing guidelines for patients who have a similar native GFR can be used. An example in a pediatric patient with a BSA of 1.2 m^2 with an effluent rate of 2000 ml/h would be ~2800 ml/1.73 m^2 divided by 60 (to convert to ml/min) which equals a total Cl of 47 ml/min. While this method has an advantage over method 2a since an estimate of CRRT dosing is made, it comes with the same shortfall mentioned above and assumes that there is negligible renal clearance (a safe assumption) and non-renal clearance which is often not the case. Additionally there is a chance of overestimating CRRT clearance since there is no adjustment made to the drug's SC. Finally drug dosing must be adjusted if the CRRT effluent rate changes.

6.9.4 Method 3: Start with Normal Dosing and Reduce It to Take Into Effect that of CRRT Clearance [10]

In this method a formal calculation is made to estimate how much CRRT (in addition to non-renal) clearance there is of the drug and that is then used to reduce the normal published dosing. Mathematically it can expressed as Dose = $\text{Dose}_{\text{normal}} \times [\text{Cl}_{\text{nonrenal}} + (\text{CRRT effluent rate} \times \text{SC})]/\text{Cl}_{\text{normal}}$. As opposed to method 2b, an attempt is made to better estimate CRRT clearance by taking into account the drug's SC. If we used small and non-protein bound drug (SC = 1) with minimal non-renal clearance, the only information needed is the effluent rate and the drug's normal clearance. A downfall of this method is that the SC is not always available and a large assumption is made that the $\text{Cl}_{\text{normal}}$ is the same in non-critically and critically ill patients.

6.9.5 Method 4: Start with Anuric Dosing and Augment It with the Drug Fraction You Expect to Be Removed Via CRRT [4]

This method uses published dosing guidelines for anuric patients (GFR <10 ml/min) and then augments it with an estimate of the fraction removed by CRRT. Mathematically it can be expressed as Dose = $\text{Dose}_{\text{anuric}}/[1 - \text{Fr}_{\text{EC}}]$ where, as described above, $\text{Fr}_{\text{EC}} = \text{Cl}_{\text{EC}}/(\text{Cl}_{\text{EC}} + \text{Cl}_{\text{NR}} + \text{Cl}_{\text{R}})$. Since it is essentially the converse approach to method 3, which takes normal dosing and then "subtracts" CRRT dosing, it has many of the same shortfalls. An additional benefit of this method is that it can be used to help with pharmacokinetics in that the dosing interval of a drug can be estimated with the following equation: Dosing interval = $\text{Dosing interval}_{\text{anuric}} \times [1 - \text{Fr}_{\text{EC}}]$.

The following presents the use of method 4:

1. Acyclovir in a 70 kg person undergoing CVVH with an Q_{eff} = 2450 ml/h
   (a) Dose = $\text{Dose}_{\text{anuric}}/[1 - \text{Fr}_{\text{EC}}]$
   (b) $\text{Fr}_{\text{EC}} = \text{Cl}_{\text{EC}}/(\text{Cl}_{\text{EC}} + \text{Cl}_{\text{NR}} + \text{Cl}_{\text{R}})$
   (c) $\text{Cl}_{\text{EC}} = \text{SC} \times Q_{\text{effluent}} = 0.85 \times 2450$ ml/h = **34.7 ml/min**
   - SC = 1-PB; Protein binding = 15%

   (d) $\text{CL}_{\text{NR}} = V_d \times K_{\text{HD}} = 56\ \text{l} \times 0.04\ \text{h}^{-1} = 2.24$ l/h = **37.3 ml/min**
   - $V_d = 0.8$ l/kg; $t_{1/2} = 19.5$ h; $K_{\text{HD}} = 0.04\ \text{h}^{-1}$

   (e) $\text{Cl}_{\text{R}} = 0$ ml/min
   (f) $\text{Fr}_{\text{EC}} = 34.7/(34.7 + 37.3 + 0) = 0.48$
   (g) CRRT dose = anuric dose/[1−0.48]
   - 5 mg/kg/day/0.52 = **9.6 mg/kg/day**

   (h) Dosing interval = $\text{Dosing interval}_{\text{anuric}} \times [1 - \text{Fr}_{\text{EC}}]$
   (i) Will change interval so would give: 5 mg/kg IV **Q12H**

References

1. Smith BS, Yogaratnam D, Levasseur-Franklin E, et al. Introduction to drug pharmacokinetics in the critically ill patient. Chest. 2012;141(5):1327–36.
2. Vincent HH, Vos MC, Akcahuseyin E, et al. Drug clearance by continuous haemodiafiltration: analysis of sieving coefficients and mass transfer coefficients of diffusion. Blood Purif. 1993;11:99–107.
3. Reetze-Bonorden P, Bohler J, Keller E. Drug dosage in patients during continuous renal replacement therapy: pharmacokinetic and therapeutic considerations. Clin Pharmacokinet. 1993;24:362–79.
4. Schetz M, Ferdinande P, Van den Berghe G, et al. Pharmacokinetics of continuous renal replacement therapy. Intensive Care Med. 1995;21:612–20.
5. Aronoff GR, Bennett WM, Berns JS, et al. Drug prescribing in renal failure: dosing guidelines for adults and children. 5th ed. Philadelphia, PA: American College of Physicians; 2007.
6. Kempke AP, Leino AS, Daneshvar F, Lee JA, Mueller BA. Antimicrobial doses in continuous renal replacement therapy: a comparison of dosing strategies. Crit Care Res Pract. 2016;2016:6.
7. Trotman RL, et al. Antibiotic dosing in critically ill adult patients receiving continuous renal replacement therapy. Clin Infect Dis. 2005;41:1159–66.
8. Pea F, et al. Pharmacokinetic considerations for antimicrobial therapy in patients receiving renal replacement therapy. Clin Pharmacokinet. 2007;46:997–1038.
9. Heintz BH, et al. Antimicrobial dosing concepts and recommendations for critically ill adult patients receiving continuous renal replacement therapy or intermittent hemodialysis. Pharmacotherapy. 2009;29:562–77.
10. Kroh UF. Drug administration in critically ill patients with acute renal failure. New Horiz. 1995;3:748–59.

Part III

RRT in a Sick Child

Acute Peritoneal Dialysis (PD)

7

Mignon McCulloch, Sidharth Kumar Sethi, Ilana Webber, and Peter Nourse

Case Study

A 10-month-old infant with severe failure to thrive weighing 6 kg presents with diarrhoea and septic shock not responsive to fluid resuscitation and requires inotropic support. After 2 days the patient remains anuric and not responsive to fluid boluses and diuretics. Examination shows that the infant is fluid overloaded with crackles in the lung bases and has an enlarged palpable liver. Potassium has been flagged as high previously and attempts have been made to treat this with conservative means. Blood results show a Na 130 mmol/l, K 8 mmol/l, Cl 110 mmol/l, urea 25 mmol/l, creatinine 200 umol/l and ABG pH 7.0 Bic 12. There is no HD or CVVH available at this institution and PD is planned. The surgeons are unable to assist and the

M. McCulloch (✉)
Paediatric Nephrology and Paediatric ICU, Red Cross Children's Hospital, Cape Town, South Africa
e-mail: mignon.mcculloch@uct.ac.za

S. K. Sethi
Pediatric Nephrology and Pediatric Kidney Transplantation, Kidney and Urology Institute, Medanta, The Medicity Hospital, Gurgaon, India

Secretary, Indian Society of Pediatric Nephrology, New Delhi, India

I. Webber · P. Nourse
Paediatric Renal Unit, Red Cross Children's Hospital, University of Cape Town, Cape Town, South Africa

S. K. Sethi et al. (eds.), *Critical Care Pediatric Nephrology and Dialysis: A Practical Handbook*, https://doi.org/10.1007/978-981-13-2276-1_7

paediatrician and nurse assistant place a PD catheter by Seldinger technique at the bed-side. PD is commenced using 1.5% Dianeal bags manually with only heparin as additives. Prescription consists of 20 ml/kg = 120 ml per cycle, fill for 10 min, dwell for 40 min and drain over 10 min. Ultrafiltrate remains poor after 12 h and the concentration of dialysis fluid is changed to 2.5%. This results in better ultrafiltration with reduction of potassium and resolution of acidosis.

After 3 days the infant starts to pass urine and the dialysis is stopped.

7.1 Introduction

By modern definitions one in three hospitalised children will develop acute kidney injury [1] (AKI). The incidence appears to be increasing in children in high-income countries [2] and is probably becoming more recognised, and hence more frequently managed in low- and middle-income countries. The management of AKI in high-income countries has moved away from the paediatric ward to the intensive care unit (ICU) setting, reflecting the alteration in the epidemiology of AKI from mainly single-organ failure, due to toxin exposure or intrinsic renal disease to AKI presenting on the basis of multi-organ dysfunction [2, 3].

In low-income countries, with the exception of developed urban centres, single entity diseases still predominate, especially in countries with limited or no ICU facilities [4, 5]. Between 7 and 66% of children with AKI will require renal replacement therapy (RRT) without which most will die [1, 6].

PD has a long and successful track record in the management of AKI in children and continues to be the most frequent form of acute RRT in children worldwide [7]. It is also the most inexpensive of all acute dialysis therapies in children [8, 9] and can be done in areas without developed infrastructure. Retrospective studies have shown that it is possible for PD to be performed safely in children with unstable haemodynamics and multi-organ failure requiring inotropic support [10]. Dialysis catheters placed at the bed-side [11] allow quick and safe initiation of therapy without the need for anticoagulation. This also allows for patients who have stable conditions to be offered dialysis outside of the PICU. Retrospective data in children show little difference in mortality when comparing dialysis modalities in children compared to the adult literature where there are some randomised control studies but still no evidence of difference in mortality between PD and extracorporeal therapies [12, 13]. Even in high-income countries, it can be challenging to insert haemodialysis catheters into premature and newborn babies and in these settings PD may still be optimal.

Overall there is enough evidence to recommend PD as an appropriate form of renal replacement therapy (RRT) in AKI in both high- and low-income settings.

7.2 Specific Indications for PD in AKI

Although PD is a suitable therapy for AKI in all settings, in the following situations it may be particularly useful:

- Small children where low gauge intravenous lines are not available or where the expertise to safely insert them are not available
- Small children where appropriate paediatric extracorporeal equipment is not available
- Haemodynamic instability (dependent on equipment available)
- In areas where there are cost constraints
- Disaster areas in remote places with underdeveloped infrastructure

7.3 Improvisation

Ideal: In the ideal setting, to commence PD one would want to have a well-trained paediatric surgeon placing a formal Tenckhoff in a theatre and then use the availability of commercial dialysis fluid via a cycling machine [14].

Less than ideal situation: Improvisation so that no child dies of acute kidney injury (AKI) without an attempt at PD first even in the absence of trained surgeons and reliable electricity.

7.4 Basic Requirements for PD

1. *Prevention of AKI* is the essence and this includes clean water supply—e.g., new innovative methods including the use of expired dialysers to clean water in Ghana (*personal communication Nathan Levin, USA*), teaching people how to resuscitate appropriately, avoid nephrotoxins.
2. *Aseptic technique*—PD has developed a bad reputation for infections in the absence of sterile handling.
   (a) For acute insertion of PD catheters—ideally in theatre but can also be done at the bed-side—use of gowns, gloves, masks and caps with aseptic technique.
   (b) Strict handwashing when inserting and dealing with any form of PD (see attached info).
   (c) Maintenance and cleaning of PD catheter while in situ.
3. *PD catheters* to be discussed in text below.
4. *Dialysis fluid* see Tables 7.1 and 7.2

PD catheters and this is where one may need to be innovative (Photos 7.1, 7.2, and 7.3):

Table 7.1 Dialysis fluid

Standard commercial dialysis fluid									
Commercial fluid	Na	K	Ca	Mg	Cl	HCO_3	Lactate	pH	Osm
Baxter									
Dianeal 1.5%									
High Ca	132		1.75	0.75	102	0	35	5.5	347
Low Ca	132		1.25	0.25	95	0	40	5.5	344
Dianeal 2.5%									
High Ca									398
Low Ca									395
Dianeal 4.25%									
High Ca									486
Low Ca									483
Physioneal	132		1.75/1.2	0.25	101	25	15	7.4	344
Extraneal Icodextrin	133		1.75	0.25	96	0	40	5.5	284
Nutrineal	132		1.25	0.25	105	0	40	6.7	365
Fresenius									
BicaVera 1.5%	134		1.75	0.5	104.5	34	0	7.4	358
BicaVera 2.3%	134		1.75	0.5	104.5	34	0		401
BicaVera 4.25%	134		1.75	0.5	104.5	34	0		511
SleepSafe 1.5% (Fresenius)	134		1.25	0.5	102.5	0	35	5.5	356

Table 7.2 Improvised fluid for PD

Non-dialysis fluid that can be used for improvisation									
Ringers lactate	131	5	1.8		112		28	6.5	270
Plasmalyte B	130	4	0	1.5	110		27	7.4	273
Hartmann's solution	131	5	2.0		111		29	7.0	278
Improvised PD fluid based on removing fluid and replacing with 50% dextrose									
30 ml 50% dextrose	1.5%								
50 ml 50% dextrose	2.5%								
85 ml 50% dextrose	4.25%								
Use *1 l Ringers lactate* with addition of dextrose to give a solution similar to commercially available *lactate-based PD* solutions available commercially									
Use *1 l Plasmalyte* with added dextrose to give a solution similar to commercially available *bicarbonate-based* solutions sold by industry									

1. Ideally a standard surgical Tenckhoff inserted in theatre by a qualified experienced surgeon. These may come as straight or curved catheters (swan-neck configuration) as well as 'pig-tail' catheters for long-term use. They may also have a single or a double cuff and which is chosen very much depends on the local protocols and surgeons.
2. Alternatively if no surgeon, then bed-side inserted PD catheter using a Seldinger technique including:
   (a) 'Peel away Tenckhoff' catheters (Kimal®, Covidien®, etc.) or
   (b) Flexible multipurpose drainage catheters in a Seldinger technique (Cook®)
3. Alternatively rigid stick catheters, venous central lines, naso-gastric tubes, chest drains, or even venous cannulae as PD catheters if nil else is available [11].

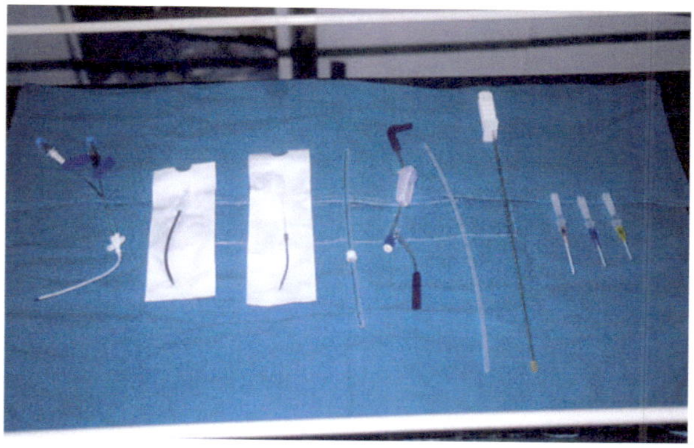

Photo 7.1 Devices used as PD catheters from left to right—central venous line (double lumen), Straight Cook® catheters (8 Fr), conventional straight Tenckhoff single cuff, rigid stick catheter and venous cannulae

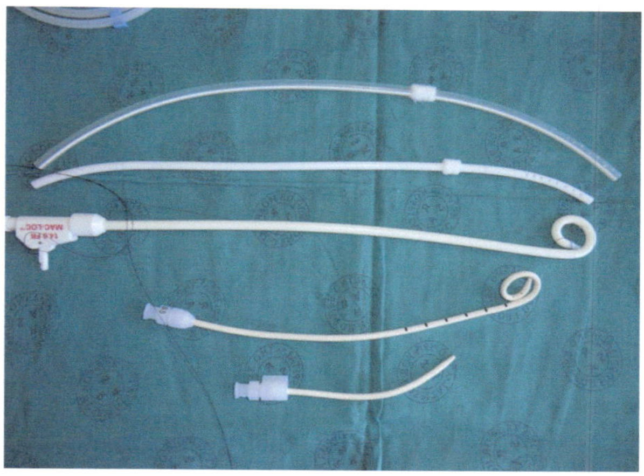

Photo 7.2 From top to bottom—Conventional straight Tenckhoff catheter, Kimal® peel-away PD catheter, Cook® catheters—multipurpose drainage catheters and straight PD catheter

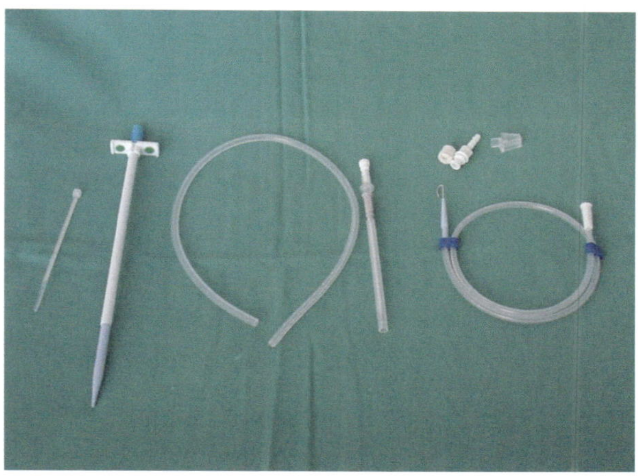

Photo 7.3 Peel away PD catheter set for Seldinger technique with uncuffed Tenckhoff (but can use cuffed catheter too)

7.4.1 'Hands-On' How to Insert a Percutaneous Acute PD Catheter at the Bed-Side

Plan to move child to a paediatric kidney facility if appropriate.
If this is not possible, request a surgical placement of a PD catheter.

If neither, prepare for placement of PD catheter at the bed-side

- Patient should be supine on a level surface. Monitoring devices should be attached to patient including oxygen saturation monitors with resuscitation equipment on standby and an assistant responsible for maintaining the patient's airway.
- The bladder should be emptied by insertion of a urinary catheter. If not already placed.
- Patient sedation as per local protocol, e.g., Midazolam (0.1 mg/kg/dose), Morphine (0.1 mg/kg/dose), or Ketamine (1 mg/kg/dose).
- Ensure sterile technique using protective personal gear (gloves, gown and mask) as well as a sterile tray.
- Chlorhexidine cleaning of the entire abdominal wall.
- Ensure that the catheter tip is positioned in the pelvis behind the symphysis pubis by marking a spot on the skin in the midline or in either flank. A PD catheter that is placed too high in the abdomen will not drain adequately.
- Use local anaesthetic to infiltrate the area of the skin and subcutaneous tissue where the catheter will be placed.
- Insert a cannula (usually size 18 Fr) through the skin at the previously marked area and advance the cannula through the skin as well as the subcutaneous tissue and the peritoneum. As the peritoneal membrane is pierced, there may be a slight resistance and then a 'give'. Pull the needle back into its plastic sheath a little in order not to pierce bowel and advance a few centimetres further before withdrawing the needle and leaving the plastic cannula in place. Ultrasound guidance can be used at this point.
- Run 20–40 ml/kg of crystalloid fluid into the abdomen to create artificial ascites until the abdomen is distended. Observe the oxygen saturations at this point in case oxygen is required. In the event of the abdomen not filling easily with fluid, the plastic cannulae will require pulling back as it may be sitting against the bowel wall.
- Ensure that fluid does not fill the subcutaneous space between the peritoneum and the skin. In event of this happening, remove and re-insert the cannula deeper with the needle again.
- Ensure respiration is not negatively affected by observing the oxygen saturations.
- Using a Seldinger approach, place the wire into the cannula and feed it into the abdominal space and place it into the pelvis. Leave the wire in situ and remove the cannula.
- Puncture the skin using a large gauge needle where the wire enters the skin.

- Ensure the skin puncture is not too large to prevent leakage.
- Thread the PD catheter (Cook or Kimal) over the wire and advance into the abdominal space by holding the catheter tip near the skin with firm downward catheter pressure using a rotating motion. The catheter should be advanced and remove the wire. Fluid should be draining easily from the top of the catheter.
- *Ensure that you do not lose the wire.*
- Other types of catheters may also be placed in this way. (Stick type catheter, Peel away Tenckhoff or any other improvised catheters, e.g., central line double lumen).
- Fluid should be collected for MC&S.
- Plastic tubing (or transfer set) with Y connection should be connected to the catheter to allow fluid drainage.
- Secure PD catheter securely to the abdominal skin.
- If possible, a formal Tenckhoff should replace the temporary catheter after 5–7 days.

7.5 Fluids

7.5.1 Commercial Fluids

Commercially available fluids are available for acute PD in 1.5%, 2.5% and 4.25% in both lactate and bicarbonate buffered solutions. In situations of worsening acidosis despite PD it may be beneficial to use a bicarbonate-based fluid. This may occur in children with liver dysfunction or in small infants with liver immaturity [15]. Because of rapid cycling potassium levels may fall in acute PD which may lead to cardiovascular instability, thus potassium should be added to the PD fluid once the blood potassium level falls to less than 4 mmol/l [16] (see prescription). Newer PD fluids including Extraneal and Physioneal are not generally used in acute PD settings.

7.5.2 Hospital Mixed/Custom Made Fluids

In low resource settings, the availability and cost of commercially made fluids may make PD often unaffordable. In these situations it is acceptable to use hospital mixed solutions [14] which can be made from physiological intravenous fluids. It is important to be aware of the risk of error in mixing the fluids and the risks of contamination which can arise during the mixing process. It is, in turn, vital that self-mixed solutions are prepared in a sterile environment using the least number of steps and additives possible. Mixing calcium and bicarbonate should be avoided because of the risk of precipitation.

Table 7.2 shows physiological intravenous fluids that can be used as alternative dialysis solutions. The comparison of the composition of these fluids to commercially manufactured dialysis solutions (Table 7.1) shows that adequate dialysis solutions can be made by supplementation of glucose and also bicarbonate. The addition of glucose will increase the ultrafiltration capacity and osmolality of the solutions. It should be noted that although magnesium and calcium are not present in some of these intravenous fluids, this is generally not a problem in the setting of acute PD; however, supplementary calcium or magnesium can be added orally or intravenously, if necessary. Some of the fluids, e.g., ringers lactate contain potassium and this may be beneficial in situations where the potassium has been lowered to less than 4 mmol/l (see above); however, caution should be used initially in hyperkalaemia.

7.5.3 Prescription

Initial prescription:

Fill volume: 10–20 ml/kg (ensure abdomen not too distended so as to cause respiratory distress)

Dwell time 45–90 min (shorter cycles for electrolyte exchange and longer for fluid removal)

Fill 1–5 min

Drain time 10–20 min

Glucose concentration: 2.5% if fluid overloaded, 1.5% if euvolaemic

Time: Continuous cycling throughout the day

Additives: Heparin 500 IU/l; KCl 4 mmol/l (once serum K below 4 mmol/l)

Medication including antibiotics: adapt to allow for removal by PD

7.5.4 Types of PD

1. Automated (Photos 7.4, 7.5, and 7.6)—these are cycling machines that are the gold standard for use in children with CKD as they can be connected at night and

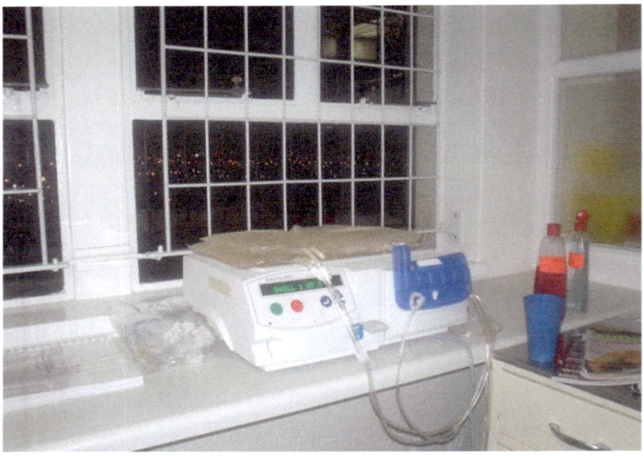

Photo 7.4 Automated PD machine—Homechoice (Baxter/Adcock Ingram)

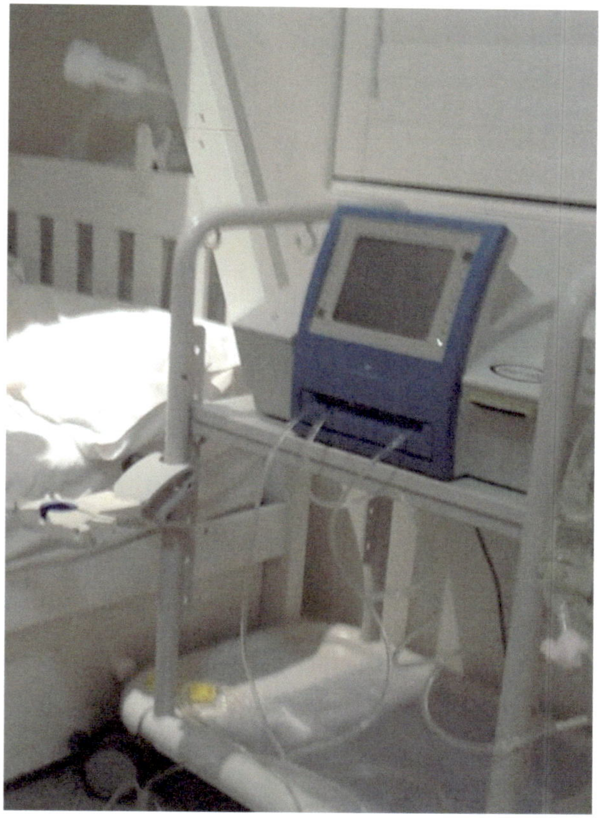

Photo 7.5 Automated PD machine—SleepSafe (Fresenius)

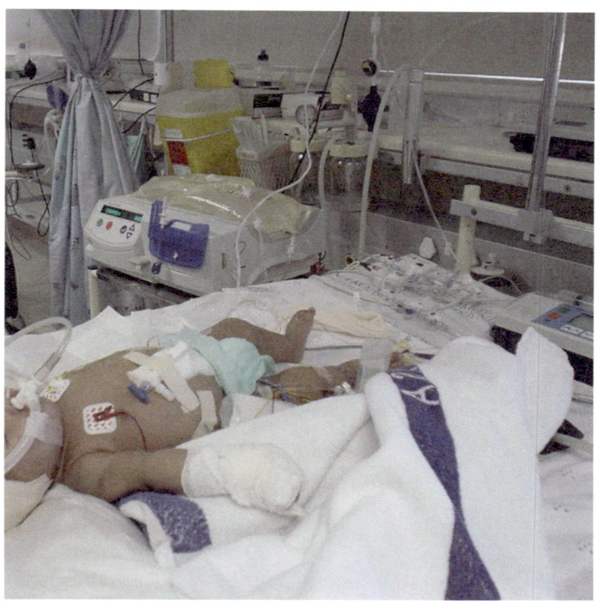

Photo 7.6 Automated PD machine in progress in PICU—assists in decreasing staff work load as compared to manual PD

be dialysed while they sleep causing minimal disturbance and allow good quality of life by going to school during the day. Currently two familiar machines are the Homechoice (Baxter) or the SleepSafe (Fresenius). Although these machines are aimed at chronic use, they can also be used in a paediatric intensive care setting to assist in the workload for the staff by its automated method of performing the cycles as well as internal record keeping of fluid volumes.

2. Manual PD (Photos 7.7, 7.8, and 7.9)
   (a) This comes manufactured as a 'closed system' either from Fresenius or Baxter with spikes which can be inserted into fluid bags, measured by buretrol to measure fluid IN and administered into the patient by a Y connector, then draining out via the other part of the Y connector into a draining buretrol which measures fluid OUT.
   (b) This can also be made manually using a dialysis fluid bag (manufactured or improvised fluid) draining into a buretrol (if available) and then via tubing* into a 3-way tap allowing fluid to fill via the PD catheter as the 'In' cycle. The three-way tap is locked off for the Dwell cycle and then for the 'Drain cycle' draining directly via tubing into a bag which can then be measured. *Any tubing can be used, e.g., intravenous fluid lines with a fluid dropper which can attach to bottom of the buretrol.
   (c) Important to record all the fluid going in and out to assess total ultrafiltration per session and cumulatively per day (Table 7.2).
3. Continuous flow PD (Photo 7.7)—this is a system which requires 2 PD catheters to be inserted at same time and for both catheters to be used to provide improved clearances. At present there is no electronic system available for this and some centres are using this in a manual format.

A useful online educational resource including knowledge guide, tactics and case studies is available: https://www.openpediatrics.org/assets/simulator/peritoneal-dialysis-simulator [17].

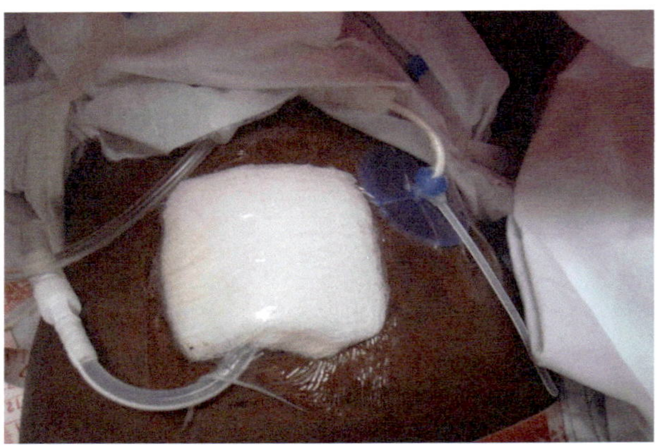

Photo 7.7 Continuous flow PD with 2 PD catheters (Courtesy Peter Nourse)

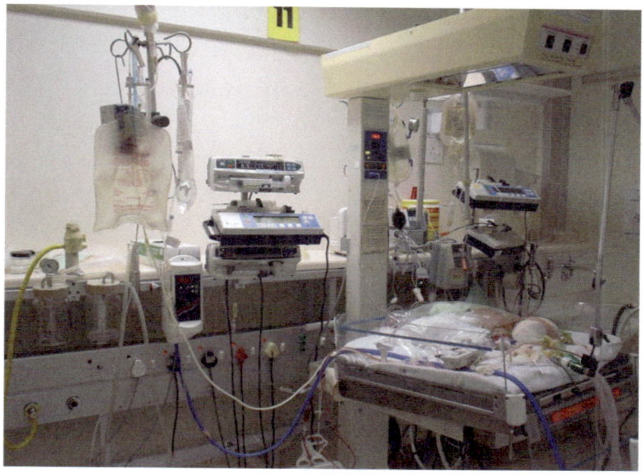

Photo 7.8 Manual PD in progress with self-constructed system including dialysis fluids hanging with buretrols attached and fluid warming tubing (optional) leading to patient PD catheter with Y connection and fluid drainage bag position under the bed

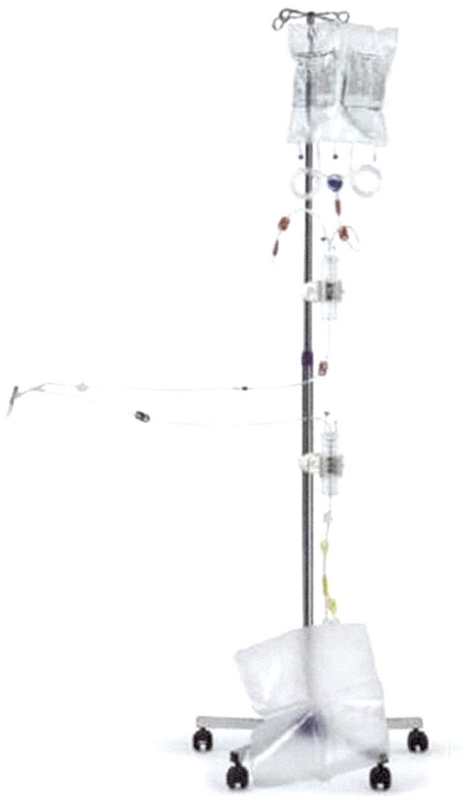

Photo 7.9 Fresenius acute PD paeds system—manufactured closed system

7.6 Record Keeping: Table 7.3

7.6.1 Complications/Troubleshooting

7.6.1.1 Peritonitis

A sterile technique with full gowning and gloves should be used at all time when inserting the PD catheter when done to prevent peritonitis. PD fluid should be sent for microscopy and culture after 3 days of PD or if peritonitis is suspected. Guidelines as for chronic PD should be used for diagnosis and therapy of peritonitis [18].

7.6.1.2 Catheter Leak

Particularly with bed-side inserted non-tunnelled catheters, catheter leak may become a problem. This can be prevented by using as small a nick in the skin at the site of the catheter placement as possible (especially in the multipurpose catheters which come with a plastic retention disc to hold the PD cath in place) and by the use of a purse string around the exit site of the catheter in Tenckhoffs. Surgical glue can be used successfully to prevent and treat catheter leak in acute and chronic PD in children [19] as well as in adults. In our experience application of surgical glue around the catheter between the tunnel wall and the catheter can be successful in treating catheter leak.

Hypernatraemia

If rapid cycling and high glucose concentrations are used the complication of hypernatraemia may occur. This is due to sodium sieving [20]. In acute PD the hypernatraemia may need to be corrected using more hypotonic IVI or oral fluids.

Hypokalaemia

If hypokalaemia is present or occurs due to too rapid clearance of potassium, then KCL can be added to the PD bags at a concentration of 3–5 mmol/l. Alternatively oral or IVI replacement can be used.

7.6.1.3 Hypernatraemic Dehydration

In children who have hypernatraemic dehydration often seen in newborns with difficulty feeding, institution of PD with standard fluids may result in too rapid

Table 7.3 PD chart recording—for 1 hourly cycles using 1.5% dialysate

Time in	Fill volume (ml)	Drain volume (ml)	Time out	Ultrafiltrate/cycle (+fluid from patient, −fluid left behind in patient) (ml)	Cumulative balance (ml)
10h00	200	230	11h00	+30	+30
11h15	200	180	12h15	−20	+10
12h15	200	200	13h15	0	+10

correction of the hypernatraemia. We advocate adding sodium to the PD fluid to make a concentration in the PD fluid of approximately 15 mmol/l less than the plasma concentration.

7.6.1.4 Pleural Effusion

Due to the connections between the peritoneal and pleural space, pleural effusions may become a problem as in the case of chronic PD. Testing the glucose concentration in the pleural fluid can be diagnostic as it will be very high if the fluid is PD fluid. If severe this may require a chest drain. If there are no other options available for dialysis, we have continued to do PD despite the pleural effusions. It is important in this situation to add the drainage from the intercostal drain to the overall fluid balance. We also advocate reducing the dialysis volumes per cycle and positioning the patient head up to allow fluid to be retained in the abdomen.

7.6.1.5 Hyperglycaemia

This complication may occur in acute PD because of rapid absorption of glucose from the peritoneal cavity especially when using 'strong' (high glucose concentration) bags. Insulin therapy may be necessary if the blood glucose is more than 15 mmol/l.

7.6.1.6 Raised Intraperitoneal Pressure

As in chronic patients this may be a problem. IPP is thought to be related to catheter leak and may also negatively impact on ultrafiltration and ventilation [21]. Raised intraabdominal pressure in critically ill children is also a mortality risk. If this expected, it can be measured by a simple manometer attached to the PD catheter or by a transducer open to the bladder catheter.

7.6.1.7 Practical

- Handwashing (Fig. 7.1)

Exit-Site Care

- Strict handwashing to prevent touch contamination and infection:
  - Wash hands with antibacterial soap and use alcohol gel
  - Dry hands completely as dampness can cause bacterial translocation
- No dressing changes in the first postoperative week
- Sterile dressing changes should be performed once weekly by an experienced health professional until the exit site is well healed
- Avoid further changes to the dressings unless there is excessive drainage, soiling or wet dressings
- Immobilise the catheter to prevent trauma to the exit site.

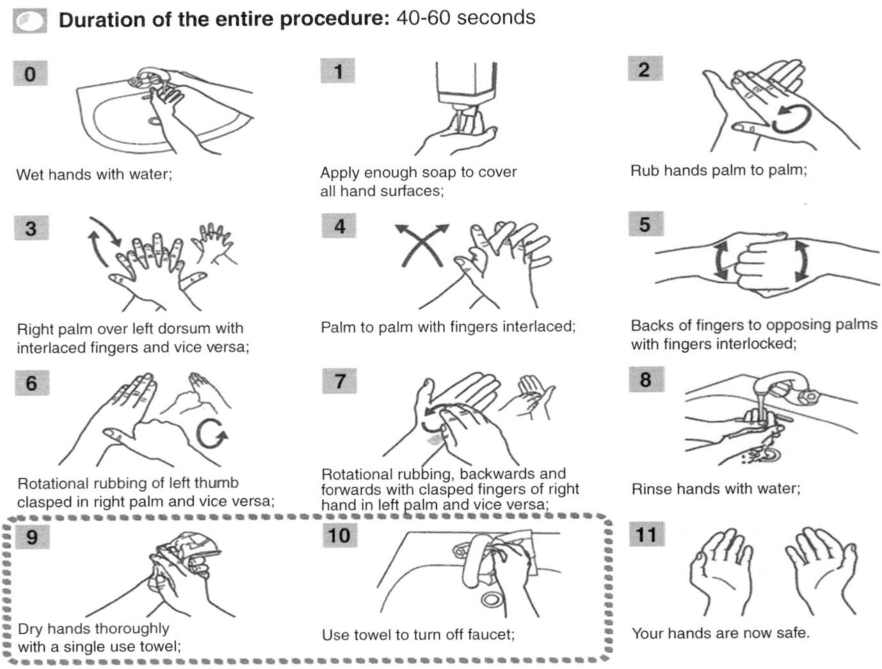

Fig. 7.1 World Health Organisation hand hygiene guidelines (2009)

Addendum: Step by Step Approach to Exit-Site Care

Follow an aseptic technique, using sterile gloves:

1. Prepare equipment:
   - Dressing trolley
   - Dressing pack
   - Normal saline/antimicrobial soap
   - Micropore/Tegaderm
   - Sterile gloves
   - Wound swab in case of discharge or redness
   - Mupirocin (Bactroban)
2. Wash hands and apply non-sterile gloves.
3. Secure catheter tip with tape, remove old dressing and take note of the condition of the exit site. If site is red or exudate/pain is present, collect a wound swab for MCS and notify renal team.
4. Wash hands, set up general field and apply sterile gloves
5. Clean around the exit site twice with sterile gauze soaked in sterile cleansing solution (N/Saline) or antimicrobial soap.

6. Crusts should not be forcibly removed.
7. Use another piece of soaked gauze to clean the tubing. Start from the exit site and work up the tubing away from the body.
8. Use gauze to gently pat the exit site dry, ensuring that it is completely dry.
9. Apply mupirocin ointment or gentamycin drops to exit site.
10. Allow the catheter to fall into its natural position from the exit site, but keep catheter tip clear of nappy area.
11. Completely cover the exit site with several layers of sterile gauze, and then secure with a dressing.
12. Immobilise the catheter below the exit-site dressing, anchoring the tube to restrict movement.
13. Document the procedure and notify any concerns

Steps to perform PD exchange:

1. Close windows and doors (no draughts or dust)
2. Cell phone on silent (no distractions)
3. Clean/wipe area with 70% alcohol spray where procedure will take place
4. Gather equipment:
   - Cassette
   - Octopus connecter
   - Drainage bag
   - K-shield (check expiry date and place with writing facing downwards)
   - Dialysis bags (fluids)
   - Alcohol spray (D-germ)
   - Soap and water
   - Dressing pack
   - Paper towel
   - Homechoice machine
5. Checking dialysis fluid (expiry date, particles, discoloration, the right fluid against prescription, holes/leaks)
6. Wash your hands and spray with alcohol. Wait for it to dry completely before carrying on.
7. Open cassette and place in machine
8. Place all lines in blue holder
9. Connect drainage bag
10. Switch machine on
11. Follow prompts
12. When machine asks for priming yourself, connect bags without touching the tips.
13. Machine will now prime the lines
14. Remove clothing/bedding to expose the PD catheter
15. Close roller clamp on transfer set
16. Wash hands thoroughly and dry completely. Spray with alcohol spray and wait until it's completely evaporated.

17. Open dressing pack and create sterile field.
18. Carefully open the K-shield onto the sterile field.
19. Carefully remove the blue cap of the patient line while still in the machine's connector without touching the tip.
20. Remove the minicap with your left hand while firmly holding the transfer set in your right hand.
21. While holding the transfer set in your right hand, remove the patient line with your left hand and carefully place the Luer connector of the transfer set into the line and screw tightly into place. *This is the most critical step in the procedure.*
22. Pick up K-shield with thumb and forefinger. Be careful not to touch iodine sponge.
23. Place the K-shield over connection with the smooth end facing the transfer set. Clip closed and rotate once.
24. Press green button on machine to start
25. Discard waste
26. Wash hands

References

1. Susantitaphong P, Cruz D, Cerda J, Abulfaraj M, Alqahtani F, Koulouridis I, Jaber B, Acute Kidney Injury Advisory Group of the American Society of Nephrology. World incidence of AKI: a meta-analysis. Clin J Am Soc Nephrol. 2013;8(9):1482–93.
2. Hui-Stickle S, Brewer ED, Goldstein SL. Pediatric ARF epidemiology at a tertiary care center from 1999 to 2001. Am J Kidney Dis. 2005;45(1):96–101.
3. Williams DM, Sreedhar SS, Mickell JJ, Chan JC. Acute kidney failure: a pediatric experience over 20 years. Arch Pediatr Adolesc Med. 2002;156(9):893–900.
4. Abdelraheem M, Ali E-T, Osman R, Ellidir R, Bushara A, Hussein R, et al. Outcome of acute kidney injury in Sudanese children—an experience from a sub-Saharan African unit. Perit Dial Int. 2014;34(5):526–33.
5. Esezobor CI, Ladapo TA, Lesi FE. Peritoneal dialysis for children with acute kidney injury in Lagos, Nigeria: experience with adaptations. Perit Dial Int. 2014;34(5):534–8.
6. Olowu WA, Niang A, Osafo C, Ashuntantang G, Arogundade FA, Porter J, et al. Outcomes of acute kidney injury in children and adults in sub-Saharan Africa: a systematic review. Lancet Glob Health. 2016;4(4):e242–50. https://doi.org/10.1016/s2214-109x(15)00322-8.
7. Cerda J, Bagga A, Kher V, Chakravarthi RM. The contrasting characteristics of acute kidney injury in developed and developing countries. Nat Clin Pract Nephrol. 2008;4(3):138–53. https://doi.org/10.1038/ncpneph0722.
8. Flynn JT, Kershaw DB, Smoyer WE, Brophy PD, McBryde KD, Bunchman TE. Peritoneal dialysis for management of pediatric acute renal failure. Perit Dial Int. 2001;21(4):390–4.
9. Reznik VM, Randolph G, Collins CM, Peterson BM, Lemire JM, Mendoza SA. Cost analysis of dialysis modalities for pediatric acute renal failure. Perit Dial Int. 1993;13(4):311–3.
10. Flynn JT. Choice of dialysis modality for management of pediatric acute renal failure. Pediatr Nephrol. 2002;17(1):61–9. https://doi.org/10.1007/s004670200011.
11. Auron A, Warady BA, Simon S, Blowey DL, Srivastava T, Musharaf G, Alon US. Use of the multipurpose drainage catheter for the provision of acute peritoneal dialysis in infants and children. Am J Kidney Dis. 2007;49(5):650–5. https://doi.org/10.1053/j.ajkd.2007.02.274.

12. Bunchman T, Smoyer W, Valentini R, Kershaw D, Gregory M, Sedman A. Modality and mortality in pediatric renal replacement therapy. Paper presented at the Journal of the American Society of Nephrology. 1994.
13. Chionh CY, Soni SS, Finkelstein FO, Ronco C, Cruz DN. Use of peritoneal dialysis in AKI: a systematic review. Clin J Am Soc Nephrol. 2013;8(10):1649–60. https://doi.org/10.2215/cjn.01540213.
14. Cullis B, Abdelraheem M, Abrahams G, Balbi A, Cruz DN, Frishberg Y, Koch V, McCulloch M, Numanoglu A, Nourse P, Pecoits-Filho R, Ponce D, Warady B, Yeates K, Finkelstein FO. ISPD Guidelines/Recommendations. Peritoneal dialysis for acute kidney injury. Perit Dial Int. 2014;34:494–517.
15. Bai ZG, Yang K, Tian JH, Ma B, Liu Y, Jiang L, et al. Bicarbonate versus lactate solutions for acute peritoneal dialysis. Cochrane Database Syst Rev. 2014;7:CD007034. https://doi.org/10.1002/14651858.CD007034.pub3.
16. Ponce D, Balbi AL, Amerling R. Advances in peritoneal dialysis in acute kidney injury. Blood Purif. 2012;34(2):107–16. https://doi.org/10.1159/000341648.
17. Olszewski, AE, Stein, D, McCulloch, M, Su, S, Hames, D, Wolbrink, TA. Virtual Peritoneal Dialysis Simulator. 2016. Online Interactive Simulator OPENPediatrics https://www.openpediatrics.org/assets/simulator/peritoneal-dialysis-simulator.
18. Warady BA, Bakkaloglu S, Newland J, Cantwell M, Verrina E, Neu A, et al. Consensus guidelines for the prevention and treatment of catheter-related infections and peritonitis in pediatric patients receiving peritoneal dialysis: 2012 update. Perit Dial Int. 2012;32(Suppl 2):S32–86. https://doi.org/10.3747/pdi.2011.00091.
19. Hisamatsu C, Maeda K, Aida Y, Yasufuku M, Ninchoji T, Kaito H, et al. A novel technique of catheter placement with fibrin glue to prevent pericatheter leakage and to enable no break-in period in peritoneal dialysis. J Pediatr Urol. 2015;11(5):299–300. https://doi.org/10.1016/j.jpurol.2015.07.005.
20. Fischbach M, Zaloszyc A, Schaefer B, Schmitt CP. Should sodium removal in peritoneal dialysis be estimated from the ultrafiltration volume? Pediatr Nephrol. 2016;32(3):419–24. https://doi.org/10.1007/s00467-016-3378-5.
21. Bunchman TE, Meldrum MK, Meliones JE, Sedman AB, Walters MB, Kershaw DB. Pulmonary function variation in ventilator dependent critically ill infants on peritoneal dialysis. Adv Perit Dial. 1992;8:75–8.

8 Vascular Access in a Child with Acute Kidney Injury

Deepa Chand and Rupesh Raina

Clinical Scenario

A 7-year-old male was admitted to the pediatric intensive care unit (PICU) after suffering internal injuries after a motor vehicle accident. Specifically, he sustained a liver laceration, from which he hemorrhaged, requiring multiple blood transfusions. His urine output has progressively decreased over the past 4 days, and now, on hospital day 5, his urine output has been less than 5 mL/h. He remains intubated and sedated, requiring ventilator support. You have been involved with his care since hospital day 2, and you have obtained a renal ultrasound which showed normal-sized kidneys with increased echogenicity and poor corticomedullary differentiation, consistent with medical renal disease. His serum creatinine on admission was 0.7 mg/dL and has progressively increased to 4.8 mg/dL at the present time. His serum chemistries at the present time are presented below.

Na^+ = 129 mEq/L
K^+ = 5.6 mEq/L
Cl^- = 97 mEq/L
CO_2^- = 18 mEq/L

You decide to initiate renal replacement therapy. The PICU team asks you what type of vascular access you would like placed.

D. Chand (✉)
University of Illinois College of Medicine, North Chicago, IL, USA

R. Raina
Department of Nephrology, Cleveland Clinic Akron General and Akron Children's Hospital, Akron, OH, USA
e-mail: RRaina@akronchildrens.org

S. K. Sethi et al. (eds.), *Critical Care Pediatric Nephrology and Dialysis: A Practical Handbook*, https://doi.org/10.1007/978-981-13-2276-1_8

8.1 Introduction

In the setting of acute kidney injury (AKI), optimizing medical management remains the first line of therapy. This often includes establishing hemodynamic stability, managing fluid and electrolyte balance, and avoiding nephrotoxic agents when possible. However, when advanced renal intervention is warranted, renal replacement therapy (RRT) may become necessary. Approximately 5% of children admitted into an ICU setting will experience AKI. With an overall mortality rate between 30 and 50% in these patients, early and appropriate RRT initiation becomes paramount and potentially lifesaving. As such, vascular access has been heralded as the cornerstone of RRT therapy [1].

While there are no published pediatric specific guidelines regarding optimal vascular access in AKI, adult guidelines are available, and some are applicable to children and adolescents. These include the Centers for Disease Control and Prevention guidelines, the KDIGO 2012 guidelines for AKI, and the 2006 National Kidney Foundation KDOQI clinical practice guidelines for vascular access [2]. However, many are not supported by strong evidence and provide general guidance, which needs to be customized to an individual patient based on the clinical circumstance. While published pediatric specific data is limited, some research consortia including the prospective pediatric continuous renal replacement therapy (ppCRRT) registry and independent studies have yielded useful, practical clinical information [3, 4].

Determination of catheter type, catheter lumen size, and catheter location are among the first decisions that need to be made when initiating CRRT. These are often determined by patient characteristics such as size, hemodynamic status, and coagulation state. In a post hoc analysis of over 1000 adult patients with AKI enrolled in the Veterans Affairs/National Institutes of Health Acute Renal Failure Trial Network Study, patient characteristics were the most influential in the type of catheter placed in adults. Clinical variables considered included body mass index, edema status, coagulation status, and age. However, among the three access sites used (subclavian vein, internal jugular (IJ) vein, and femoral vein), complication rates were low and occurred with similar frequencies (p-values >0.05 on all parameters).

In children, clinical variables impacting access location are also significant and may include prior use of central venous catheter, which may have resulted in vessel stenosis or thrombosis, hemodynamic status with possible compromise of lower extremity/femoral perfusion, edema status which may create technical challenges, and available catheter sizes as shorter catheters may not be feasible to obtain the desired central access. Location of catheter placement in children is predominantly the femoral vein (70%), internal jugular vein (16%), or subclavian vein (8%). While femoral vessels are used more frequently, catheters placed in the IJ vessels have been reported to result in significantly longer circuit life. If long-term dialysis needs are anticipated, the subclavian vein should be avoided to preserve the associated limb vessels for future arteriovenous fistula placement [5].

Catheter length can also be a significant variable in catheter functionality. Due to right atrial proximity, catheters placed in the internal jugular vein can be shorter than those placed in the femoral or subclavian veins. Noteworthy, longer catheters are associated with increased resistance that can potentially increase catheter malfunction. Furthermore, longer catheters are more prone to kinking, again potentially delivering less adequate clearances. In these vessels, larger bore catheters may be desirable in order to overcome resistance issues.

Many catheter options are available for use for RRT in children. These can include single-, double-, or triple-lumen catheter. In general, double-lumen catheters remain the mainstay to provide for the greatest exchange. Single-lumen catheter use is usually reserved for younger children, often <5 kg in size. These are often placed in two separate central veins with one catheter serving as a blood withdrawal line and the other as a return line. These catheters can also be placed in the umbilical veins if needed. Due to poorer circuit life, the use of small-bore, single-lumen catheters should be avoided unless absolutely necessary. With triple-lumen catheters, the additional port may be used for infusions. Although recirculation of medications may occur, this is not often of clinical concern, but medication response should be monitored and, if inadequate, recirculation considered as a possible etiology [6].

The mantra "the bigger, the better" often holds true in the choice of catheter size, as optimization of blood flow enhances clearance. It is important to note that in the ppCRRT registry, circuit survival was extremely poor in those using two 5-French single-lumen catheters, yielding circuit survival of less than 10 h with no circuits surviving longer than 20 h. Similarly, 48-h circuit survival was significantly better with 8-French catheters (76%) than with 7-French catheters (26%). In another single-center, prospective study of over 100 children treated with RRT, catheters larger than 6.5-French were associated with significantly longer circuit life. While catheters ≥8-French are preferred, they may not be practical in younger children with smaller vessel sizes. Alternatively, too large a catheter may result in impairment of venous drainage, with resultant decrease in circuit life. As such, a balanced, weight-based approach should be utilized and is outlined in Table 8.1.

8.2 Complications

While proper vascular access placement is crucial, complications are possible and should be anticipated. Potential complications during placement may include accidental arterial puncture, pneumothorax, hemothorax, air embolism, or cardiac arrhythmia (Figs. 8.1 and 8.2) [7]. Catheter placement is often performed by the intensivist at the bedside due to the acuity of the situation and is preferred. However, in a child with complicated anatomy or possible vessel compromise, surgical or interventional specialist consultation should be obtained. As these

Table 8.1 Acute hemodialysis catheters

Catheter	Site	Length (cm)	Pt wt (kg)	Availability	Oracle
7F Medcomp DL T74M	IJ, Fem	10	<6	CSP 147-B-07 Prentiss OR	003706
8F Arrow DL AK-11802-F	IJ, Fem	11	6–10	GS 20-C-03 Prentiss OR-CWA	058842
8F Mahurkar DL 8832539002	IJ	12	8–20	Prentiss OR-CWA	017702
9F Medcomp DL T94M	IJ, Fem	12	10–30	CSP 147-B-03 Prentiss OR-CWA	021740
10F Mahurkar DL	IJ, Fem	12	30–40	GS 20-D-02	56556
10F Mahurkar DL	IJ, Fem	15	30–40	GS 20-H-04	56557
11.5F Medcomp DL Pre-curved	IJ	20	>40	GS 172-B-03 Prentiss OR-CWA	014015
11.5F Raulerson DL	IJ, Fem	12	>40	CSP 101-E-01 POR implant room	014017
11.5F Raulerson DL	IJ, Fem	15	>40	CSP 101-E-02 POR implant room	002343
12F Arrow TL	IJ, Fem	16	>40	GS 114-B-05 PICU	017814
12F Arrow TL	IJ, Fem	20	>40	GS 114-C-03 PICU	009647

Note: It is preferable to place an acute dialysis catheter in the *right internal jugular vein with the distal tip in the right atrium*. Subclavian catheters may be considered in the acute situation but should be avoided for chronic access because of the possibility of vessel stenosis. Femoral catheters may be used; however, disadvantages include (1) reduced blood flow with patient movement and (2) inability to ambulate as patient recovers. StatLock devices are routinely used to secure acute pediatric hemodialysis catheters. If StatLock device is not securely attached, hemodialysis staff may carefully replace it.

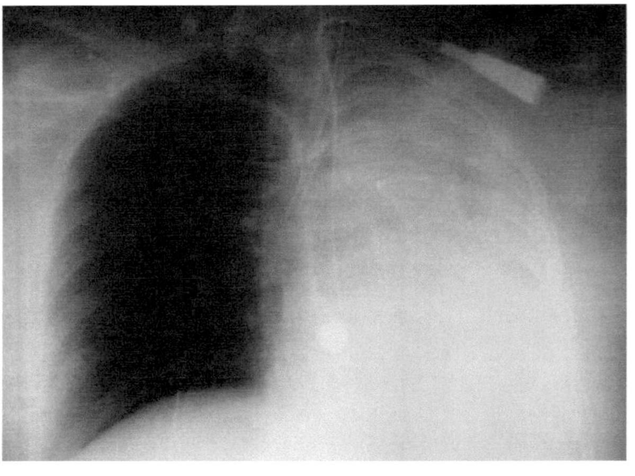

Fig. 8.1 Hemothorax, a complication of acute dialysis catheter insertion

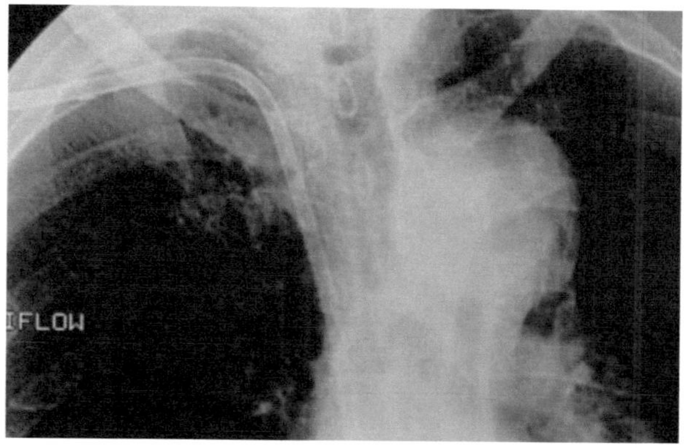

Fig. 8.2 Kinked dialysis catheter

children are critically ill and likely have hemodynamic instability, minimizing vascular trauma in order to preserve vessels is of paramount importance. An important caveat is to avoid peripherally inserted central catheter (PICC) lines whenever possible to preserve the vessels as well. Finally, an arteriovenous access should be considered and utilized in those undergoing extracorporeal membrane oxygenation (ECMO) as this access will already be in place and a circuit can be added, utilizing the existing access.

Catheter-related bloodstream infection and vascular thrombosis can potentially impact the quality of CRRT delivered and should be monitored. Factors that may impact the risk of clotting and infection include catheter location, duration of catheter placement, possible coagulopathies, and associated comorbidities [7]. Femoral catheters may pose a higher infectious risk, while subclavian catheters possess a higher risk of vessel thrombosis. Furthermore, subclavian catheters are highly associated with vessel stenosis, which is often permanent. Prolonged use of femoral catheters may result in deep venous thrombosis, which may negatively impact lower extremity circulation. For these reasons, several recommendations regarding catheter use for AKI in adults exist, which can be applied to children. The CDC recommends avoidance of femoral catheters, while the KDOQI guidelines recommend that femoral catheter use be restricted to 5 days in immobile patients and IJ catheters not be used for longer than 1 week.

When monitoring for infection, usual signs such as fevers may not occur [7]. As the blood is being circulated extracorporeally, the patient's temperature may be low at baseline. Signs and symptoms consistent with hemodynamic instability such as a widened pulse pressure should raise suspicion for infection. The catheter exit site should be covered and cared for regularly, with routine inspection for erythema and drainage. Exit site infections should be addressed promptly, and if catheter-related bloodstream infection is suspected, appropriate laboratories including a complete blood count and culture should be obtained. Empiric antibiotic pending culture results should be considered and tailored to regional microbial presence. If infection persists or fungal etiologies are of concern, catheter removal should be considered.

If poor clearances result, one should consider recirculation as a possible etiology. Additionally, femoral catheters have been reported to under-deliver dialysis doses in adults, especially when providing intermittent hemodialysis. This may necessitate adjustment of the dialysis prescription to provide adequate dialysis delivery.

8.3 Circuit Life

Once CRRT has been initiated, prolonging circuit life is critical to achieve the desired ultrafiltration and clearances. Multiple access-related factors have been identified that can impact circuit life. In the ppCRRT registry, variables including catheter site and catheter characteristics were collected [8]. Of note, catheter position can impact vessel resistance. For example, catheter tip malposition outside of the right atrium can increase vascular resistance, thereby decreasing catheter life. Further, internal jugular catheters have been associated with longer circuit life, which may be in part due to the relatively shorter catheter length but also possibly due to a decreased likelihood of catheter kinking or compression with patient movement. Similarly, patient movement can cause the dialysis/CRRT machine to alarm and pump to stop, increasing the risk of clotting. As such, it is important to keep the patient immobile, especially if a femoral catheter is in place. This may require heavy sedation and possibly medical paralysis while the treatment is provided.

Also, if the patient is disconnected for a prolonged period of time, known as "downtime" (i.e., for procedures), circuit life can be negatively impacted. In adult patients, Uchino et al. described a significant decrease in ultrafiltration rate from 35 mL/kg/h to 23 mL/kg/h if downtime was ≥8 h/day. Of note, an ultrafiltration rate of less than 20 mL/kg/h has been associated with higher mortality (DO-RE-MI study). Furthermore, in children, an ultrafiltration rate of >35 mL/kg/h has been associated with an increased circuit life of >24 h. However, this may not be practical in younger children with lower circulating volume. Irrespectively, if downtime is necessary, the line should be filled with a heparin solution or continuously infused to maintain patency.

8.4 Clinical Approach to Catheter Malfunction

Catheter malfunction can be challenging to manage; however, a poorly functioning catheter yields suboptimal results. The first step in troubleshooting includes obtaining imaging to ensure the catheter is in the appropriate location and has not migrated. Once this has been ascertained, a thrombolytic agent such as tissue plasminogen activator or urokinase can be instilled. The agent can be administered continuously or instilled into the catheter, allowed to dwell, and then removed. The optimal dwell duration if instilled should be determined by the pharmacologic properties of the agent itself. Unlike long-term catheters, which may develop fibrin sheath formation requiring mechanical stripping, this is often not desirable in acute use catheters due to hemodynamic instability. If medical management is unsuccessful, catheter replacement becomes necessary. Depending on the etiology, catheter replacement over a guidewire in the same vessel is possible; however in some circumstances, placement in a new vessel is necessary. This is true in the case of inherent vascular compromise with the former being possible if a mechanical catheter-related issue is the etiology.

8.5 Neonatal Nuances

While peritoneal dialysis is preferred in neonates due to small intravascular blood volumes, up to 30% of neonates with AKI may require hemodialysis or CRRT due to comorbidities such as abdominal surgery. While hemodialysis is not preferred due to rapid solute and fluid shifts, CRRT can be an option in these children. CAVH has been utilized successfully in this age group since 1985; however, advances over the past two decades have allowed for the use of a veno-veno access in this age group as well. While a catheter can be placed in the internal jugular, femoral, or subclavian veins using either a Seldinger or cutdown technique, an important alternative to consider is the umbilical vessels: both the artery and vein can be utilized, ideally with a 5- or 7-French catheter [6]. When initiating therapy, a blood prime may be required, and careful attention must be given so as to prevent catheter clotting. Various protocols for blood administration are available, and care must be individualized. When initiating CRRT, hypotension and bradycardia may occur and possibly cause severe hemodynamic instability.

8.6 Summary

The care of children with AKI must be individualized based on the child's circumstance. Once medical management has been deemed inadequate to serve the patient's need, RRT may become necessary. If hemodialysis or CRRT is utilized, optimizing vascular access becomes essential. Several decisions need to be made, including choice of catheter type, location of catheter placement, and anticipation of possible consequences and complications. In general, catheters should be double lumen, of appropriate caliber in relationship to patient vessel size, and placed in the internal jugular vein if possible. Infection and thrombosis remain the most frequent complications and should be diligently monitored and addressed. With the hope of renal recovery, catheters should be left in place only for the duration necessary to avoid short- and long-term vessel damage.

In the child presented in the initial vignette, a 9- or 10-French right internal jugular double-lumen catheter should be placed by the intensivist at the bedside using Seldinger technique. A chest radiograph should be obtained after placement to ensure the tip of the catheter is situated in the right atrium.

References

1. Chand DH, Brandt ML. Hemodialysis vascular access in children. In: Warady BA, Schaefer F, Alexander SR, editors. Pediatric dialysis. 2nd ed. Dordrecht: Springer; 2012. p. 275–85.
2. Goldstein SL. Advances in pediatric renal replacement therapy for acute kidney injury. Semin Dial. 2011;24:187–91.
3. Garzotto F, Zanella M, Ronco C. The evolution of pediatric continuous renal replacement therapy. Nephron Clin Prac. 2014;127:172–5.
4. Hackbarth R, Bunchman TE, Chua AN, Somers MJ, Baum MA, Symons JM, Brophy PD, Blowey D, Fortenberry JD, Chand D, Flores FX, Alexander SR, Mahan JD, McBryde KD, Benfield MR, Goldstein SL. The effect of vascular access location and size on circuit survival in pediatric continuous renal replacement therapy: a report from the PPCRRT registry. Int J Artif Organs. 2007;30(2):1116–21.
5. Ng YN, Ganta K, Davis H, Pankratz VS, Unruh M. Vascular access site for renal replacement therapy in acute kidney injury: a post hoc analysis of the ATN study. Front Med. 2017;4(40):1–7.
6. Ponikvar R, Kandus A, Urbancic A, Kornhauser AG, Primozic J, Ponikvar JB. Continuous renal replacement therapy and plasma exchange in newborns and infants. Artif Organs. 2002;26(2):163–8.
7. Chand DH, Ramage IJ. Hemodialysis vascular access: complications and outcomes. In: Geary DF, Schaefer F, editors. Comprehensive pediatric nephrology. 1st ed. Philadelphia: Mosby Elsevier; 2008. p. 855–65.
8. Del Castillo J, Lopez-Herce J, Cidoncha E, Urbano J, Mencia S, Santiago MJ, Bellon JM. Circuit life span in critically ill children on continuous renal replacement treatment: a prospective observational evaluation study. Crit Care. 2008;12:R93.

Hemodialysis Treatment Prescription

9

Rupesh Raina and Vinod Krishnappa

9.1 Case: 1

A 16-year-old female with end-stage renal disease due to diabetic nephropathy is scheduled to start hemodialysis next week. She has poorly controlled blood sugars, along with moderate obesity (weight of 42 kg, body mass index of 34 kg/m^2). Her blood pressure and proteinuria have been reasonably well controlled with lisinopril and atenolol. She is moderately hypoalbuminemic (serum albumin of 3.4 g/dL [34 g/L]) and anemic (hemoglobin of 9.6 g/dL [96 g/L]), while her serum potassium and bicarbonate levels have been normal on alkali supplementation. She had dialysis catheter insertion into her right internal jugular vein and a creation of arteriovenous fistula simultaneously this past week, after her blood urea nitrogen level surpassed 94 mg/dL (33.9 mmol/L) the week prior. Factors that need to be considered while writing hemodialysis prescription are summarized in (Table 9.1).

9.1.1 What Is the Principle of Blood Purification via Hemodialysis?

Concentration gradient-driven diffusion process is the main principle underlying blood purification in hemodialysis (HD), which effectively eliminates small

R. Raina (✉)
Department of Pediatric Nephrology, Akron Children's Hospital, Akron, Ohio, USA

Department of Nephrology, Cleveland Clinic Akron General, Akron, Ohio, USA
e-mail: rraina@akronchildrens.org; raina@akronnephrology.com

V. Krishnappa
Department of Nephrology, Cleveland Clinic Akron General/Akron Nephrology Associates, Akron, Ohio, USA

Northeast Ohio Medical University, Rootstown, Ohio, USA

S. K. Sethi et al. (eds.), *Critical Care Pediatric Nephrology and Dialysis: A Practical Handbook*, https://doi.org/10.1007/978-981-13-2276-1_9

Table 9.1 Hemodialysis prescription

Dialyzer type	Determined by patient size, clearance, and UF needs
Tubing type	Neonatal tubing—in patients <10 kg blood pump set at 2.6 mm Pediatric tubing—in patients 10–20 kg blood pump set at 6.4 mm
Priming of system	For circuits with extracorporeal volume >10% of patient blood volume (>80 mL/kg), diluted PRBC, or whole blood circuit priming
Dialysate composition	Composition determined on a per-patient basis
Dialysate flow	Flow <200 mL/min for infants/small children
Dialysate temperature	To avoid hypothermia, temperature may be elevated to 37.5 °C To prevent hypotension, temperature may be lowered to 35 °C
Blood flow rate	Gradually increase over first 3–5 treatments First treatment, BF = 2–3 mL/kg/min Second treatment, BF = 3–4 mL/kg/min Third treatment, BF = 4–5 mL/kg/min
Urea reduction	30% reduction in the first session 50% reduction in the second session 70% afterward
UF goals	No >5% of child's body weight removed during 3–4-h session
Anticoagulation	For continuous heparinization of patients <10 kg, consider loading dose of 10–15 units/kg, with a maintenance dose of 10–25 units/kg/h For routine heparinization of all low-risk dialysis patients, consider total heparin dose of 25 units/kg/h of dialysis For patients at slight to moderate risk of bleeding (such as those with recent surgery with low bleeding risk, pericarditis, and/or Coumadin therapy), consider total heparin of 10 units/kg/h of dialysis
Medications	Administered via infusion pump connected to venous port or IV push
Blood transfusion	Transfuse blood during dialysis to reduce volume overload and hyperkalemia risk
Patient monitoring	– Vital signs should be recorded at least every 30 min (q 15 min in PICU patients) in patients <15 kg – Staff members performing dialysis must remain within visual and auditory range of the patient/dialysis machine – Crit-Line monitoring and/or sodium modeling may help prevent intradialytic hypotension

UF ultrafiltration, *PRBC* packed red blood cell, *BF* blood flow, *IV* intravenous

molecules such as urea. The rate of blood flow correlates directly with HD clearance (K_{HD}) [1]. It is a passive transfer of solute across a semipermeable membrane. There is no net transfer of solvent, mainly driven by concentration gradient, much like a tea bag in water. Factors that affect mass transfer are [2]:

- Concentration gradient (*dC*)
- Dialyzer surface area (*A*)
- Dialyzer diffusivity (*KO*) for particular solute
- Sum of resistances (Rb + Rm + Rd) ~ (d*x*/KO) where Rb is mass transfer resistance of blood, Rm is mass transfer resistance of membrane, and Rd is mass transfer resistance of dialysate
- Countercurrent flow
- Time

$$\text{Mass Transfer} = \text{Driving Force} / \text{Resistance}\left(J = KOA \times dC / dx\right)$$

where J is diffusive mass transfer rate (mg/s) and dC/dx is the change in concentration of the solute in relation to distance.

9.1.2 What Is the Terminology Used to Decide the Prescription?

The low-flux and high-flux F-series Fresenius Polysulfone membrane dialyzers are available with a very good performance, larger endotoxin retention capability, and superb hemocompatibility. These hemodiafilters are manufactured specifically for high-volume hemodiafiltration (HDF) to handle more than 15 L of fluid exchange per treatment [3]. These hemodiafilters use new variant of the Helixone membrane with sophisticated housing design and enable [3]:

- Increased fluid exchange rates during HDF (>15 L/treatment)
- Increased elimination of low-molecular-weight substances such as phosphate
- Better elimination of middle molecules

The benefit of high-flux steam dialyzer is the integration of safe sterilization technique with blood-compatible membrane [3]. Its advantages are:

- Exceptional compatibility with blood.
- Best performance.
- Broad range of the products (0.7–2.4 m^2).
- Good for HD, hemofiltration (HF), and HDF.
- Efficient elimination of β_2-microglobulin.
- Enhanced capability for endotoxin retention.
- Exclusive steam sterilization in-line (without sterilization of by-products/residues and dry).
- Rinsing is not required prior to treatment.

Factors to keep in mind during the blood flow rate prescription for a HD are the relation between the specific solute clearance rate, dialysis membrane type, and rate of the blood flow [4]. Clearance of small solutes such as urea (molecular weight, 60) is highly flow dependent as linear relationship is observed between urea clearance and blood flow rates. Furthermore, property of the dialysis membrane is the limiting factor as clearance rates gradually reduce at higher blood flow rates [4]. The dialyzer efficacy in urea elimination (KoA) is dependent on the surface area of dialyzer, pore size, and membrane thickness. By increasing the rate of blood flow, clearance rate of urea can be augmented further by using high-efficiency membrane (KoA >600 mL/min). On the contrary, there is no notable difference in urea clearance between high-efficiency and conventional membranes at low blood flow rates since the rate of blood flow is the main factor affecting clearance, not the membrane [4].

Dialysis Clearance Clearance is a function of dialyzer efficiency. Clearances are routinely reported for urea (small solutes), β_2-microglobulin (middle molecule), and vitamin B12 (large solute).

Flux Flux is a measure of ultrafiltration capacity. The coefficient of ultrafiltration (Kuf) differentiates low flux from high flux. Kuf less than 10 mL/h/mm Hg is considered as low flux, whereas Kuf greater than 20 mL/h/mm Hg is considered as high flux [5].

Permeability Permeability is the capability of the dialyzer to eliminate middle molecular weight substance such as β_2-microglobulin (middle molecule clearance). With usual clinical flow and ultrafiltration, the correlation between permeability and flux is; permeability is low when the clearance of β_2-microglobulin is <10 mL/min (*low-flux membrane*), whereas the permeability is high when the clearance of β_2-microglobulin is >20 mL/min (*high-flux membrane*) [6, 7].

Efficiency It is the dialyzer's capability to remove urea (urea clearance). Low-efficiency dialyzer has KoA less than 500 mL/min, whereas high-efficiency dialyzer has KoA greater than 600 mL/min [6].

Surface Area Larger surface area dialyzer usually has higher clearance for urea, but the dialyzer efficiency (KoA) is vital in attaining optimal urea clearance, independent of a dialyzer's surface area.

The Mass Transfer Area Coefficient of the Dialyzer for Urea (KoA) KoA is the measure of dialyzer efficiency in removing urea and other small molecular weight solutes. At infinite dialysate and blood flow rates for a particular solute, KoA of the dialyzer is the highest theoretical clearance measured in milliliters/minute. Usually the surface area of any given dialyzer membrane will be proportional to KoA; however, drop in KoA occurs when the surface area becomes very large [8]. Small patients should be dialyzed with low-efficiency dialyzers with KoA <500 mL/min. Routine treatments are done with moderate-efficiency dialyzers with KoA of 500–700 L/min. Large-size patients with the need for >4-h dialysis session should be dialyzed with high-efficiency dialyzers of KoA >700 mL/min. KoA increases with increase in flow rate of the dialysate from 500 to 800 mL/min because of good dialysate penetration into hollow-fiber bundle at higher dialysate flow resulting in higher efficacy of dialysis due to expansion of effective surface area of the dialyzer [9, 10]. However, change in blood flow rates does not affect KoA.

Ultrafiltration Coefficient (Kuf) Kuf is the fluid volume (mL/h) transported through the membrane per mmHg of pressure gradient. It is the measure of dialyzer's permeability relative to water [2]. A low Kuf (near zero) denotes low permeability and low flux, whereas high Kuf (near 1.0) denotes near-complete permeability and high flux. The lower the permeability to water, the higher the transmembrane pressure (TMP) needed to achieve ultrafiltration. High-flux dialyzers achieve desired ultrafiltration (UF) volumes at lower TMPs. Volumetric machines control TMP based on the desired UF rate.

Kuf-UF Coefficient It is the volume of plasma filtered in mL/h for each mmHg of TMP. UF/h = Kuf × TMP. For example, for 100 ml UF/hr, you need 2 Kuf and 500 mmHg TMP, and for Kuf 8, you need TMP 125 mmHg. Minor error in TMP setting will lead to major error in the UF amount when Kuf is high.

9.1.3 What Is an Ideal Dialyzer?

9.1.3.1 Characteristics of High-Efficiency Dialysis

Both high-flux and high-efficiency membranes are similar with respect to clearance of solutes with low molecular weight (urea) and KoA (>600 mL/min). Larger pore size in high-flux membranes results in remarkably higher clearance rates for solutes with high molecular weight such as β_2-microglobulin, which is not cleared with low-flux membranes (Kuf less than 10 mL/h/mm Hg) [4]. As much as 400–600 mg/week of β_2-microglobulin can be cleared with some high-flux membranes. The following are the typical high-efficiency dialysis characteristics [5–7]:

The rate of urea clearance is normally >210 mL/min.
The dialyzer KoA for urea is normally >600 mL/min.
The Kuf and the clearance of middle-molecular-weight molecules may be high or low.
Cellulosic or synthetic membrane dialyzers can be used for dialysis.

High Flux Kuf >14 mL/min/mmHg (hydraulic or fluid removal)
β_2-Microglobulin clearance >20 mL/min (clearance of large molecules) [11]

High Efficiency KoA > 500 L/min at 500 mL/min of dialysate flow rate (Qd)

9.1.4 What Is Dialysis Adequacy and Why Is *KT/V* >1.4 Important?

The main part of dialysis prescription is providing sufficient amount of dialysis. Sudden decrease in urea levels occurs during dialysis followed by a slow rise during the interdialytic period. The three main factors that drive fall in urea concentration during dialysis are clearance rate of the dialyzer for urea (*K*), duration of dialysis (*t*), and urea distribution volume (*V*) [12]. Dialysis membrane properties (KoA), convective urea flux during ultrafiltration, rate of blood, and dialysate flow influence the dialyzer clearance rate for urea (*K*). In a stable patient, interdialytic urea rise depends on the dietary protein intake, volume of urea distribution, and residual kidney function.

Urea kinetic modeling (UKM) consists of *KT/V* and the urea reduction ratio (URR). *KT/V* is a measure of dialysis sufficiency determined by the dialyzer efficiency, dialysate and blood flow rates, HD frequency and duration, and volume of body water in which urea is distributed. The goal for *KT/V* is ≥1.4 and an acceptable *KT/V* is ≥1.2 [13]. A value of <1.2 denotes inadequate hemodialysis. The URR is also calculated to assess dialysis adequacy using blood urea nitrogen (BUN) before and after dialysis. Desirable URR is ≥65%. No outcome studies exist for pediatric HD patients and require advanced computational capability, which is not available to many pediatric dialysis units. A simple and reliable *Kt/V* estimation method is needed for month-to-month comparison of *Kt/V* in a single unit and across multiple units.

KT/V represents *fractional urea clearance*

K = dialyzer clearance (blood water) in mL/min or L/h
T = time in minutes or hours
V = urea distribution volume in milliliters or liters
Dimensionless

$$\mathrm{URR} = \left(\mathrm{BUN}_{\mathrm{PRE}} - \mathrm{BUN}_{\mathrm{POST}}\right) / \mathrm{BUN}_{\mathrm{PRE}}$$

URR is not precise as urea cleared by ultrafiltration is not taken into account. URR of 65% may have varying sp*Kt/V* (single pool) of 1.1–1.35 based on ultrafiltration volume. Also, URR does not give information about nutrition status (nPCR).

If measurements of dialysis adequacy (*KT/V* and URR) fall below the minimum acceptable levels, the following measures must be taken:

1. Evaluate for errors in prescribed HD dose delivery.
2. Increase the dose of HD prescription:
   - Increase dialyzer size.
   - Increase treatment time.
   - Increase dialysate flow.
   - Increase blood flow.
3. Increase the heparin dose.
4. Correct the dialysis access site if inadequate.

KT/V = 0.5—associated with uremic symptoms, hospitalization, & death

0.7—associated with EEG abnormalities
1.0—associated with good short-term outcome
1.2–1.4—associated with good long-term outcome
>1.4—associated with better outcome

9.1.5 How to Write Initial Prescription in Acute on Chronic Hemodialysis Case?

Equation for Initial HD prescription

$$Kt / V \sim -In\left(C1 / C0\right)$$

K = urea clearance of the dialyzer (mL/min)
t = duration of treatment (minutes)

V = total body water estimation (600 mL/kg)
$C0$ = BUN before dialysis (mg/dL)
$C1$ = BUN after dialysis (mg/dL)
ln = natural log

1. Determine the amount of urea to be removed (e.g., 50%).
2. Select dialyzer size appropriately and enter K.
3. Calculate V (600 mL/kg).
4. Get BUN before dialysis ($C0$), perform dialysis for prescribed duration (t), and get BUN after dialysis ($C1$).
5. Estimate V from K, t, and measured $C0$ and $C1$.
6. Repeat steps 1–5 using estimated V.

9.1.5.1 Let's Write Perception?

Desired clearance of urea is 50%.

Choose 1.3 m^2 surface area dialyzer.
(K_{urea} = 210 mL/min at 250 mL/min blood flow rate (Qb))
Weight of the patient is 42 kg before dialysis.
Using the equation: $Kt/V \sim -\ln(C1/C0)$
210 mL/min × t/(42 kg × 600 mL/kg) = −ln (50/100)
Leading to t = 83 min
Example of initial HD prescription and refinement
Hemodialysis performed
BUN before dialysis ($C0$) = 94 mg/dL
BUN after dialysis ($C1$) = 65 mg/dL
HD duration = 83 min
Using the equation: $Kt/V \sim -\ln(C1/C0)$
210 mL/min × 83 min/V = −ln (65/94)
Leading to V = 47.2 L

Acute HD should be delivered in a dialysis center or in pediatric or neonatal ICU with support from the multidisciplinary team that provides integrated and individualized care.

1. *The following must be specified in all pediatric hemodialysis treatment orders:*
   (a) Dialyzer type
   (b) Tubing type (adult, pediatric, or neonatal)
   (c) Priming of system (blood, 5% albumin)/amount to administer
   (d) Dialysate composition
   (e) Dialysate flow
   (f) Dialysate temperature
   (g) Blood flow rate
   (h) Duration of treatment
   (i) Ultrafiltration goal
   (j) Anticoagulation
   (k) Medications
   (l) Blood transfusion
   (m) BP and pulse parameters/management of hypotension

2. *Machine specifications*: Fresenius 2008K machines will be used.
   (a) For blood flow <120 mL/min, use the pediatric mode. If normal mode is used with low blood flows, UF will automatically be set at 70 mL/h.
   (b) Selection: Move arrow on display to MENU, and then push SET. Move arrow to DIALYSIS OPTIONS, and then push SET. Move arrow to PEDIATRIC, and then push SET to change “NO” to “YES.” Move arrow to DIALYSIS, and then push SET to go back to DIALYSIS screen.
   (c) To change back to normal mode, move arrow to MENU, and then push SET. Move arrow to DIALYSIS OPTIONS, and then push SET. Move arrow to PEDIATRIC, and then push SET to change “YES” to “NO.” Move arrow to DIALYSIS, and then push SET to return to DIALYSIS screen.
3. *Dialyzer*
   (a) Determined by patient’s size and the patient’s clearance and UF needs.
   (b) Consult the specification sheets for the clearance and UF capacities of specific dialyzers (Table 9.2).
4. *Tubing*
   (a) Patients <10 kg—*neonatal tubing* with blood pump set at 2.6 mm
   (b) Patients 10–20 kg—*pediatric tubing* with blood pump set at 6.4 mm
   (c) Patients >20 kg—*adult tubing* with blood pump set at 8 mm
5. *Priming of system*
   (a) Extracorporeal volume (tubing volume + dialyzer volume) >10% of the estimated blood volume of the patient (>80 mL/kg), blood priming of the circuit should be done especially in patients <10 kg to prevent intradialytic hypotension [2, 14].
   (b) One unit of *diluted packed red blood cells* (PRBCs) (hematocrit 35%) should be ordered which has been typed and crossmatched with the patient.
   (c) Prime the circuit with normal saline.
   (d) Add two units of heparin/mL into the diluted PRBCs.
   (e) Prime the circuit with diluted PRBCs.
   (f) Wait for 5 min to recirculate and heparinize the system and to warm the blood to an adequate level for the patient.

Table 9.2 Specifications of different dialyzers [14]

Dialyzer	Membrane	SA (m^2)	Prime volume (mL)	Kuf	Patient weight (kg)
F3	PS	0.4	28	1.7	10–15
F4	PS	0.7	42	2.8	15–25
F6	PS	1.3	82	5.5	25–35
F160	PS	1.5	83	50	35–80
F180	PS	1.8	99	48	>80
B 190 Xebium	PES	1.9	114	75	
B 150	CET	1.5	95	3.15	(Hypoallergenic)

PS polysulfone, *PES* polyethersulfone, *CET* cellulose triacetate, *SA* surface area, *Kuf* ultrafiltration coefficient of a dialyzer

(g) Entire blood priming should be done by connecting the arterial and venous lines concurrently.
(h) Caution should be exercised in deciding about giving half or the entire prime in children who weigh 10–15 kg or hemodynamically unstable.
(i) No prime is given in children >15 kg who are hemodynamically stable.

6. *Dialysate*
   (a) Dialysate is ordered based on patient's lab reports.
7. *Dialysate flow rate (Qd)*
   (a) Standard Qd of 500 mL/min is adequate for most patients [2].
   (b) In infants and small children during initial HD, decreased flow of <500 mL/min should be considered to prevent disequilibrium syndrome.
   (c) To attain adequate clearance in larger children, higher flow of 800 mL/min may be needed [2].
8. *Dialysate temperature*
   (a) To avoid hypothermia in infants, dialysate temperature is increased to 37.5 °C [2].
   (b) In children with hypotension, dialysate temperature is decreased to as low as 35 °C to improve cardiovascular stability [14].
9. *Blood flow rate (Qb)*
   (a) The rate of blood flow is increased slowly during the initial three to five treatments [2, 14]:
      - First treatment: Qb 2–3 mL/kg/min (start at 200 mL/min in adult-size patients)
      - Second treatment: Qb 3–4 mL/kg/min
      - Third treatment: Qb 4–5 mL/kg/min
   (b) Minimum Qb is 25 mL/min and maximum Qb is 500 mL/min.
   (c) Blood flow may be limited by catheter size/position.
   (d) Monitor for any problems with outflow or high venous resistance.
10. *Duration of treatment*
   (a) First dialysis treatment in uremic patients should be limited to 2 h.
   (b) Subsequent dialysis treatments may be slowly increased to 3–4 h (30–60 min/treatment).
   (c) If serum osmolality >300 mOsm, BUN > 100 mg/dL, or first dialysis in chronic patient, intravenous mannitol 0.25 g/kg/dose should be considered at the beginning of dialysis.
   (d) The duration of treatment is estimated based on serum ammonia levels in children with hyperammonemia or intoxication (in PICU/NICU) as the duration is not known at onset.
11. *Ultrafiltration goal*
   (a) General rule is no >5% of the child's body weight should be removed during a 3–4-h HD session [14].
   (b) Fluid removal is usually better tolerated in a shorter period of time in an isolated UF session.
   (c) UF goal adjustments are done by referring Crit-Line monitoring protocol.

12. *Anticoagulation*
    (a) Usually, heparin is given as bolus (patient >10 kg) or by constant infusion (patient <10 kg).
    (b) Monitor machine pressure readings for signs of elevation, which indicates clotting.
    (c) If the pressures increase and the access is patent, stop the dialysis before the system completely clots, and return as much blood as possible to the patient (unless system was primed with blood).
    (d) In children with increased risk for bleeding, non-heparin-based dialysis (normal saline flushes) may be considered [2].
13. *Medications*
    (a) All medications should be given as intravenous push or through infusion pump connected to the venous port.
    (b) Alarm may go on as the venous dialysis bloodline pressure is usually more than that of the infusion pump due to small volume and low infusion rate.
    (c) Medication should be given via a different access if the infusion pump continues to alarm for high pressures.
14. *Blood transfusion*
    (a) Risks of volume overload and hyperkalemia are decreased if blood is transfused during dialysis.
    (b) Order type and crossmatch for 15–20 mL/kg PRBCs (and premedication if needed).
    (c) Transfusion should be done over a period of at least an hour and via blood administration tubing and, if possible, should be extended over the entire duration of the treatment to prevent acute hypertension.
    (d) Only RN should transfuse the blood, and the technician may assist RN about connecting the blood administration line to the saline port of the dialysis tubing and by monitoring vital signs.
    (e) RN should transfuse blood to children in the PICU, including blood verification, control of transfusion rate, and assessment of the patient's response.
    (f) UF goal should include volume of the blood to be transfused.
    (g) Monitor for any transfusion reaction.
    (h) Posttransfusion CBC should be done at the time of the next dialysis treatment to assess response to transfusion.
15. *Patient monitoring/management of hypotension*
    (a) Vital sign parameters are very different in children compared to adults and vary with the age and size of the child.
    (b) Vital signs must be recorded at least every 30 min (every 15 min in PICU or children <15 kg), and the nephrologist should be informed of any significant variations [14].
    (c) Intradialytic hypotension may be prevented by Crit-Line monitoring and/or sodium modeling.
    (d) Before beginning dialysis, orders should be in place for treatment of hypotension unresponsive to adjustment in UF goal per Crit-Line [2]:

- Saline bolus, 5 mL/kg
- 25% albumin 0.25 g/kg, maximum 12.5 g
- Mannitol 0.25 g/kg, maximum 12.5 g

(e) Albumin and mannitol are given no more than every 1 h and should not to be given during the last hour of treatment.

(f) In PICU, vasopressor support may be considered to correct dialysis-associated hypotension.

(g) Dialysate cooling may be considered to increase vascular tone and support BP [14].

16. *Patient monitoring*

(a) In PICU treatments, the technician performing dialysis must be within visual and auditory range of the patient/dialysis machine.

(b) If the technician wants to leave the area, even for a few minutes, another staff member must supervise the treatment.

(c) Patient should be taken off dialysis if another staff member is not available and set up again when the staff member returns.

(d) To avoid these circumstances, any supplies that might even rarely needed should be taken to the PICU.

17. *Completion of dialysis treatment*

(a) In children without a blood prime, blood in the system should be returned. Decrease the blood flow rate by 50% when returning the blood to prevent acute hypertension in children <20 kg.

(b) Discard the entire setup with the blood in it to avoid acute increase in blood volume in whom blood prime was used.

(c) The nephrologist should be notified of any blood loss.

References

1. Gulati S, Lall N. Hemodialysis in children: a simplified approach. J Int Med Sci Acad. 2012;25(2):101–5.
2. Sethi SK, et al. Unique considerations in renal replacement therapy in children: core curriculum 2014. Am J Kidney Dis. 2014;63(2):329–45.
3. Hemodialysis: Dialysers and Filters (Fresenius Medical Care). 2007. Available from: http://www.fmc-ag.dk/files/Filterbrochure.pdf.
4. Dialysis as treatment of end-stage renal disease: considerations in choice of membranes. [cited 2018]. Available from: https://www.cybernephrology.ualberta.ca/cn/Schrier/Volume5/ch6/ADK5-06_4-6.ccc.QXD.pdf.
5. Cheung AK, Leypoldt JK. The hemodialysis membranes: a historical perspective, current state and future prospect. Semin Nephrol. 1997;17(3):196–213.
6. Ambalavanan S, Rabetoy G, Cheung AK. Dialysis as treatment of end-stage renal disease: high-efficiency and high-flux hemodialysis. Available from: https://www.kidneyatlas.org/book5/adk5-03.ccc.QXD.pdf.
7. Leypoldt JK, et al. Hemodialyzer mass transfer-area coefficients for urea increase at high dialysate flow rates. The hemodialysis (HEMO) study. Kidney Int. 1997;51(6):2013–7.
8. Daugirdas JT, Blake PG, Ing TS. Chronic haemodialysis prescription: a urea kinetic approach. In: Handbook of dialysis. Boston: Little Brown; 1994. p. 92–120.

9. Leypoldt JK. Effect of increasing dialysate flow rate on KoA and dialyzer urea clearance. Semin Dial. 1998;11(3):195–6.
10. Leypoldt JK, Cheung AK. Increases in mass transfer-area coefficients and urea Kt/V with increasing dialysate flow rate are greater for high-flux dialyzers. Am J Kidney Dis. 2001;38(3):575–9.
11. Eknoyan G, et al. Effect of dialysis dose and membrane flux in maintenance hemodialysis. N Engl J Med. 2002;347(25):2010–9.
12. NIDDK: Hemodialysis Dose & Adequacy. 2014. Available from: https://www.niddk.nih.gov/health-information/kidney-disease/kidney-failure/hemodialysis/dose-adequacy.
13. Locatelli F, et al. Dialysis dose and frequency. Nephrol Dial Transplant. 2005;20(2):285–96.
14. Raina R, et al. Hemodialysis in neonates and infants: a systematic review. Semin Dial. 2018;31(3):289–99.

Prolonged Intermittent Renal Replacement Therapy in Pediatric AKI

10

Sidharth Kumar Sethi

10.1 Introduction

Acute kidney injury in children in intensive care is often secondary to shock and multi-organ dysfunction syndrome. These children are often on inotropes, are hypotensive, and are fluid overloaded. Continuous renal replacement therapy (CRRT) often used in developed world requires expertise, expensive machinery, consumables, trained staff and is labor intensive. Sustained low-efficiency dialysis (SLED) refers intermittent renal replacement therapy over an extended period of time. There is now evidence in favor of this therapy especially in adults, with few case series from pediatric literature [1–6].

Case Scenario

A 2-year-old child (weight = 16 kg; body surface area 0.6 m^2) is admitted in pediatric intensive care with dengue shock syndrome. The child is on dopamine 10 μg/kg/min, with a blood pressure 90/60 mmHg. The child is intubated and is 15% fluid overloaded. The child is anuric since the last 4 h.

Blood urea: 120 mg/dl
Serum creatinine: 4 mg/dl
Na/K (meq/l): 135/5.5
Venous blood gas: pH 7.25/HCO_3 15/BE −7
Prothrombin time/INR: 14.5 s/1.5
Activated partial thromboplastin time: 54 s

S. K. Sethi (✉)
Pediatric Nephrology and Pediatric Kidney Transplantation, Kidney and Urology Institute, Medanta, The Medicity Hospital, Gurgaon, India

Secretary, Indian Society of Pediatric Nephrology, New Delhi, India

S. K. Sethi et al. (eds.), *Critical Care Pediatric Nephrology and Dialysis: A Practical Handbook*, https://doi.org/10.1007/978-981-13-2276-1_10

A Typical SLED Prescription

- Fresenius 5008S machine; SLED-f (SLED with convection)
- F4/FX40 dialyzer (if convection is planned)
- Qb (blood flow rate) = 5 ml/kg/min = 80 ml/min
- Qd (dialysate flow rate) = 2 × Qb
- [If convection planned] Q replacement flow rate = 25 ml/min (can be increased if increased convective dose is planned); pre-dilution
- Duration = 6 h
- Dialysate potassium = 3 meq/l
- Ultrafiltration rate = 200 ml/h
- Anticoagulation = heparin free

10.2 Definitions

Sustained low-efficiency dialysis is mostly defined as an extracorporeal mode of renal replacement therapy given intermittently over a prolonged session (i.e., ≥6 h). In the present era, both diffusive and convective methods of extended extracorporeal therapies are being used in these settings. The terminologies used in the hybrid therapies are mostly SLED (sustained low-efficiency dialysis), S-HDF (sustained hemodiafiltration), ED (extended dialysis), EDD (extended daily dialysis), E-HFD (extended high-flux hemodialysis), PIRRT (prolonged intermittent renal replacement therapy), PDIRRT (prolonged daily intermittent renal replacement therapy), or SLED-f (sustained low-efficiency dialysis with convection) [1, 2].

10.3 Importance of a Prolonged Therapy in Critically Sick Children

Critically ill children have increased nutritional needs but on the other hand are fluid overloaded due to receiving large fluid volumes. They receive large fluid volumes due to the need for blood products, multiple antibiotics, and inotrope infusions. A prolonged intermittent renal replacement therapy has the advantage of continuous renal replacement therapy (CRRT) being continuous and being well tolerated in sick patients. It also gives the advantage of ancillary procedures "downtime" when the patient is off circuit, in addition to being cheaper. Recent surveys among pediatric and adult nephrologists show SLED to be used commonly in ICUs in sick patients [1, 2].

10.4 Setup Required and Prescription for PIRRT

The setup is classically similar to intermittent hemodialysis machine with few modifications.

Machines for PIRRT Any hemodialysis machine with the ability to lower the Qb/Qd and increase the duration of the therapy can be used for SLED.

Fresenius Medical Care company machines are commonly used for these therapies. These machines are of two types: single pass (uses dialysate generated online from reverse osmosis purified water and bicarbonate proportionating system) or batch machine (dialysate generated from prepackaged salts and sterile water which is stored in the machine). The single pass machines such as 2008, 4008, and newly available 5008 series or the batch dialysate machine such as Genius machine have been commonly used. Batch dialysate machines are more user-friendly and use ultrapure dialysate, and there is no need for on-the-spot water purification, as ultrapure water is not readily available in most ICUs. The Genius (batch dialysate) machine has a dual-headed roller pump for both blood and dialysate flows; hence the ratio of blood flow rates and dialysate flow rates [Qb/Qd] is 1 in this machine. The ARrt plus, 5008 series, and the AK200 Ultra machines possess additional unique feature of cold sterilization or ultrafiltration of the dialysate leading to a reduction of bacteria and endotoxins, producing a sterile pyrogen-free fluid suitable for intravenous infusion to the patients [1, 2].

Extracorporeal Circuit Similar to hemodialysis, it should to be ensured that the extracorporeal volume (volume of blood tubing + dialyzer) should be less than 10% of the child's total blood volume, else the circuit should be primed with albumin or blood.

Dialyzers The dialyzer surface area should be approximated to the body surface area of the child. High-flux dialyzers or hemofilters (AV series-Fresenius) should be used for adding the convection component.

Qb/Qd The Qb and Qd should be decided keeping the hemodynamic stability in mind. The Qd is kept low (usually $\leq 2 \times$ Qb). The blood flow rates are usually 3–5 ml/kg/min. Duration varies between 6 h and 18 h and is individualized. The blood flow may have to be adjusted according to the replacement fluid rate so that the filtration fraction does not exceed 25–30%, to avoid filter clotting.

Adding Convection Adding convective clearance (though not allowed in the United States) to the predominant diffusion clearance of SLED has been the latest innovation in this technology. Sustained low-efficiency daily diafiltration (SLEDD-f) is commonly employed with the ARrT plus, 5008S, and AK 200 Ultra machines. The prerequisite is ultrapure water and sterile dry powder concentrates for making the dialysate preparation. High-flux dialyzers or hemofilters, having UF coefficients >20 ml/mm Hg/h, are required for adding the convective component of this treatment. Replacement fluid component should be delivered prefilter, and the blood flow has to be proportionally higher in order to avoid a filtration fraction >20%, which predisposes to filter loss due to clotting of the filter. These machines display the online filtration fraction on the screen to help in prescription. The convective dose in Fresenius 5008 series machine has an online substitution rate of minimum 25 ml/min.

Dialysate Fluid Standard hemodialysis dialysate fluid consists of sodium, potassium, calcium, and bicarbonate, the concentration of which can be varied as per the clinical requirement. A dialysate potassium of 3 meq/l and bicarbonate around 28–30 mmol/l should be preferred for prolonged sessions to avoid metabolic alkalosis and hypokalemia. These children may also require phosphate supplements, especially those requiring daily and prolonged sessions.

Anticoagulation The incidences of extracorporeal circuit clotting in various studies have been reported between 26 and 46% with no anticoagulation and 10 and 26% with heparinization/citrate, respectively.

No Anticoagulation Anticoagulation can be avoided in SLED with frequent flushing of extracorporeal circuits with saline, thus preventing the risk of bleeding. There have been adult studies on heparin-free anticoagulation in SLED with the incidence of extracorporeal circuit clotting between 26% and 29%. We have recently published in *PLOS One* the data on SLED with convection – herein called SLED-f in sick children. Between 2012 and 2017, a total of 242 sessions of SLEDD-f were performed on 70 children. There were 21 sessions (8.6%) terminated due to hypotension and 2 sessions (0.8%) terminated due to circuit clotting. It is suggested that if planning for anticoagulation-free session, then blood flow rate may be increased by 20–25%, provided it can be hemodynamically tolerated [6].

Unfractionated Heparin The use of unfractionated heparin in PIRRT reduces the incidence of extracorporeal circuit clotting, but this has to be weighed against the higher risk of bleeding and thrombocytopenia.

Regional Citrate Anticoagulation or Prostacyclin There have been very few studies on citrate or prostacyclin anticoagulation in SLED, and there is a need to have more studies on this aspect.

10.5 Evidence

Adults The recent systematic review by Zhang et al. primarily in adults had conclusions in favor of PIRRT. In their review of 17 studies comparing outcomes of PIRRT versus CRRT, they demonstrated a favorable mortality trend for PIRRT. PIRRT was found to be similar in efficacy to CRRT for fluid removal, solute clearance (urea, creatinine, phosphate), need for escalating vasopressors, mortality, or renal outcomes. PIRRT also showed a definite cost advantage over CRRT which should be of great interest for any resource-constrained setup [4].

Pediatrics Lee et al. published their experience on SLED-f (i.e., EDD along with hemodiafiltration) among 14 critically ill children totalling 60 sessions. SLED-f provided good hemodynamic tolerance and correction of fluid overload, pH, and electrolyte imbalance. In addition they also showed a significant drop in inflammatory cytokines [5].

We did a multicentric retrospective study across four centers in India, published in *Hemodialysis International*, on 68 children on whom 211 sessions of SLED were performed. Most of the patients had one or more organ systems involved in addition to renal (n = 64; 94%). Heparin-free sessions were achievable in 153 sessions (72%). Intradialytic hypotension or need for inotrope escalation was seen in 31 (15%) sessions, but termination of the session for drop in BP was required in only 20 (9%) sessions [1].

We recently did a retrospective data analysis of our sessions of SLED-f at our center from 2012 to 2017, using the Fresenius 5008S machine. A total of 242 sessions of SLEDD-f were performed on 70 patients. SLEDD-f sessions were well tolerated, with marked improvement in fluid status and acidosis. Premature terminations had to be done in 23 (9.5%) of the sessions. There were 21 sessions (8.6%) terminated due to hypotension and 2 sessions (0.8%) terminated due to circuit clotting [6].

10.6 Conclusion

Although there is a need to have more evidence supporting superiority SLED, current evidence does support outcomes of SLED being at least equivalent to CRRT in adults. There is now more evidence coming in support for its use in children as well. There is a need to have a prospective multicentric SLED database, and the authors are currently in process of formulating a prospective database.

References

1. Sethi SK, Sinha R, Jha P, Wadhwani N, Raghunathan V, Dhaliwal M, Bansal SB, Kher V, Lobo V, Sharma J, Raina R. Feasibility of sustained low efficiency dialysis in critically sick pediatric patients: a multicentric retrospective study. Hemodial Int. 2017. https://doi.org/10.1111/hdi.12605.
2. Sinha R, Sethi SK, Bunchman T, Lobo V, Raina R. Prolonged intermittent renal replacement therapy in children. Pediatr Nephrol. 2017. https://doi.org/10.1007/s00467-017-3732-2.
3. Raina R, Chauvin AM, Bunchman T, Askenazi D, Deep A, Ensley MJ, Krishnappa V, Sethi SK. Treatment of AKI in developing and developed countries: an international survey of pediatric dialysis modalities. PLoS One. 2017;12(5):e0178233. https://doi.org/10.1371/journal.pone.0178233.
4. Zhang L, Yang J, Eastwood GM, Zhu G, Tanaka A, Bellomo R. Extended daily dialysis versus continuous renal replacement therapy for acute kidney injury: a meta-analysis. Am J Kidney Dis. 2015;66(2):322–30.
5. Lee CY, Yeh HC, Lin CY. Treatment of critically ill children with kidney injury by sustained low-efficiency daily diafiltration. Pediatr Nephrol. 2012;27(12):2301–9. https://doi.org/10.1007/s00467-012-2254-1.
6. Sethi SK, Bansal SB, Khare A, Dhaliwal M, Raghunathan V, Wadhwani N, Nandwani A, Yadav DK, Mahapatra AK, Raina R. Heparin free dialysis in critically sick children using sustained low efficiency dialysis (SLEDD-f): a new hybrid therapy for dialysis in developing world. PLoS One. 2018;13(4):e0195536.

CRRT in a Sick Child

11

Timothy E. Bunchman

11.1 Scenario

A 30 kg child with leukemia develops septic shock with multi-organ system failure including the need for intubation, vasopressor support for hemodynamic compromise, as well as progressive oliguria with both solute and fluid retention. Current ventilator settings include a FIO_2 delivery of 70%, a PEEP of 10. Blood pressure is currently 98/45 with 1 mic/kg/min of norepinephrine adjustment to keep at systolic >110 mmHg. The child is febrile with a temperature of 39 °C. Fluid overload calculations reveal that the child is 15% above dry weight with insufficient urine output to allow for adequate room for medications, nutrition, and overall medical care. Labs reveal a BUN of 69 mg/dL, a cr of 2.3 mg/dL, and a K of 5.9 meq/dL.

Questions are:

1. What is the optimal way to deliver renal support?
2. What is the impact of renal support on medical (and vasopressor) clearance?
3. What is the optimal location of vascular access?
4. What is the optimal prescription?
5. How much fluid can be removed safely?

T. E. Bunchman (✉)
Children's Hospital of Richmond at Virginia Commonwealth University, Richmond, VA, USA
e-mail: timothy.bunchman@vcuhealth.org

S. K. Sethi et al. (eds.), *Critical Care Pediatric Nephrology and Dialysis: A Practical Handbook*, https://doi.org/10.1007/978-981-13-2276-1_11

11.2 Background

The use of continuous renal replacement therapy (CRRT) has become commonplace over the last two decades in children who require renal replacement therapy (RRT). CRRT is often used in an intensive care setting in patients who have hemodynamic compromise, hypermetabolic syndrome, fluid overload, or ongoing need for fluid management [1]. CRRT can be used as a standard or in conjunction with extracorporeal membrane oxygenation (ECMO) if needed. The purpose of this section is to describe the technical aspects of CRRT in a critically ill child.

11.3 Definition

The definition of CRRT is any form of RRT that is used 24 h a day. In theory then that would include both extracorporeal therapies that are commonly used called CRRT but also could include PD. For the purpose of this discussion, we will limit ourselves to CRRT.

CRRT can be performed as continuous veno-venous hemofiltration (CVVH), continuous veno-venous hemofiltration with dialysis (CVVHD), or a combination of continuous veno-venous hemofiltration with dialysis (CVVHD).

CVVH is using a convective form of dialysis, whereas CVVHD is using a diffusive form of dialysis with CVVHD as a combination of both.

Convection occurs by mass transport. This is essentially a concept of placing a physiologic fluid into a vascular space and forcing across a membrane mass solute for improved clearance.

Diffusion is commonly used in CVVHD, peritoneal dialysis, hemodialysis, as well as slow low-efficiency dialysis (SLED).

Historically, programs that have been ICU initiated commonly use convective clearance, whereas programs that are nephrology initiated often use diffusion clearance.

The question is always is one superior to the other.

If one looks at a paper by Maxvold et al., a perspective study was done looking at small-molecular-weight clearance (urea) and looking at clearance by CVVH versus CVVHD [2]. Using identical blood flow rates, surface areas of membranes, as well as fluid exposure, one identified in that paper that there is no difference in solute clearance. One though has to look at the concept of the sieving coefficient. The sieving coefficient is that which decides the rate at which something comes across a membrane. Things that are a small molecular weight and low protein-bound (e.g., urea, citrate) have a sieving coefficient of 1 in both convection and diffusion. Essentially that means they come across the membrane at roughly a one-to-one relationship.

Things that are a large molecular weight and highly protein-bound (e.g., vancomycin, molecular weight of around 1450 kDa, and a protein-bound of 75%) have a superior clearance on convection (sieving coefficient of 0.84) versus diffusion (sieving coefficient of 0.74) (Fig. 11.1).

Solute (MW)	Convective Coefficient	Diffusion Coefficient
Urea (60)	1.01 ± 0.05	1.01 ± 0.07
Creatinine (113)	1.00 ± 0.09	1.01 ± 0.06
Uric Acid (168)	1.01 ± 0.04	0.97 ± 0.04*
Vancomycin (1448)	0.84 ± 0.10	0.74 ± 0.04**
Calcium (protein bound)	0.67 ± 0.1	0.61 ± 0.07
Cytokines (large)	adsorbed	minimal clearance

*P<0.05 **P<0.01

Fig. 11.1 Examples of sieving coefficients

Experience would suggest that in highly cytokine inflammatory patients, such as stem cell transplants and septic patients, there may be an advantage of doing convection over diffusion. This was identified by Flores et al. in a retrospective data base analysis of patients with stem cell transplants. Looking at roughly 51 patients with stem cell transplants who underwent CVVH or CVVHD, the patients who underwent CVVH had a superior survival rate over CVVHD. This data may be the style of practice or may be that of outcome [3].

11.4 Equipment

Equipment for CRRT would include the machine, vascular access, solutions, as well as anticoagulation protocols.

Over the last few decades, many machines have come and gone. The standard machines are made by the Baxter, B. Braun, and Bellco, as well as the machines in the Asian and Eastern European area. Newcomers to the areas that are currently in clinical trials include the CARPEDIEM in Italy as well as the NIDUS in the UK [4, 5].

The commonality of these present machines is that they have blood flow rate controllers, dialysate flow rate controllers, convective flow rate controllers, as well as heating sources.

All machines currently used throughout the world have an error rate of ultrafiltration; therefore there needs to be a very close attention to detail of the volume status.

Access for CVVH or CVVHD is important. Work by Hackbarth et al. has demonstrated the optimal location and size of access based on the age and size of the patient [6]. In their clinical observation in greater than 300 children, a right IJ vein is superior to any other location for consistent flow rates. They also demonstrated that the largest vascular access with the shortest length of the access would give superior flow rate and low resistance with less clotting sources (Fig. 11.2).

Solutions in CRRT have changed dramatically over the last two and a half decades. In North America prior to the year 2000, lactate-based solutions were

PATIENT SIZE	CATHETER SIZE & SOURCE	SITE OF INSERTION
NEONATE	Dual-Lumen 7.0 French (COOK/MEDCOMP)	Femoral vein
3-6 KG	Dual-Lumen 7.0 French (COOK/MEDCOMP)	Internal/External-Jugular, Subclavian or Femoral vein
6-30 KG	Dual-Lumen 8.0 French (KENDALL/ARROW)	Internal/External-Jugular, Subclavian or Femoral vein
>15-KG	Dual-Lumen 9.0 French (MEDCOMP)	Internal/External-Jugular, Subclavian or Femoral vein
>30 KG	Dual-Lumen 10.0 French (KENDALL, ARROW)	Internal/External-Jugular, Subclavian or Femoral vein
>30 KG	Triple-Lumen 12 French (KENDALL/ ARROW)	Internal/External-Jugular, Subclavian or Femoral vein

Fig. 11.2 Suggestions of vascular access for size of child

commonly used. Lactate-based solutions would deliver lactate to the patient, and it would be hard to discriminate whether the lactate in the blood was related to the patient or the machine. Since 2000 work by Normocarb Dialysis Solutions Inc., which is no longer on the market, as well as other companies all now have bicarbonate-based replacement solutions for convection and dialysis solutions for diffusion.

FDA will identify that convective solutions are considered a drug and can be placed in the vascular space but that diffusive solutions are considered a device and should only be placed in the extravascular space. Many programs will utilize a single solution for convection and use it also for diffusion which is within the constraints and law of the FDA.

Anticoagulation protocols have commonly been based around heparin. This is because heparin is being used commonly throughout the world for dialysis. Heparin-based protocols have a common source of a bolus, and then it continues the infusion of heparin targeting a clotting time or an activated clotting time of roughly twice normal at bedside. Other programs do not have the ability to do ACT at bedside; therefore they often will send it to the lab for a much slower turnaround time but targeting a partial thromboplastic time or a PTT of nearly twice normal.

In the latter part of the 1980s and early 1990s, Mehta and Ward identified the concept of citrate anticoagulation [7]. Work done by our group has identified in 2000 that citrate anticoagulation can be used easily in pediatrics [8]. Citrate utilizes calcium chelation, and by dropping the calcium out of the blood, it will actually have a low clotting circuit. Citrate has to occur by putting the citrate in post-patient prefilter, but the patient needs calcium back independent of the dialysis or the CRRT line in order to recover any complications from hypocalcemia.

Recent work by Deep et al. identified the use of prostacyclin used predominantly in liver failure patients as another source of anticoagulation [9].

The source of anticoagulation is a style of practice and should best be consistent within the individual program.

11.5 Prescriptions for CRRT

Historically blood flow rates for CRRT have been identified as 3–5 mL/kg/min. This historical data was done in the 1990s. The style of practice at present though suggests that blood flow rate is probably optimally based on the maximum blood flow rate that the vascular access will allow. The only exception to this is in patients with very high osmolar situations where one does not want to dialyze them rapidly in order to bring the osmos down slowly. So we will often begin at 5 mL/kg/min and adjust upward to as high as 8–10 mL/kg/min as long as our arterial access which is our vascular access is −150 or closer to 0 and our return access is +150 or closer to 0. This will give us the flexibility of maximum blood flow with less clotting.

Whether one does dialysis or replacement fluid, two papers should be brought to mind. One is Maxvold's paper that suggests that 2000/1.73 m^2/h will give us optimal clearance per urea, and the other paper is by Ronco et al. in the Lancet that identified 35–45 mL/kg/h on convective solutions [2, 10]. Roughly, Maxvold's 2–2.5 liters/1.73 m^2/hr is similar to Ronco's 40 mL/kg/h of convective clearance.

11.6 Anticoagulation Protocols

As mentioned, heparin is commonly used. Standard protocol would be bolusing the patient with 10–20 units/kg of unfractionated heparin and starting the child on roughly 10–20 units/kg/h of unfractionated heparin. One would then check a post-membrane ACT or activated clotting time to target an ACT of roughly 200, normal being 100. Risk of heparin use would include heparin-induced thrombocytopenia, which is a rare event in children, as well as bleeding in the patient.

Once heparin is discontinued, the half-life is roughly 4 h; therefore procedures need to be thought about in the context of having the patient systemically heparinized. Heparin can also be revered with protamine if necessary by knowing that the protamine has a shorter half-life than the heparin itself.

Citrate anticoagulation has become more common since the early 2000s. Citrate works by chelating the calcium by making the circuit hypocalcemic. Essentially, as the blood comes out of the patient, the citrate mixes into the blood, and the circuit has a citrated or hypocalcemic circuit. One can then target the ionized calcium of the circuit post-membrane. One then needs to deliver calcium chloride or calcium gluconate back to the patient in order to rescue them from the citrate.

A standard protocol for citrate would be a blood flow rate of 5 mL/kg/min, a dialysate or replacement flow rate of roughly 2.5 L/1.73 msq/h, and a citrate rate of roughly 1.5 times the blood flow rate. Therefore, if the blood flow rate is at 100, the citrate rate goes at 150, and the calcium chloride (8 g/L saline) or calcium gluconate (23 g/L saline) can run at roughly 0.6–0.8 the blood flow rate. So essentially if the blood flow rate is 100, the citrate rate starts at 150 using ACDA, and the calcium replacement is roughly between 60 and 80/h.

One then targets post-membrane ionized calcium of roughly one-third physiologic in patients' ionized calcium back to physiologic. Therefore in our hospital, normal ionized calcium is 1.1–1.3 mmol/L, and one would adjust upward or downward the calcium back to the patient for that target. Using that same data, we would target our post-membrane ionized calcium levels to 0.25–0.5 in order to have a hypocalcemic circuit.

Prostacyclin is commonly used in the liver failure patient at King's Hospital in London. Their protocol is essentially starting the prostacyclin at no greater than 5–6 Ng/kg/h and adjusting upward.

Complications of heparin as mentioned are HIT as well as bleeding. Complications of citrate can be hypocalcemia or metabolic alkalosis secondary to the citrate metabolizing to bicarbonate [11]. Complications of prostacyclin can be vasodilatation and bleeding.

All these protocols need to be watched carefully at bedside in order to assure there are no complications.

11.7 Benefits of CRRT

In a patient who is quite inflamed and who is hyperthermic, CRRT will often allow for extracorporeal cooling as well as for clearance of solute. The standard protocol would allow for the patient to become hemodynamically stable and then slowly take fluid off over time.

From the practical setting if one starts someone on CRRT using pressor agents, the goal for the first 4–6 h should not be to take fluid off but to make the patient at lease fluid even. Once hemodynamics are under control, then one can slowly start targeting 1–2 mL/kg/h of net fluid off.

To be practical about this, if one has total IV fluids in roughly 300 mL/h that would include the calcium, the TPN, the meds, as well as the citrate in a 20 kg child, then your goal for the first 3–4 h is to have your net fluid removal at 300 to keep the child even. After a few hours of hemodynamic stability and if necessary turning up the norepinephrine or vasopressor agents, one can slowly start taking off 20–40 mL or roughly 1–2 mL/kg/h net fluid removal from that patient.

The temptation is to try to get off all the fluid in the first 24 h that one has accumulated over 5 days, but one has to understand that fluid will come off slowly and it is really based on hemodynamic situations.

It is important to have a high level of communication on medications and nutrition on patients on continuous dialysis. It is important to understand how much potassium is in the foods or in the TPN and how much potassium is in the dialysate and replacement in order to ensure there is no hyper or hypokalemia.

Many protocols have a phosphorous-free solution; therefore it is important to maximize phosphorous in TPN in order to prevent problems with hypophosphatemia.

11.8 Complications of CRRT

The first complication one has to think about is membrane reactions [12]. In the Baxter M60 and M100 series, this membrane does not react well to acidotic plasma. Blood bank blood has a pH of roughly 6.2–6.4. Therefore if one does a blood prime with this membrane because of a small child and a large extracorporeal circuit, then one will actually induce anaphylaxis as the blood goes back into the patient. Protocols by Brophy et al. as well as Hackbarth et al. have mitigated these side effects. Brophy protocol uses blood transfusions into the patient with a saline prime and this dump of a saline prime in order to maintain euvolemia and avoid having the acidotic plasma into the patient. That protocol still requires 3–4 meq/kg as initial bolus of bicarb to the patient to offset the metabolic acidosis.

Hackbarth's paper identifies dialyzing the blood containing circuit from a blood bank in order to pH normalize and cytokine normalize the patient. This protocol takes about an hour [13]. If one uses the Hackbarth's protocol, one realizes that citrate will be dialyzed off because of the sieving coefficient of 1 and heparin must be added to that circuit in order to avoid clotting.

Other complications are thermic control. In children less than 25 kg, hypothermia is a relatively common even and needs to be paid attention to in patients on extracorporeal therapy. In larger children thermic normalization may occur masking that of a fever. Therefore one will lose the normal findings of thermic changes if one is looking for fever. Many programs will do daily blood cultures routinely on patients on CRRT because of this mask effect.

Nutrition is lost during CRRT. In Maxvold's paper in 2000 in Critical Care Medicine, she pointed out that roughly 30% of amino acids are lost in CRRT [2]. In further workup by Zappitelli both as part of a consortium study and individual study, he pointed out that many programs do not target their protein to more than 2 g/kg/day and one probably needs to target to 4 g/kg/day on CRRT [14]. Further things that Zappitelli has identified are that water-soluble vitamins are easily cleared on CRRT and need to be given back to the patient.

Vasopressor agents are typically low protein-bound and low molecular weight; therefore they are cleared easily. Therefore epinephrine, norepinephrine, dopamine, and dobutamine are commonly cleared and may need to be adjusted upward in patients as one initiates CRRT. It is not an unusual finding though that after a few hours of CRRT these vasopressor agents can be slowly turned down because of hemodynamic stability.

In summary, CRRT has become now the standard of care for renal replacement therapy in ICU patients with critical illness. In patients with sepsis, in patients with fluid overload, and in patients who are hypermetabolic, it is a common practice that can be done easily at bedside.

Programs have gone through learning curves but have markedly improved the outcome with the use of this therapy. Further, industry is improving access, solutions, protocols, as well as machinery to work with medical systems in order to overall improve healthcare.

References

1. Barletta GM, Bunchman TE. Acute renal failure in children and infants. Curr Opin Crit Care. 2004;10(6):499–504.
2. Maxvold NJ, Smoyer WE, Custer JR, Bunchman TE. Amino acid loss and nitrogen balance in critically ill children with acute renal failure: a prospective comparison between classic hemofiltration and hemofiltration with dialysis. Crit Care Med. 2000;28(4):1161–5.
3. Flores FX, Brophy PD, Symons JM, et al. Continuous renal replacement therapy (CRRT) after stem cell transplantation. A report from the prospective pediatric CRRT Registry Group. Pediatr Nephrol. 2008;23(4):625–30.
4. Lorenzin A, Garzotto F, Alghisi A, et al. CVVHD treatment with CARPEDIEM: small solute clearance at different blood and dialysate flows with three different surface area filter configurations. Pediatr Nephrol. 2016;31(10):1659–65.
5. Coulthard MG, Crosier J, Griffiths C, et al. Haemodialysing babies weighing <8 kg with the Newcastle infant dialysis and ultrafiltration system (Nidus): comparison with peritoneal and conventional haemodialysis. Pediatr Nephrol. 2014;29(10):1873–81.
6. Hackbarth R, Bunchman TE, Chua AN, et al. The effect of vascular access location and size on circuit survival in pediatric continuous renal replacement therapy: a report from the PPCRRT registry. Int J Artif Organs. 2007;30(12):1116–21.
7. Mehta RL, McDonald BR, Aguilar MM, Ward DM. Regional citrate anticoagulation for continuous arteriovenous hemodialysis in critically ill patients. Kidney Int. 1990;38(5):976–81.
8. Bunchman TE, Maxvold NJ, Barnett J, et al. Pediatric hemofiltration: Normocarb dialysate solution with citrate anticoagulation. Pediatr Nephrol. 2002;17(3):150–4.
9. Deep A, Zoha M, Dutta KP. Prostacyclin as an anticoagulant for continuous renal replacement therapy in children. Blood Purif. 2017;43(4):279–89.
10. Ronco C, Bellomo R, Homel P, Brendolan A, Dan M, Piccinni P, La Greca G. Effects of different doses in continuous veno-venous haemofiltration on outcomes of acute renal failure: a prospective randomised trial. Lancet. 2000;356(9223):26–30.
11. Brophy PD, Somers MJ, Baum MA, et al. Multi-centre evaluation of anticoagulation in patients receiving continuous renal replacement therapy (CRRT). Nephrol Dial Transplant. 2005;20(7):1416–21.
12. Brophy PD, Mottes TA, Kudelka TL, et al. AN-69 membrane reactions are pH-dependent and preventable. Am J Kidney Dis. 2001;38(1):173–8.
13. Hackbarth RM, Eding D, Gianoli Smith C, et al. Zero balance ultrafiltration (Z-BUF) in blood-primed CRRT circuits achieves electrolyte and acid-base homeostasis prior to patient connection. Pediatr Nephrol. 2005;20(9):1328–33.
14. Zappitelli M, Goldstein SL, Symons JM, et al. Protein and calorie prescription for children and young adults receiving continuous renal replacement therapy: a report from the Prospective Pediatric Continuous Renal Replacement Therapy Registry Group. Crit Care Med. 2008;36(12):3239–45.

Renal Replacement Therapy for Patients Requiring ECMO Support

12

Anna Maslach-Hubbard, Raoul Nelson, and
Jamie Furlong-Dillard

12.1 Introduction

Extracorporeal membrane oxygenation (ECMO) is an advanced mode of support for critically ill patients with life-threatening respiratory and/or cardiovascular failure who have failed conventional management. It is a temporary support most commonly implemented as a bridge to organ function recovery or definitive intervention (e.g., congenital heart defect repair, ventricular assistant device implantation, or heart or lung transplant).

Patients who require ECMO are at high risk of developing multi-organ failure (MOF) including acute kidney injury (AKI). The pathophysiologic features of AKI and ECMO are multifactorial and complex. Progression of a pre-existing disease, pre-ECMO management, and hemodynamic alterations leading to decreased renal oxygen delivery, activation of pro-inflammatory mediators, hemolysis, coagulation abnormalities, and iatrogenic nephrotoxic medications use may all lead to the development of AKI on ECMO. Patients who develop an AKI before or during ECMO support have notable higher risk of mortality [1]. The

A. Maslach-Hubbard (✉)
University of Utah SOM, Pediatric Critical Care Division, Salt Lake City, UT, USA
e-mail: anna.hubbard@hsc.utah.edu

R. Nelson
University of Utah SOM, Pediatric Nephrology Division, Salt Lake City, UT, USA
e-mail: raoul.nelson@hsc.utah.edu

J. Furlong-Dillard
University of Louisville SOM, Pediatric Critical Care Division, Louisville, KY, USA
e-mail: jamie.furlong-dillard@louisville.edu

S. K. Sethi et al. (eds.), *Critical Care Pediatric Nephrology and Dialysis: A Practical Handbook*, https://doi.org/10.1007/978-981-13-2276-1_12

incidence of AKI in neonatal and pediatric population is reported to be up to 70% depending on the patient's age, primary illness, indication for ECMO, and definition used to define AKI.

Renal replacement therapies (RRT) are commonly used as a concomitant treatment with ECMO support to provide renal replacement and fluid management. Approximately 25–68% of patients on ECMO require a form of RRT depending on the specific population of patients [2–4]. Patients who require RRT while on ECMO have an overall higher mortality than those who require ECMO alone. The most common indications for RRT while on ECMO are similar to the indications for all critically ill patients and include fluid overload, acidosis, electrolyte imbalance, or inadequate renal clearance. AKI may evolve into chronic renal insufficiency or end-stage renal disease as a consequence of critical illness in ECMO patients. However, in pediatric patients who survive extracorporeal life support (ECLS), this outcome is not common, and the greatest risk for development is preexisting renal disease [5].

This chapter introduces the basic characteristics of ECMO types, strategies for management of renal insufficiency and fluid overload, and technical aspects of RRT incorporation into an ECMO support system.

12.2 Basics of ECMO Support

ECMO is a potentially lifesaving advanced technology that provides sufficient gas exchange and perfusion for patients with acute, reversible cardiac or respiratory failure. Deoxygenated blood is drained from patient's venous system and then moved forward by an external pump through a membrane gas exchange unit (oxygenator), where gas exchange occurs. Oxygenated blood is then returned to the patient's venous or arterial system depending on which type of ECMO support the patient requires (Fig. 12.1). Two main types of ECMO are utilized to provide respiratory and/or cardiovascular support.

12.2.1 Venovenous (VV) ECMO

VV ECMO was developed almost exclusively for the support of patients with severe respiratory failure. In a VV ECMO configuration, the blood is drained from the venous system (major central veins and/or the right atrium (RA)) and returned to a large vein or the RA where mixing of oxygenated and deoxygenated blood occurs. The net oxygen saturation of arterial blood is usually 75–95% depending on a patient's residual lung function and the degree of ECMO flow recirculation. Recirculation is a phenomenon that occurs on VV ECMO where reinfused oxygenated blood is withdrawn through the drainage cannula without passing through the systemic circulation.

This system "bypasses" the lungs; therefore a patient must have adequate cardiovascular system function for this type of support to work sufficiently. Multiple

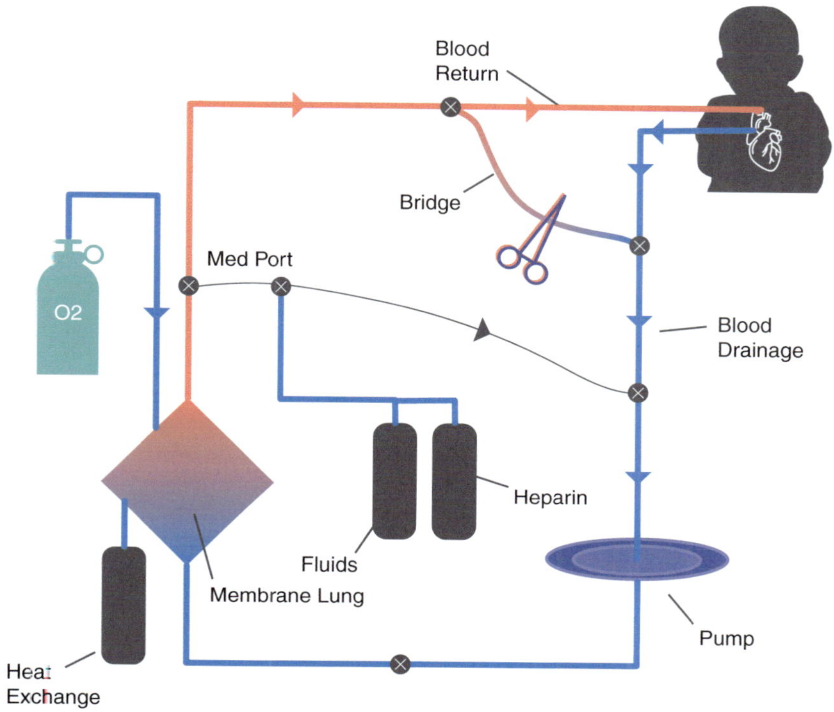

Fig. 12.1 Basic ECMO configuration

advantages have been identified in regard to VV support, and those associated with renal function include preservation of pulsatile renal blood flow and a lower risk of arterial embolic events (unless an intracardiac shunt is present).

12.2.2 Venoarterial (VA) ECMO

Complete support of cardiovascular and respiratory system is possible with VA ECMO. The blood is drained from a large central vein or the RA and returned directly to the arterial circulation (e.g., aorta or femoral artery). The rate of oxygenated ("arterial") blood return and patient's residual intrinsic cardiac function will determine mean arterial pressure and perfusion in patients with cardiovascular collapse.

ECMO pumps provide constant, non-pulsatile flow, which, in the case of VA support with decreased cardiac intrinsic function, leads to suppression or complete loss of pulsatile blood flow. Lack of pulsatile blood flow may affect end-organ function. This may impair renal function, but more importantly VA ECMO is associated with an increased risk of systemic thrombotic or air microembolisms, potentially further compromising renal perfusion.

12.3 Anticoagulation on ECMO

For all types of ECMO, systemic anticoagulation is necessary to prevent thrombi formation. The blood is exposed to foreign non-endothelial materials as it travels through the ECMO circuit, and through complex immune mechanisms, this can trigger acute inflammatory responses and promote coagulation. Anticoagulation is most commonly achieved with continuous infusion of unfractionated heparin (UFH).

Anticoagulation is monitored by frequent measurement of activated clotting time (ACT) and anti-factor Xa levels for UFH. Newer anticoagulants including direct thrombin inhibitors as well as factor Xa and XIIa inhibitors may also be used for systemic anticoagulation but are less well validated and therefore used less frequently.

12.4 Pathophysiology of Renal Dysfunction on ECMO

Pathophysiology of renal injury during ECMO support is complex and still not clearly understood. Although renal dysfunction is often related to hemodynamic instability of critically ill patients and associated with patient's pre-existing disease(s), ECMO may contribute to the exacerbation of AKI and development of significant fluid overload (FO). Since non-ECMO-related factors are described in details in previous sections of this book (Table 12.1), this chapter will concentrate mainly on ECMO-related factors contributing to the development of AKI and fluid overload (Tables 12.2 and 12.3).

Physiological features intrinsic to the initial phase of ECMO may contribute to the development of AKI. Relative intravascular volume depletion and the increased

Table 12.1 Overview of major non-ECMO-related factors contributing to the development of renal injury and fluid overload in critically ill patients

Non-ECMO factors associated with AKI (patient and primary illness related)
1. Severe respiratory and/or cardiovascular failure prior to ECMO initiation leading to hypoperfusion and decreased O_2 delivery to the peripheral organs
2. Compromised vascular autoregulation
3. Systemic inflammation
4. Hormonal dysregulation compromising fluid and renal homeostasis
5. DIC-related microthrombi formation leading to compromised microvascular blood flow and organ perfusion
6. Vasopressor therapy causing vasoconstriction and potentially compromising peripheral organ perfusion
7. Nephrotoxic medications use
8. Pre-existing chronic renal disease prior to ECMO initiation
9. Primary renal disease, e.g., glomerulonephritis prior to ECMO initiation

Table 12.2 Major ECMO-related factors contributing to the development or exacerbation of renal injury

ECMO support-related factors contributing to AKI
1. Altered and/or compromised organ perfusion (a) Non-pulsatile flow compromising renal cortical perfusion (b) Inability to achieve sufficient level of ECMO support for adequate renal perfusion, especially during initial phase of ECMO (c) Fluctuation in hemodynamic status causing ischemia-reperfusion-related AKI (d) Hemorrhagic events leading to hypovolemia and hypoperfusion
2. Exacerbated systemic inflammation (a) Exposure to artificial surface during initiation of ECMO (b) Addition of extra components to circuit (hemofilter, dialysis machine) (c) Blood shear stress
3. Hypercoagulation and thrombi formation (a) VA system—risk for arterial thrombotic and/or air embolic events (b) VV system—risk for pulmonary emboli (thrombi, air) or systemic emboli if intracardiac shunt is present
4. Hemolysis (a) Shear injury of red blood cells at the pump level and other circuit components (b) Excessive negative or positive pressures of venous or arterial limb of circuit
5. Cannula position-related complications (a) Extremity ischemia with femoral artery cannulation causing tissue ischemia, compartment syndrome, rhabdomyolysis, and hypermyoglobinemia contributing to AKI (b) IVC cannulas causing renal vein flow alterations (c) Descending aorta retrograde dissection due to cannulation

Table 12.3 Major factors contributing to the development or exacerbation of fluid overload on ECMO

Factors leading to fluid overload on ECMO
1. Exacerbation of inflammatory state requiring significant volume resuscitation during initial phase of support (a) Relative intravascular volume depletion due to vasodilatation (b) Vascular leak and "third spacing"
2. Alteration of RA volume load and distending pressure by drainage of venous system to the ECMO circuit (a) Inaccurate CVP assessment as reflection of volume status (b) Alteration of patient's intrinsic mechanisms of volume regulation (c) Inadequate ANP release
3. Significant blood product transfusions (a) Hemorrhagic complications are frequent on ECMO requiring frequent blood product infusions (b) Platelet count and correction of coagulopathy with FFP are needed to mitigate increased risk for bleeding
4. Altered renin-angiotensin-aldosterone axis by altered perfusion to the renal system
5. ECMO and primary illness exacerbation of AKI leading to oliguria/anuria
6. Necessity for nutrition and medications

inflammatory state with resulting systemic vasodilation may contribute to an inability to achieve sufficient level of circulatory support for adequate end-organ perfusion and oxygen delivery. Exposure to artificial surfaces during initiation of ECMO or addition of extra components to the circuit like an ultrafiltrate or dialysis machine further exacerbates the body's inflammatory response. Fluctuation in hemodynamic status and significant fluid shifts after ECMO cannulation may lead to ischemia-reperfusion renal injury, and the non-pulsatile flow on VA ECMO may further contribute to the worsening of AKI. Perfusion is usually better in patients supported with VV ECMO as long as native cardiovascular function remains adequate.

Other risk factors contributing to the development or worsening of AKI include the ineluctable hypercoagulable state making patients more prone to embolic events and hemolysis caused by shear injury to RBCs from the ECMO centrifugal pumps as well as excessive negative or positive pressures of venous or arterial limbs of the circuit. Hemolysis is one of the most frequently described complications related to ECMO support resulting not only in decreased oxygen carrying capacity and delivery to organs but also leading to free hemoglobin release, potentially further exacerbating renal damage by causing renal tubular obstruction.

Certain cannula positioning may lead to pathology exacerbating renal injury. Arterial femoral cannulation may compromise lower extremity perfusion resulting in severe tissue ischemia and even at times the development of compartment syndrome, resulting in worsening renal injury from rhabdomyolysis and hypermyoglobinemia. With arterial femoral cannulation, retrograde dissection of the aorta may occur, further significantly compromising renal blood flow. The position of cannulas in the inferior vena cava may lead to stasis of blood flow with an inflammatory response and result in renal vein thrombosis and flow alteration at the level of renal veins.

12.5 Pathophysiology of Fluid Overload on ECMO

Severe FO is frequently reported in critically ill patients, and it is usually significantly aggravated during the first 24–48 h after ECMO initiation [6–9]. FO has been associated with increased mortality and longer ECMO duration, creating potential for more complications. Some patients with MOF who achieved dry weight after implementation of RRT had improved survival and shorter time to decannulation.

Etiology of FO on ECMO is multifactorial (Table 12.3) with the most contributing risks being systemic inflammation leading to vasodilatation and capillary leak as well as relative intravascular volume deficit requiring volume replacement in order to achieve adequate venous drainage. Fluid and blood product resuscitation is very common within the first 24 h of ECMO support leading to worsening FO. Necessity for adequate nutrition and medication infusions further adds to FO. These risks are increased in a state of oliguric or anuric renal failure.

The position of venous drainage or infusion cannula in the vena cava/RA system significantly affects intrinsic regulatory mechanisms of volume control by altering downstream blood flow and "sensing" of true volume status in patients supported with ECMO. Reduction of ANP release was described in patients supported with

ECMO, negatively affecting not only cardiorespiratory-renal system interactions but also leading to decreased renal-protective and anti-inflammatory benefits of ANP. Other hormonal changes cause dysregulation of the renin-angiotensin-aldosterone (RAA) axis. In some studies upregulation of the RAA system was thought to be responsible for the hypertensive state commonly seen on ECMO and possibly in response to non-pulsatile blood flow.

12.6 Renal Support Strategies Utilized in ECMO Patients

Due to the well-known associated negative outcomes for patients with AKI and FO during ECMO support [4, 8, 9], careful strategies to avoid excessive fluid administration should be undertaken. Balance must be achieved between FO and the volume of necessary infusions for medications, nutrition, and blood products and the volume need for "circuit resuscitation" during the first 24 h on ECMO. It is unclear if early fluid removal on ECMO is beneficial, but patients who tolerate net fluid loss while supported with ECMO are thought to have lower risk of death.

Diuretics are commonly instituted as an initial management option to facilitate fluid removal after stable hemodynamic status is achieved with ECMO support. Effective diuresis may not be possible during the early hyper-acute inflammatory state due to significant vascular leak, relative intravascular volume deficit, and fluid infusions necessary to maintain adequate ECMO flows. In addition, it may create secondary electrolyte and acid/base imbalances. With diuretic therapy precise rate of fluid removal is difficult to predict and control. If instituted, continuous infusion of diuretics is preferred over intermittent doses to avoid more abrupt intravascular volume alterations, which may affect ECMO flow.

For patients supported on ECMO with significant FO and/or AKI, not responding to conventional management, continuous renal replacement therapy (CRRT) is frequently utilized. Major indications for initiation of CRRT on ECMO are listed in Table 12.4. There is no standard of care developed regarding

Table 12.4 General indications for the use of CRRT for patients on ECMO

Indication for renal replacement therapy use in patients supported with ECMO
1. Fluid overload (a) Inadequate urine output due to compromised renal function (b) Large-volume fluid resuscitation to assure adequate ECMO flows and organ perfusion (c) Necessity to provide adequate nutrition, medications, and blood product transfusions
2. Refractory acidosis
3. Electrolyte imbalance
4. Azotemia
5. Toxin removal
6. Decreased renal clearance
7. In some institutions, early institution of CRRT is utilized as mode of stabilization of inflammatory response

the choice and superiority of one specific RRT modality over another, and it depends on the patient's condition and reason RRT is required. In choosing the mode of RRT, specific institutional practices and renal support team availability have to be taken into consideration. CRRT ranges from slow continuous ultrafiltration (SCUF) with in-line hemofilter use to continuous venovenous hemodiafiltration (CVVHDF) with dialysis device incorporated into ECMO circuit. Multiple different methods of CRRT implementation into the ECMO circuit are described by various authors; however, there are no comparative studies available to assess the superiority of one method over another, and clinical practices are based on expert opinions and institutional experiences (Table 12.5). An example of initial approach to patient with fluid overload and AKI is illustrated in Fig. 12.2.

12.7 Modalities of RRT and Technical Aspects of Implementing CRRT Devices into ECMO Support

12.7.1 Ultrafiltration (UF) with In-Line Filter Use

SCUF is utilized frequently in patients for whom only net fluid removal is desired and native kidney function is able to regulate electrolytes, acid, and base and assure adequate renal clearance. This system is easy to incorporate into the ECMO circuit, requires lower blood prime volume, and is lower in cost. It functions as a "shunt" within an ECMO circuit causing total pump flow to be higher than rate of blood return to the patients. A flow probe reader on the arterial limb of the ECMO circuit will indicate the difference between total pump flow and decreased flow returning to the patient. Limitations include less precise fluid balance control and lack of pressure monitoring in the hemofiltration circuit, potentially delaying detection of filter failure (rupture, clotting).

The hemofilter is placed in-line on the ECMO circuit's higher-pressure arterial limb pre- or post-oxygenator after the pump, and blood returns to the venous, pre-pump ECMO circuit limb (Fig. 12.3). A pressure gradient from the arterial to venous side ensures flow through the hemofilter. Flow of 100–200 ml/min can be achieved via hemofilter which creates a relatively high ultrafiltrate rate due to significant transmembrane pressure. Smaller patients usually need only 30–50 ml/min flow for adequate therapy. To achieve a more precise fluid removal, a standard IV infusion pump can be incorporated post-filter which will limit the UF flow rate by setting the IV pump flow rate as the desired hourly fluid removal rate, and UF will empty into a reservoir. Even with the use of an IV pump, inaccuracies in measurement may occur. In patients who have a significant rate of ultrafiltration, electrolyte imbalance may occur requiring vigilant monitoring and appropriate fluid replacement.

Table 12.5 Examples of different connection options for incorporation of CRRT device into ECMO circuit. Modified from: Seczynska et al. [3]

Type of CRRT used	CRRT device INLET "arterial" connection to ECMO circuit	CRRT device OUTLET "venous" connection to ECMO circuit	Advantages	Disadvantages	Potential complications specific to the type of connection	Troubleshooting
In-line hemofilter placement	*Always* post-pump, pre- or post-oxygenator	– Pre-centrifugal ECMO pump – To the bladder or any pre-pump connector if roller pump is in use	– Easy to set up – Less blood prime necessary – Low cost	– Requires external IV pump for UF control – No TMP monitoring – Less precise UF removal	– Excessive UF removal leading to electrolyte imbalance – Delayed detection of filter failure	– Increase IV pump resistance on outlet tubing of filter – Visual monitoring of filter
CRRT machine incorporation into ECMO circuit	Pre-pump	Post-pump, pre-oxygenator	Oxygenator works as a trap for microemboli or entrained air	– Low-pressure arterial access alarm – High venous pressure alarm	– Entrainment of air into the circuit via pre-pump connection	– Maintenance of adequate intravascular volume for adequate ECMO circuit feeling – Reduction of flow through CRRT device
	Post-pump	Pre-pump closer to drainage cannula or the bladder	– Unrestricted flow to CRRT arterial line – Low-resistance return flow from CRRT	– High-pressure "arterial" alarms – "Access disconnection" alarms due to low venous outflow resistance	– Frequent disruption of CRRT flow with potential for system clotting – Risk for thrombus formation, hemolysis	– Flow restriction using clamp or stopcock or smaller caliber of connecting tubing to increase resistance – Change alarm setup on CRRT device
	Outlet of oxygenator port	Inlet of oxygenator port	– Simple to integrate with ECMO circuit – Less risk of air entering circuit – Good pressure profile for CRRT flow	– High-pressure alarms on both sides of CRRT circuit interrupting flow	– Circuit clotting due to frequent flow interruption	– Change to positive access pressure on setup for arterial and venous lines
	Pre-pump (for roller pump)	Pre-pump to the bladder or closer to drainage cannula		– Low-pressure arterial access alarm – "Circuit disconnect" on outlet side of CRRT	– Frequent disruption of CRRT flow with potential for system clotting	– Flow restriction using clamp or stopcock to increase outflow resistance and minimize the risk for thrombus and hemolysis

UF ultrafiltration, *TMP* transmembrane pressure

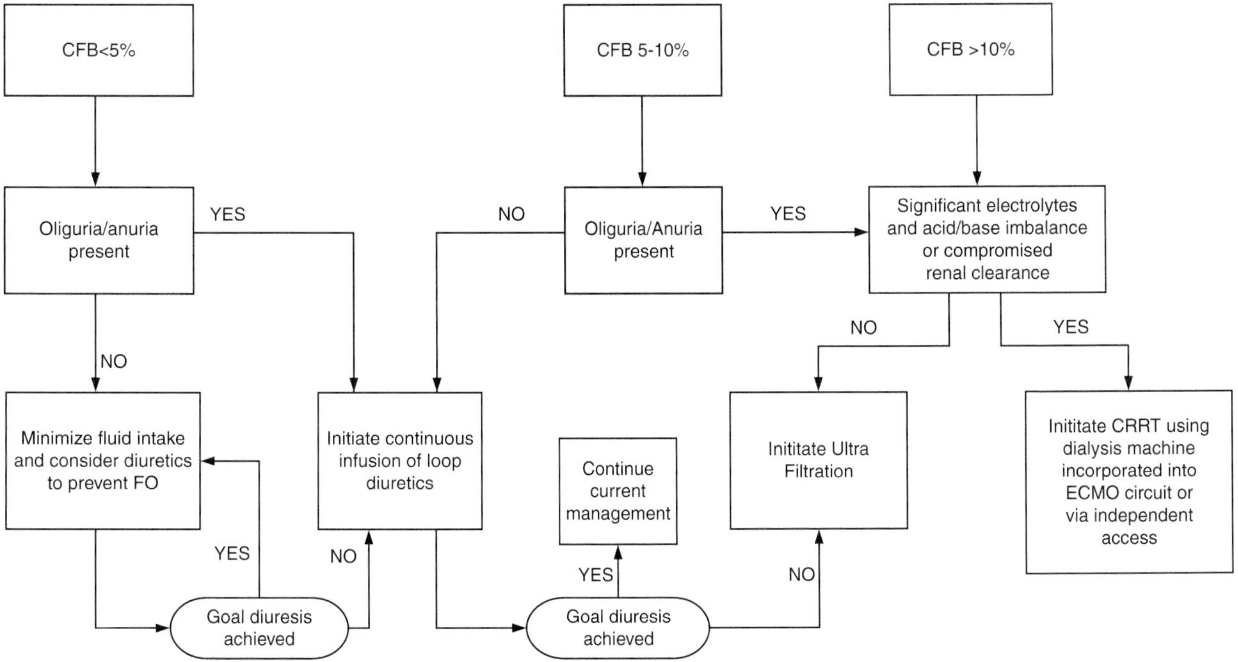

Fig. 12.2 Suggested approach to initial management of patients with fluid overload and AKI. Since there is no standard of care established, the guideline needs to be modified to institutional approach and resources. *CFB* cumulative positive fluid balance, *AKI* acute kidney injury, *CRRT* continuous renal replacement therapy, *FO* fluid overload

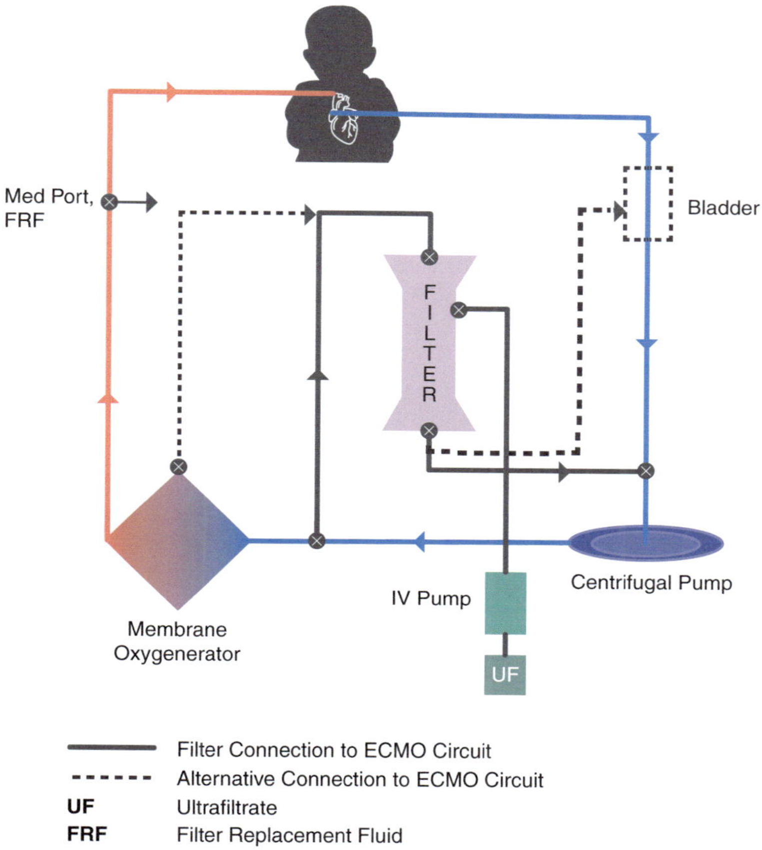

Fig. 12.3 Example of in-line hemofilter connection within ECMO circuit. Modified from: Seczynska et al. [3]

12.7.2 Continuous Venovenous Hemodialysis (CVVHD)

There are different methods used to achieve hemodialysis on ECMO. There is an option to provide hemodiafiltration with the use of in-line hemofilter, which requires dialysate infusion via designed access port. Due to the inability to control accurate UF rates and solute balance, this technique is used less frequently. More advanced techniques require the use of a CRRT machine concomitantly with the ECMO circuit. This method provides higher rate of solute clearance with lower risk of hypovolemia, electrolytes shifts, and more accurate fluid balance. It also requires CRRT trained staff.

There are no standard guidelines regarding which technique should be used to provide CRRT on ECMO and which method of combining CRRT and ECMO is most efficient and safest. Two main methods include independent utilization of CRRT machine via separate dialysis access or incorporation of CRRT machine into the ECMO circuit. The ECMO circuit is a stable platform for incorporation of hemofilter or CRRT device into the system making the option of independent dialysis less appealing although safe as no access to ECMO circuit is necessary. With any external system introduced "in series" into the ECMO circuit, there is a risk of complications including the risk of introduction of air during placement, increased hemolysis, thrombosis at connector sites, hemorrhage, and additional inflammatory response with contact of blood with the new filter membrane.

12.7.2.1 Independent CRRT Technique via Separate Dialysis Access

This method may be utilized in patients with a dialysis catheter in place before ECMO was initiated. It is more challenging in children less than 15–20 kg as the commonly used vessel for a dialysis catheter (right internal jugular vein) also serves as main access site for venous cannula placement in this sized population. Dialysis catheters could be potentially placed in a femoral vein, but as a general principle, attempts of any invasive procedure, including dialysis catheter placement, should be avoided once a patient is on ECMO to minimize the risk of bleeding.

12.7.2.2 CRRT Device Connected to the ECMO Circuit

There are many different ways to incorporate CRRT equipment into an ECMO circuit (Figs. 12.4 and 12.5). Frequently inlet or "arterial" line of the CRRT system is

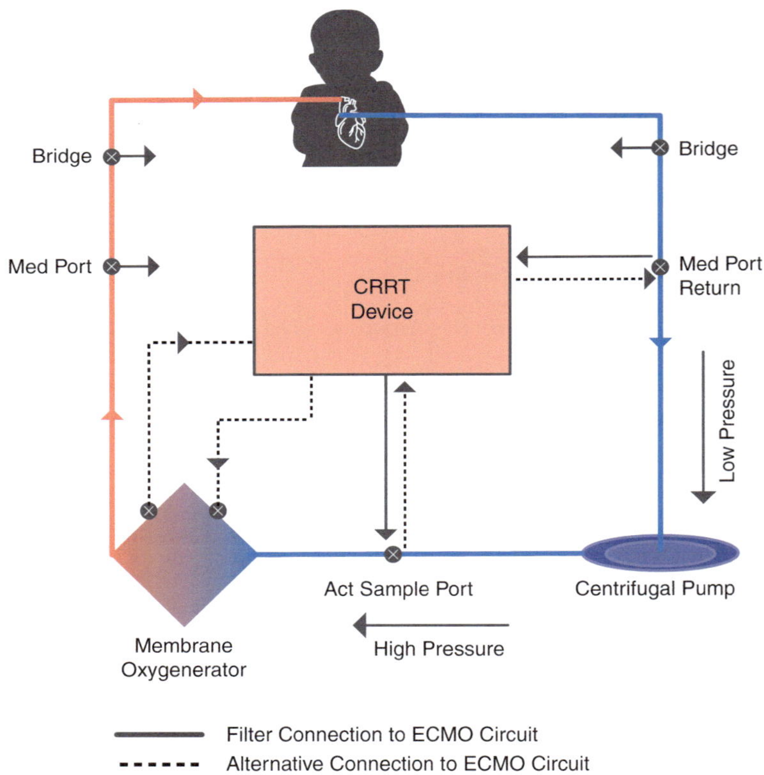

Fig. 12.4 Example of CRRT device incorporation into ECMO circuit. ECMO system with centrifugal pump

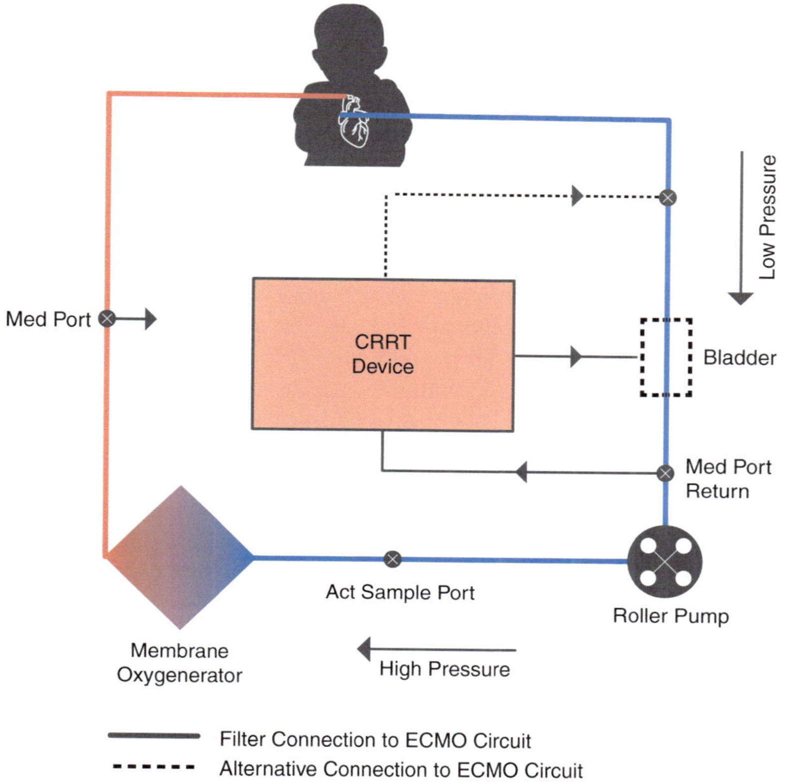

Fig. 12.5 Example of CRRT device incorporation into ECMO circuit. ECMO system with roller pump

connected to the low-pressure, pre-pump ECMO limb via a three-way stopcock, and the return CRRT "venous" line is connected to the high-pressure, post-pump, pre-oxygenator ECMO tubing via "ACT sample port." This method poses a risk of entraining air into ECMO circuit. Pre-oxygenator return of purified blood from CRRT machine to the ECMO circuit will minimize the risk of air or thrombotic emboli, as the oxygenator will serve as a "trap." The other frequent method is the exact opposite—"arterial" inlet CRRT line connecting to high-pressure, post-membrane ECMO site and returning to low-pressure, pre-pump ECMO site. Depending on which configuration is used, there are various issues with internal CRRT machine alarms. For example, if the "return high-pressure" alarm occurs while the CRRT device is connected exclusively to a venous, low-pressure side of ECMO, evaluation needs to be done looking for occlusion or clot in the tubing. Another frequent alarm described "access disconnection" may be related to low return pressures if the venous outflow line of CRRT is connected to pre-pump low-pressure ECMO limb. This may be mitigated but turning access stopcock by 90° (1/4 of cycle) to allow CRRT machine to have more accurate pressure reading—this may cause higher hemolysis or thrombus formation, and caution is advised with this approach. Smaller connector tubing may be used instead as well (e.g., 4" small-bore IV connector). The CRRT/ECMO connection options are described in Table 12.5.

12.8 Management of the Patient on CRRT and ECMO

Management related to CRRT for a patient requiring ECMO is similar to those who are not on ECMO, with the main exceptions being the anticoagulation method. Systemic anticoagulation with heparin to prevent ECMO circuit clotting is often satisfactory for the CRRT circuit as well, and no additional anticoagulation is needed in the majority of cases especially with plain hemofilter use in line. The additional use of regional anticoagulation for the CRRT circuit may still be needed, especially if goals for systemic anticoagulation levels are decreased in patients who are at high risk for bleeding or if heparin was stopped in patients with severe bleeding.

More precise fluid management, including early prevention of FO, can be achieved with CRRT during ECMO. It is not clear when CRRT should be initiated, but earlier and more intensive CVVHD was associated with improved mortality in certain patients. Fluid goals should be established early and usually a return to dry weight is desired, however may be very challenging due to the previously stated factors. Electrolyte and acid/base management is similar to patients not requiring ECMO. Regarding medication infusions, dosing, clearance, patient and ECMO circuit volume of distribution, and interaction of medications with the ECMO oxygenator membrane all need to be taken into consideration. Medication dosing needs to be carefully adjusted after a patient is separated from ECMO. In patients who have ongoing renal injury and will require CRRT after transitioning off ECMO, a dialysis catheter may need to be placed at the time of decannulation. If a patient was cannulated via the right internal jugular (RIJ) vein, the ECMO cannula can be exchanged for a dialysis catheter. If the patient was cannulated via groin vessels, a separate dialysis catheter needs to be placed preferentially into the RIJ location.

References

1. Fleming GM, et al. A multicenter international survey of renal supportive therapy during ECMO: the Kidney Intervention During Extracorporeal Membrane Oxygenation (KIDMO) group. ASAIO J. 2012;58:407–14.
2. ELSO ECLS Registry Report: International Summary. Extracorporeal Life Support Organization, Ann Arbor MI. 2017.
3. Seczynska B, et al. Continuous Renal Replacement Therapy During ECMO in Patients Treated in Medical Intensive Care Unit: Technical Considerations. Therapeutic Apheresis and Dialysis 2014;18(6):523–34.
4. Chen H, et al. Combination of extracorporeal membrane oxygenation and continuous renal replacement therapy in critically ill patients: a systemic review. Crit Care Open Access. 2014;18:675.

5. Paden ML, et al. Recovery of renal function and survival after continuous renal replacement therapy during extracorporeal membrane oxygenation. Pediatr Crit Care Med. 2011;12:153.
6. Villa G, et al. Extracorporeal membrane oxygenation and the kidney. CardioRenal Med. 2016;6:50–60.
7. Kilburn DJ, et al. The complex relationship of extracorporeal membrane oxygenation and acute kidney injury: causation or association? BioMed Res Int. 2016;2016:1–14.
8. Askenazi DJ, et al. Renal replacement therapy in critically ill patients receiving extracorporeal membrane oxygenation. Clin J Am Soc Nephrol. 2012;7:1328–36.
9. Selewski DT, et al. Fluid overload and fluid removal in pediatric patients on extracorporeal membrane oxygenation requiring continuous renal replacement therapy. Crit Care Med. 2012;40:2694.

Part IV

Special Situations

13 Plasmapheresis in Pediatric Renal Disease

Daniella Levy-Erez and Haewon C. Kim

13.1 Case Vignette

A 10-year-old boy with no significant past medical history presents to the emergency department with severe respiratory distress and hemoptysis which started and progressed a week prior. His mother notes his urine had become darker color with a "tea-colored urine." His evaluation included a serum creatinine of 2 mg/dl and minimal urine output and noted to have a blood pressure of 140/90. His urine analysis is significant for +3 protein and +4 RBC with notable RBC casts visible on microscopy. A renal ultrasound shows echogenic kidneys without hydronephrosis and a normal bladder. Serologies: antinuclear antibody (ANA) negative, anti-neutrophilic cytoplasmic antibody (ANCA) negative. Over the course of the following week, his urine output declines, his blood pressure worsens, and his serum creatinine rises to 4.8 mg/dl. The differential diagnosis included a range of causes for rapidly progressive glomerulonephritis (GN) including post-infectious, ANCA-associated GN, anti-GBM disease. He underwent a kidney biopsy which pathology findings were consistent with positive anti-glomerular basement membrane (GBM) on immunofluorescence and crescentic glomerulonephritis. Despite

D. Levy-Erez
Division of Nephrology, The Children's Hospital of Philadelphia, Philadelphia, PA, USA

Perelman School of Medicine at the University of Pennsylvania, Philadelphia, PA, USA

H. C. Kim (✉)
Perelman School of Medicine at the University of Pennsylvania, Philadelphia, PA, USA

Department of Pediatrics, The Children's Hospital of Philadelphia, Philadelphia, PA, USA

Department of Pathology and Laboratory Medicine, The Children's Hospital of Philadelphia, Philadelphia, PA, USA
e-mail: kimh@email.chop.edu

S. K. Sethi et al. (eds.), *Critical Care Pediatric Nephrology and Dialysis: A Practical Handbook*, https://doi.org/10.1007/978-981-13-2276-1_13

pulse steroids he developed progressive renal function deterioration and persistent hemoptysis with the need of mechanical ventilation. Due to clinical deterioration with acute respiratory and renal failure, TPE was initiated. After a few treatments, his clinical symptoms were improving; he was weaned off mechanical ventilation, and creatinine gradually was down trending. This case illustrates one of the cases where TPE can have major impact on outcome and should be considered an important treatment modality.

13.2 Introduction

Kidney disease in children encompasses a wide range of diseases which can either be congenital or acquired. In younger children below 5 years of age, structural anatomic diseases are the common etiologies such as renal dysplasia and hypoplasia. In older children the acquired diseases increase in prevalence and include glomerular diseases, tubular disease, as well as genetic disease with a later age onset such as cystic kidney disease. The various kidney diseases can progress with the development of chronic kidney disease, and some will develop end-stage renal disease (ESRD). In addition to conventional initial treatments including antihypertensive medications and diuretics, many of them require disease-modifying medications, such as immunosuppressive agents, and in ESRD renal replacement therapy, including dialysis and kidney transplantation. Another form of immunomodulation includes removal of pathogenic substances in the circulation by therapeutic plasma exchange (TPE) or plasmapheresis. In glomerular diseases, either immune mediated or inflammatory, at pre- or post-renal transplantation with an abrupt progression, TPE has been reported successful either as a first-line treatment or a second-line therapy. Data is limited in children, and the vast of the data is extrapolated from adult-based evidence. Of the many kidney diseases in children, TPE may be beneficial in a small number of diseases. These include glomerular disease with a rapidly progressive form, such as ANCA-associated rapidly progressive glomerulonephritis; anti-glomerular basement membrane (anti-GBM) disease (Goodpasture's syndrome); nephrotic syndrome such as focal segmental glomerulosclerosis (FSGS), specifically after recurrence in kidney transplant; thrombotic microangiopathy (primary or secondary); and ABO incompatible kidney transplant or antibody-mediated rejection. In resistant cellular rejection, a newer modality such as extracorporeal photopheresis (ECP) may be beneficial since ECP modulates immune function by activation of the circulating regulatory T cells. This leads to increased immune tolerance, particularly in cellular rejection, although it appears to affect both the cellular and humoral immune response to the allograft. TPE is not a benign procedure, and complications in children are higher compared with adults. However, continuous improvement in techniques of apheresis procedures and instrument and availability of various types of central venous catheters and ports encourage the use of apheresis and allow apheresis procedure to be performed safely in children. This chapter has primarily two objectives: (1) to provide the overview of therapeutic apheresis with emphasis on special technical considerations unique to pediatric patients, including securing adequate vascular access, maintaining desired intravascular volume and circulating red cell mass, and preventing complications by early recognition of adverse reactions; and (2) to provide clinical applications of plasmapheresis in pediatric patients with renal diseases on the basis of evidence utilizing the American Society for Apheresis (ASFA) guidelines [1]. We suggest the readers to also go through previously published literature on pediatric apheresis which consists of excellent reviews [2–6].

13.3 Overview of Therapeutic Apheresis

The term "apheresis" is originated from a Greek word, *aphairesis*, meaning removal. Apheresis is defined as any procedure in which whole blood is withdrawn from a donor/patient, one or more components (plasma, platelets, or white blood cells) are separated from the blood and retained/discarded, and the remainder is reinfused into the donor/patient. Apheresis procedures are divided into exchange and collection procedures. Exchange procedures are performed with therapeutic goals of removing pathogenic plasma constituents or abnormal red blood cells (RBC) from the circulation in exchange for normal plasma constituents or healthy donor RBC. There are two types of exchange procedures: plasma exchange (plasmapheresis) and RBC exchange (erythrocytapheresis). Collection procedures are performed for two purposes: to collect a desired normal blood component, such as granulocytes, platelets, RBC, or plasma, from healthy blood donors for transfusion purpose, and to deplete cellular blood components, such as an excess number of white blood cells (WBC) or platelets from a patient for therapeutic purposes. Apheresis collection procedures in pediatrics are limited exclusively to leukocytapheresis, performed primarily (1) to harvest peripheral blood hematopoietic progenitor/stem cells (HPC) for autologous or allogeneic HPC transplantation or T cells for chimeric antigen receptor (CAR) T-cell therapy and, rarely, (2) to reduce an excess number of WBC or leukemic blast cells from patients with leukemia and hyperleukocytosis to treat or prevent complications due to leukostasis. Therapeutic plateletpheresis (or platelet depletion) is rarely used as a therapy, even in adults, to deplete platelets from patients with thrombocythemia or thrombocytosis to prevent thrombosis.

13.4 Types of Apheresis

13.4.1 Erythrocytapheresis or Red Cell Exchange (RCE) [7]

The primary goal of therapeutic RCE is to remove abnormal RBC or an excess number of RBC from a patient. There are three indications: (1) polycythemia or erythrocytosis with resultant hyperviscosity of whole blood with altered blood rheology, (2) hemochromatosis, and (3) the presence of abnormal RBC due to intrinsic or acquired RBC disorders. For the first two reasons cited above, RCE is done to deplete the red cells or iron stores. For this purpose, non-red cell replacement solution such as saline (0.9%) or albumin (5%) may be used. For removing abnormal RBCs such as those due to intrinsic or acquired RBC disorders, RCE aims to remove abnormal RBC and replace them with normal ones from the donor. RCE is most commonly utilized in treating acute and chronic complications of sickle cell disease (SCD) and is rarely used in non-SCD disorders. ASFA classifies the indications for RCE for complications of SCD as follows: acute stroke, Category I (grade 1C); stroke prophylaxis/iron overload prevention, Category I (grade 1A); severe acute chest syndrome, Category II (grade 1C); and multiorgan failure, Category III (grade 2C). Other non-acute complications of SCD including vaso-occlusive pain crisis, preoperative management, and pregnancy are classified as Category III (grades 2A–2C) [1].

13.4.2 Leukocytapheresis [1, 8–10]

There are primarily two goals for leukocytapheresis: (1) to harvest granulocytes, HPC, or T lymphocytes for the purpose of transfusion, hematopoietic stem cell transplantation, or chimeric antigen receptor T-cell (CAR T-cell) therapy for malignant cancers, respectively, and (2) to remove an excess number of white blood cells, such as leukemic blast cells. Hyperleukocytosis is defined as a circulating WBC or blast cell count >100 × 10^9/L. When the WBC count is greater than 100 × 10^9/L in acute myeloid leukemia (AML) and greater than 400 × 10^9/L in acute lymphoblastic leukemia (ALL), respectively, there is an increased risk of developing tumor lysis syndrome (TLS), disseminated intravascular coagulopathy (DIC), and thrombotic and/or hemorrhagic complications primarily due to leukostasis. Leukostasis results in end-organ complications such as CNS abnormality (blurred vision, confusion, and coma), pulmonary hemorrhage with respiratory failure, and multiorgan failure including renal failure as a result of WBC aggregates forming in microvessels, increase in viscosity, impaired blood flow, and reduced tissue perfusion leading to infarction. The rigidity of the cell and its size along with its rheological properties and cytoadhesive interactions (with myeloid blasts being larger and more rigid than lymphoid blasts) and releasing large quantities of cytokine products. Therapeutic leukocytapheresis quickly removes excessive number of WBC/blast cells resulting in reduction of whole blood viscosity and prevention of leukostasis with prevention or improvement of pulmonary and CNS manifestations.

Prophylactic leukocytapheresis can reduce early mortality but does not improve overall or long-term survival in patients with AML and hyperleukocytosis [11]. Symptomatic hyperleukocytosis is classified as ASFA Category II indication (grade 1B) for leukocyte depletion, whereas prophylactic or secondary hyperleukocytosis is as Category III indication (grade 2C) [1].

13.4.3 Plasmapheresis or Therapeutic Plasma Exchange (TPE)

TPE reduces the pathogenic substance from the plasma; thus it has been used to treat a variety of diseases in both children and adults. Readers are referred to the Sect. 13.5.2 for details.

13.4.4 Technical/Procedural Considerations for Pediatric Apheresis [2, 3, 5, 6]

Apheresis equipment that is available is designed primarily for adults, not for children. To be able to perform the procedure safely in children using currently available device, it is of utmost importance to be well versed with physical characteristics of apheresis equipment. In particular, careful consideration should be given primarily to three areas to provide a safe and effective apheresis treatment for pediatric patients: intravascular volume red cell mass, anticoagulation, and vascular access. While automated exchange using apheresis equipment is attractive, it should be noted that for infants weighing less than 5–10 kg, a manual whole blood exchange might be a reasonable alternative to an automated procedure.

13.5 Technical Considerations for Pediatric Apheresis

13.5.1 Intravascular Volume and Circulating Red Cell Mass Shifts [5, 6]

The apheresis procedure starts with withdrawal of whole blood into the apheresis circuit while diverting the priming normal saline to the waste bag, which results in a reduction of the patient's blood volume and red cell volume. This degree of volume deficit persists throughout the procedure until almost all of the content of the centrifuge chamber is rinsed back into the patient at the end of the procedure. Intravascular volume depletion during the procedure is mainly due to extracorporeal circuit, i.e., the disposable set of the equipment, which is referred to as extracorporeal volume (ECV).

Each instrument has a fixed ECV, and it may vary with type and make of same equipment, depending on the type of procedure. For example, the ECV of the leukocytapheresis set is larger than that of red cell or plasma exchange set. Irrespective of the type of equipment, the ECV of any given instrument would represent a larger fraction of total blood volume when used for a child as compared to that of an adult resulting in a greater volume depletion in children than in adults. A child may become symptomatic if there is an ECV shift greater than 15%; therefore, the maximum safe ECV shift should be established in each patient beforehand. If this shift is predicted to be greater than 15% or a critically sick child who is in ICU and may not tolerate any shift in volume, the procedure should be modified to ensure that volume shifts are limited to less than 15% of TBV.

It is equally important to maintain RBC volume to maintain adequate tissue delivery. This deficit of RBC volume occurs when, for example, the centrifuge chamber is filled with patient's blood, and such a deficit would persist till the end of the procedure, when the red cells in the chamber are returned to patient at the end of procedure. Patients with anemia and others with low red cell volume would not be able to tolerate this reduction in circulating red cell mass. Again the extent to which this volume depletion would occur depends on the type of equipment used and procedure performed.

Continuous-flow apheresis devices such as the Spectra Optia systems (Terumo BCT, Lakewood, CO) and Amicus system (Fenwal, Inc., Lake Zurich, IL) are preferred over intermittent-flow devices for pediatric use because of the smaller ECV. Membrane separators, e.g., Prisma TPE (Terumo BCT, Lakewood, CO) which also has a relatively small ECV, may be used in pediatric applications.

To estimate the degree of volume shift in each child, the total blood volume (TBV) of the child should be estimated before the procedure [5, 6]. Automated apheresis devices use more complex algorithms to calculate TBV on the basis of patient sex, height, and weight. In children weighing <25 kg, TBV calculated by automated apheresis equipment is not accurate, and the Spectra Optia system does not even calculate TBV. Thus, a weight-based TBV should be calculated in children weighing <25 kg. The calculated TBV is used to evaluate the patient's ability to tolerate the intravascular shifts of fluid and red cells that occur during apheresis.

13.5.2 Anticoagulation

Of anticoagulants, e.g., citrate, heparin, or both, used to prevent thrombotic occlusion of the extracorporeal circuit [2, 3, 6], citrate is the most commonly used anticoagulant at most institutions [12–14]. When heparin is considered for anticoagulation, the patient must be evaluated clinically for active bleeding or a history of bleeding disorder as well as laboratory evidence for coagulopathy by ordering at least a CBC with platelet count, prothrombin time (PT), activated partial thromboplastin time (aPTT), and fibrinogen assay.

The use of citrate may be associated with citrate toxicity, ranging from paresthesias to even arrhythmia or tetany, which primarily result from hypocalcemia (reduced ionized calcium) due to chelation of calcium by citrate. Children may not exhibit typical symptoms and signs of hypocalcemia, such as acral and circumoral paresthesias, but often present with abdominal pain, emesis, pallor, and hypotension [2, 3, 7].

The citrate toxicity is higher with the use of fresh frozen plasma (FFP) than with the 5% albumin replacement, primarily due to the fact that FFP contains approximately four times more citrate than 5% albumin. The citrate toxicity may be more common particularly in subjects with slow citrate metabolism due to hepatic or renal dysfunction. Since only ionized calcium is physiologically important, the ionized calcium level must be monitored frequently during the procedure when FFP is used as the replacement fluid. Intravenous calcium supplementation should be instituted to prevent serious adverse reactions due to hypocalcemia depending upon ionized calcium level.

Primarily, two types of solutions are used as a replacement solution (RS) for plasmapheresis: normal serum 5% albumin (albumin) and fresh frozen plasma (FFP). Albumin is readily available and does not transmit infectious diseases but lacks clotting factors, natural anticoagulants, and most of functioning proteins. In addition, albumin contains less citrate then FFP as stated above. There are almost no side effects other than very mild urticarial reactions. However, they are quite expensive. On the other hand, FFP contains clotting factors, natural anticoagulants, and almost all functioning proteins. However, FFP does transmit infectious diseases and often cause allergic reactions and citrate reactions compared to albumin. In general, albumin is the primary RS for most of TPE procedures. However, empiric plasma therapy using FFP is indicated or highly recommended as a RS in the following situations:

- TTP or TMA where replacing ADAMTS 13 protease activity or replacing absent or defective complement regulators
- Presence of active bleeding or coagulopathy
- A minimum 2–5 days or longer pre- and post-surgery depending upon the type of surgery
- For daily, multiple closely spaced (e.g., every other day) or sequential TPEs with albumin replacement which result in a dilutional coagulopathy

13.5.3 Vascular Access

Adequate vascular access is essential to maintain the rate of blood flow required for apheresis procedures. Every effort should be made to use the peripheral venous access. However, peripheral access is not an option in infants and young children and those who require long-term apheresis. Central venous access device (CVAD) may be preferable to peripheral access for these young children and some adolescents as well. Proper type of CVAD should be selected for patient safety and effective TPE procedure depending on the urgency of the clinical situation, the expected duration of apheresis treatment, and easy care. The catheter must be rigid enough to withstand the negative pressure required to draw blood into the apheresis device. In general, hemodialysis catheters are frequently used for pediatric apheresis because of their large bore, double lumen, and ability to support the required blood flow rates during apheresis procedures. In general, ports are easier to care for than central venous catheters, requiring only a monthly heparin flush when not in use.

Some catheters and ports, such as the Infusaport (Uromed, Yverdon-les-Bains, Switzerland) or peripherally inserted central venous catheters (PICCs), can be used for returning replacement solutions during apheresis procedures; these types of catheters do not typically provide sufficient flow rates needed for drawing blood from a patient into the apheresis machine. Complications associated with central venous lines include vessel damage, bleeding, infection, and thrombosis. The implanted ports have the lower rates of failure and central line-associated

Table 13.1 Pediatric guidelines for central venous access devices for acute or short-term (<14 days) and chronic (>14 days) apheresis[a] [6]

Patient weight (kg)	Catheter/port size (French)[b]	
	Acute or short term (<14 days) (non-cuffed)	Chronic (>14 days) (cuffed)
<10	Single-lumen, 5 Fr Turbo-flo PICC[c]	Double-lumen, 6 Fr[d]
	Double-lumen, 7 Fr	
11–19	Single-lumen, 5 Fr Turbo-flo PICC[c]	Double-lumen, 6 Fr[d]
	Double-lumen, 8 Fr	Double-lumen, 8 Fr
20–29	Double-lumen, 8 Fr	Double-lumen, 8 Fr
		Single-lumen, 7.5[e], 6.6[f], 8[f] Fr port
30–39	Double-lumen, 9 Fr	Double-lumen, 8 Fr
		Single-lumen, 8 Fr port[f]
41–50	Double-lumen, 9 Fr	Double-lumen, 10 Fr
	Double-lumen, 11.5 Fr	Double-lumen, 11.4 Fr port[e]
		Single- lumen, 9.6 Fr IV Port[g]
>50	Double-lumen, 11.5 Fr, 12 Fr, or 13.5 Fr	Double-lumen, 10 Fr
		Single- lumen, 9.6 Fr IV Port[g] Double-lumen, 11.4 Fr port[e]

[a]Updated guidelines used at the Children's Hospital of Philadelphia
[b]Any hemodialysis or apheresis catheters are acceptable
[c]Cook Medical, Inc, Bloomington, IN. Because this is a single-lumen catheter, a second line is required for replacement, such as a Broviac catheter (CR Bard, Murray Hill, NJ), other types of PICCs, or an Infusaport (Uromed, Yverdon-les-Bains, Switzerland)
[d]Medcomp Pro-Line (Harleysville, PA)
[f]Medcomp Dignity (Harleysville, PA) gBard IV port (Tempe, AZ)
[e]Vortex ports (AngioDynamics, Latham, NY)

bloodstream infection (CLABSI) than central venous catheters. Line placement, maintenance, and risks associated with CVDA should be weighed against the expected benefits of the apheresis procedures. The updated guidelines for the types and sizes of catheters and ports based on the weight of the patient at the authors' institution are given in Table 13.1 [6].

13.6 Indications for Therapeutic Apheresis

13.6.1 ASFA Indication Categories

In this chapter, indications for therapeutic apheresis in renal diseases are derived from the evidence-based ASFA guidelines [1]. ASFA has developed guidelines on the use of therapeutic apheresis in clinical practice by categorizing indications for therapeutic apheresis, with each disease entity being categorized as Category I through IV and having a grade of recommendation [1]. The category assignments and recommendation grades were based upon the strength of evidence and quality

Table 13.2 ASFA category definitions for therapeutic apheresis

Category	Description
I	Disorders for which apheresis is accepted as first-line therapy, either as a primary stand-alone treatment or in conjunction with other modes of treatment
II	Disorders for which apheresis is accepted as second-line therapy, either as a stand-alone treatment or in conjunction with other modes of treatment
III	Optimum role of apheresis therapy is not established Decision-making should be individualized
IV	Disorders in which published evidence demonstrates or suggests apheresis to be ineffective or harmful

Table 13.3 Grading recommendation for therapeutic apheresis [1]

Recommendation	Description	Quality of supporting evidence
Grade 1A	Strong recommendation, high-quality evidence	RCT without important limitations or overwhelming evidence from observational studies
Grade 1B	Strong recommendation, moderate quality evidence	RCT with important limitations or exceptionally strong evidence from observational studies
Grade 1C	Strong recommendation, low-quality or very low-quality evidence	Observational studies or case studies
Grade 2A	Weak recommendation, high-quality evidence	RCTs without important limitations or overwhelming evidence from observational studies
Grade 2B	Weak recommendation, moderate-quality evidence	RCTs with important limitations or exceptionally strong evidence from observational studies
Grade 2C	Weak recommendation, low-quality or very low-quality evidence	Low quality or very Low-quality evidence Observational studies or case series

of data to support recommending use of apheresis as a treatment modality and determined by consensus of all writing committee members. ASFA category definitions for therapeutic apheresis are described in Table 13.2 [1].

Table 13.3 describes grading the level of clinical recommendation on the basis of quality of supporting evidence [1].

13.6.2 Plasmapheresis for Kidney Disease

TPE or plasmapheresis efficiently removes pathogenic antibodies, immune complexes, plasma proteins, cytokines, lipoproteins, protein-bound drugs, and metabolic toxins from the plasma. Consequently, TPE has been used to treat a variety of diseases including renal diseases in both children and adults. In certain kidney

Table 13.4 ASFA category indications for plasmapheresis in kidney disease, with grading recommendations [1]

Disease	Indication	Category	Recommendation (grade)
ANCA-associated rapidly progressive glomerulonephritis (RPGN)	Dialysis dependent	I	Strongly recommended (1A)
	Diffuse alveolar hemorrhage (DAH)	I	Strongly recommended (1C)
	Dialysis independent	III	Weakly recommended (2C)
Anti-GBM glomerulonephritis	Diffuse alveolar hemorrhage (DAH)	I	Strongly recommended (1C)
	Dialysis dependent, no DAH	III	Weak recommendation (2B)
	Dialysis independent RPGN	I	Strongly recommended (1B)
Kidney transplant	FSGS recurrence	I	Strongly recommended (1B)
	Antibody-mediated rejection (AMR)	I	Strongly recommended (1B)
	Pretransplant ABO incompatible, desensitization (living donor)	I	Strongly recommended (1B)
Thrombotic microangiopathy (TMA)	HSCT	III	Weak recommendation (2C)
	Factor H autoantibodies	I	Weak recommendation (2C)
	TTP	I	Strongly recommended (1A)
Sepsis with multiorgan failure		III	Weak recommendation (2B)

disorders, especially with glomerular diseases, immune-mediated mechanisms play a major role in pathogenesis of diseases. TPE may be beneficial in reducing immune-mediated injury by rapid depletion of an antibody or immune complexes from the plasma, such as anti-GBM in alveolar hemorrhage or ABO or HLA antibodies in antibody-mediated rejection or an undefined substance removal such as in FSGS. Standard immunosuppressive therapies including corticosteroids may take a time to exert their immunosuppressive effects, but TPE results in not only a rapid reduction in the concentration of offending antibodies and immune complexes but may also result in immunomodulation by reducing T helper type-1/T helper type-2 (Th1/Th2) cytokine ratio [15].

However, TPE could stimulate synthesis of the autoantibodies by reducing negative feedback control. In Table 13.4 we summarized ASFA category indications for plasmapheresis in kidney disease with grading recommendation [1].

13.6.3 Disease Descriptions and Management

Plasmapheresis treatment plan for kidney diseases is summarized in Table 13.5 along with postulated or offending antibody or pathologic substance in the plasma which can be removed by plasmapheresis.

Table 13.5 Plasmapheresis treatment plan and postulated mechanisms for kidney diseases

Disease	Indication	Postulated mechanism	TPE treatment: Dose and frequency	TPE treatment: Duration	Replacement solution
ANCA-associated rapidly progressive glomerulonephritis (RPGN)	A. Dialysis dependent	ANCA autoantibody	1–1.5 TPV daily for a few days or during rapidly progressive period, then every other day	Total 6–9 TPEs or until pulmonary hemorrhage is under control	Albumin or plasma
	B. Diffuse alveolar hemorrhage (DAH)				FFP[a] is the first choice when DAH present
	C. Dialysis independent				For daily TPE, a mixture of albumin with FFP to prevent bleed
Anti-GBM glomerulonephritis	A. Diffuse alveolar hemorrhage (DAH), RPGN, dialysis independent	Ant-GBM antibody	1–1.5 TPV daily for a few days or for rapidly progressive period, then every other day	10–20 days until antibody level decreases or	Albumin or plasma
	B. Dialysis dependent, no DAH			Continue until resolution of ongoing glomerular or pulmonary injury	FFP[a] is the first choice when DAH present
	C. Dialysis independent RPGN				For daily TPE, a mixture of albumin with FFP

(continued)

Table 13.5 (cotinued)

Disease	Indication	Postulated mechanism	TPE treatment: Dose and frequency	TPE treatment: Duration	Replacement solution
Kidney transplant	FSGS recurrence	Plasma factor of unknown origin	1–1.5 TPV daily for a few days then every other day	Acute recurrence: 9 TPEs over 2 weeks until proteinuria decreases/resolved	Albumin or plasma
				Maintenance TPE: following initial daily TPEs, gradually taper as indicated, e.g., 3/week for the first 3 weeks, 2/week for 3 weeks, 1/week until month 3, and so on	For daily TPE, a mixture of albumin with FFP maintenance TPE, albumin
	Antibody-mediated rejection (AMR)	HLA antibodies	1–1.5 TPV daily or every other day	For desensitization: daily or every other day until negative crossmatch	Albumin or plasma
				Posttransplant: a minimum of 3 TPEs	FFP should be used for at least 3–5-day pre-/posttransplant surgery
	Pretransplant ABO incompatible, desensitization (living donor)	Isoagglutinins (anti-A or anti-B)	1–1.5 TPV daily or every other day	Continue until antibody titer < critical threshold (both IgG and IgM < 1:16) prior to transplant	Albumin or plasma FFP should be used for at least 3–5-day pre-/posttransplant surgery and be compatible with both the recipient and donor ABO type

Thrombotic microangiopathy (TMA)	HSCT	Undefined	1–1.5 TPV daily	Undefined Daily until a clinical and/or hematologic response	Plasma
	Factor H autoantibodies	Anti-factor H	1–1.5 TPV daily	Dependent on patient condition and stable Hct and platelet count	Plasma
	TTP	Anti-ADAMTS13 autoantibody	1–1.5 TPV daily: initially 1.5 TPV daily for a few days, then 1 TPV	Daily until the platelet count >150 × 10^9/L and LDH = near normal for 2–3 consecutive days	Plasma
Sepsis with multiorgan failure		Inflammatory and antifibrinolytic mediators	1–1.5 TPV daily for 2–14 days	2–14 treatments or until improvement in organ function	Plasma

[a]*FFP* fresh frozen plasma

13.7 Antineutrophilic Cytoplasmic Antibody (ANCA)-Associated Glomerulonephritis (GN)

13.7.1 Brief Description

ANCA-associated GN is a rare form of GN which typically can be divided into three subtypes: GPA (granulomatous polyangiitis or Wegener's), MPA (microscopic polyangiitis), and eosinophilic polyangiitis. The incidence of ANCA-associated GN has been reported to be 46–184 per million population with a peak age between 50 and 70 years old [16, 17]; the prevalence of ANCA-associated GN in children is unknown but is much rarer than in adults [18].

Any of these three entities are associated with ANCA either PR3 (anti-proteinase 3) or MPO (myeloperoxidase antibody). However, MPO is more often associated with MPA, whereas PR3 ANCA is more common. Most studies collectively studied these entities together. In all three diseases, the pathology of the kidney is characterized by pauci-immune necrotizing glomerulonephritis.

In a recent study published in 2017 [19] reported a single-center experience with pediatric ANCA GN among 22 children over a period of 22 years with a slight female prevalence of 59% and a median age of 13.7 years. Most of these children (20/22) presented with systemic manifestations which included respiratory symptoms (55%), fever (41%), abdominal pain (41%), and joint pain (36%). The median creatinine level was 2.7 mg/dl with 100% of children presenting with hematuria and proteinuria. 8/22 (36%) of the children needed renal replacement therapy at the time of initial presentation; 7/22 (32%) of these children progressed to end-stage renal disease (ESRD). Two of the children who progressed to ESRD did not need dialysis at initial presentation.

13.7.2 Current Management

The cornerstone of ANCA-associated GN management includes immunosuppressive therapy. For severe GN, induction therapy with pulse steroid therapy is the first line in combination of either cyclophosphamide (Cytoxan) or rituximab followed by a long course of oral and maintenance therapy. In a recent RCT comparing Cytoxan and rituximab, Stone et al. demonstrated a non-inferiority of rituximab compared to Cytoxan in induction therapy with possible long-term remission [20]. Besides immunosuppression these patients receive medications to control electrolytes disturbances, hypertension, and anemia which are either a sequela of their acute inflammatory illness or chronic kidney disease (CKD). If disease rapidly progresses with concurrent rapid kidney deterioration or severe pulmonary involvement, this should prompt consideration of plasmapheresis (or TPE).

13.7.3 Plasmapheresis Management

The rationale of using TPE is removal of ANCA antibodies which are involved in the pathogenesis of the disease. In the European Dialysis and Transplant Association (EDTA) recommendations published in 2016 for management of ANCA-associated GN, TPE was considered for patients with an elevated creatinine (above 5.7 mg/dl) due to rapidly progressive glomerulonephritis (RPGN) in the setting of a new or relapsing disease with level of evidence of 1B as well as severe diffuse alveolar hemorrhage. The ASFA guidelines published in 2016 provided similar indications with a level of recommendations 1A and 1C based on current evidence [1]. In a meta-analysis of Walsh et al. in 2011 of 387 patients from 9 trials, his study reported that plasma exchange may decrease the composite end point of ESRD or death in patients with renal vasculitis [21]. The largest trial published so far, the MEPEX study that recruited 137 patients (adults) with an elevated creatinine above 5.7 mg/dl or on dialysis. Plasmapheresis increased the rate of renal recovery in ANCA-associated systemic vasculitis when compared with intravenous methylprednisolone. ;all patients recieved cyclophosphamide) although patient survival and severe adverse event rates were similar in both groups [22]. TPE should be considered as the first-line therapy in conjunction with immunosuppressive treatment for acute and life-threatening complications, such as DAH. The recommended TPE dose is daily for severe cases for at least 2–3 days with initial starting does of 1.5× TPV daily and subsequently at 1.0× TPV every 2–3 days for a total of 6–9 procedures (Table 13.5).

13.8 Anti-glomerular Basement Membrane (Anti-GBM) Glomerulonephritis

13.8.1 Brief Description

Anti-GBM GN (Goodpasture's syndrome) is a small vessel vasculitis which affects glomerular and pulmonary small vessels [23]. This disease results in a necrotizing rapidly progressive GN as well as pulmonary manifestations including diffuse alveolar hemorrhage (DAH). Patients with this disease have circulating antibodies against the non-collagenous domain of alpha3 chain of collagen type 4. The antibody has been found present both in the kidney as well as in the blood. Serum from patients with anti-GBM disease reacts with the epitope, and these antibodies have been shown already in 1967 by Lerner and his group to produce a crescentic GN after administered to nonhuman primers confirming the pathogenicity of these antibodies [24]. Anti-GBM disease accounts for 10% of crescentic GN in kidney biopsies in a large cohort [25], but its specific incidence is not known in adults (suggested to be 0.5–1 cases per million) or in children; US renal data system (USRDS) reports that 0.4% of ESRD cases in children (2002–2006) were attributed to anti-GBM disease. There are multiple hypothesis and triggers which have shown to induce exposure of this epitope resulting in antibody production and disease manifestation, but still there is little known given this is a rare entity. Most patients presenting with anti-GBM GN will present with a rapidly progressing form (80–90%) with about half having simultaneous pulmonary hemorrhage [23]. Levy et al. reported the outcome of 71 adults presenting with anti-GBM disease; in patients who presented with dialysis-dependent renal failure (39/71), patient survival was 65% at 1 year and 8% renal survival at 1 year and 36% and 5%, respectively, at follow-up. All patients with dialysis dependency remained on dialysis [26]. Bayat et al. reviewed 23 pediatric cases described in English literature over a 25-year period. Most children (91%) survived; but in many cases, renal disease progresses to end stage, requiring maintenance therapy on dialysis, and some undergo kidney transplantation. However, no case was identified with signs of relapse after remission [27]. A larger retrospective analysis included 123 patients between 1986 and 2015 from 6 centers; results demonstrated a correlation between histopathologic class and degree of fibrosis/crescents, anti-GBM titer and dialysis dependency at presentation, and kidney outcome [28]. Two to three percent of patients can present with no detectable anti-GBM in the serum but will be detected in kidney biopsy. There have been multiple studies demonstrating a correlation between antibody titer and avidity with disease outcome [29, 30], leading to the conception that removing these antibodies utilizing TPE should have an impact on outcome.

13.8.2 Current Management

Without treatment anti-GBM GN is a life-threatening disease, and there have been studies demonstrating that early therapy has a large impact on outcome. Due to the grave prognosis, patients presenting with RPGN are treated with aggressive management which includes immunosuppressive agents including steroids and cyclophosphamide, and plasmapheresis is included as first-line therapy for these patients. Williams et al. reported a 25-year experience in pediatric anti-GBM in a large pediatric center in the USA. The report includes four children with anti-GBM disease which all needed renal replacement therapy and one child who had renal recovery and did not remain on dialysis [31].

13.8.3 Plasmapheresis Management

The rationale behind TPE is the concept of removing the pathogenic antibody targeted against the GBM. The grave outcome of this disease led to treatment with TPE in the 1970s. Without conclusive evidence [26] and given the rarity of this disease, there is only one underpowered RCT study evaluating plasmapheresis in anti-GBM disease among adults. In this study 17 patients (mostly young males under 25 years of age) were randomized to one arm of steroids and cyclophosphamide alone or concurrent with plasmapheresis. The study demonstrated an advantage of combining plasmapheresis and immunosuppressive with patients with crescentic GN secondary to anti-GBM compared to only immunosuppression although there was a difference in disease severity among the two groups prior to allocation which may have impacted the results [32]. Zhang et al. compared double-filtration plasmapheresis (DFPP) with immunoadsorption (IA) therapy in 28 patients which consisted of 13 males and 15 females, of median age 44.5 years (range, 22.5–57 years). The clinical and pathological features of the DFPP and IA groups were similar. Efficacy of clearing anti-GBM antibody was similar in the two groups, although fewer patients in the DFPP group experienced reduced IgG (62.7 vs 83.5%, $p = 0.002$). At the end of follow-up, patient survival and renal survival were similar in the DFPP and IA groups. In most patients treated with immunosuppressive therapies and TPE, anti-GBM antibody levels become undetectable within 2 weeks [33]. The course of TPE is usually at least 2–3 weeks duration. Given there are patients which their antibody levels are negative at the initiation of TPE, this should not dictate the timing for initiation or stopping TPE, and the decision should be focused on active renal or pulmonary disease progression. TPE should be considered as the first-line therapy in conjunction with immunosuppressive treatment for acute and life-threatening complications, such as DAH or a rapidly progressive disease. Since anti-GBM antibodies do not directly correlate with disease severity, TPE should continue until resolution of evidence of ongoing glomerular or pulmonary injury rather than the presence of antibody. In patients with DAH, replacement with fresh frozen plasma (FFP) is indicated to avoid dilutional coagulopathy and potential bleeding.

13.9 Kidney Transplant

13.9.1 ABO Incompatible Kidney Transplant or Highly Sensitized Patients

13.9.1.1 Brief Description

Kidney transplant offers multiple advantages over chronic dialysis including lower morbidity, lower rates of mortality, and an improved quality of life [34]. Gillen et al. report similar results in children compared to adults; transplanted children have a lower mortality rate (13.1 deaths/1000 patient-years) compared to patients on the transplant waiting list on dialysis (17.6 deaths/1000 patient-years). After 6 months, the risk of death was found to be significantly lower among children who received a kidney transplant compared to children who remained on dialysis [35]. As the demand for organs continues to increase beyond the deceased donor supply, the number of days spent waiting for a kidney transplant increases exponentially. Renal transplant for pediatric patients in the USA from a previous study conducted between 2005 and 2010 reports a waiting time of 284 days. In the recent USRD report as of December 31, 2014, the kidney transplant waiting list increased by 3% over the previous year to 88,231 candidates, of which 83% were awaiting their first kidney transplant. With fewer than 18,000 kidney transplants performed in 2014, the active waiting list was 2.8 times larger than the supply of donor kidneys [36]. In patients who are difficult to match secondary to having broadly reactive human leukocyte antigen (HLA)-specific alloantibodies or less common blood groups such as blood group B have longer waiting times on the deceased donor list and await much longer for a kidney transplant with significant morbidly. ABO incompatible kidney transplantation is a growing possibility resulting from a shortage of compatible organs, which can offer children more expanded options with the current limited allografts. The presence of natural antibodies (isoagglutinins) like anti-A or anti-B, in the recipient's plasma against donor's, is referred to as major ABO incompatibility. As A and B antigens are expressed on vascular endothelium on the graft, the presence of these antibodies may lead to hyperacute rejection and acute antibody-mediated rejection. TPE is therefore used to reduce anti-A and/or anti-B titers in patients nearing transplant with a goal of preventing rejection and facilitating survival of the graft.

Any level of sensitization poses a challenge for successful transplantation due to the strong immune response of preformed anti-HLA antibodies, anti-ABO antibodies, and immunologic memory T cells. Desensitization protocols for highly sensitized patients and ABO (blood group)-incompatible patients [37] have improved renal survival and offer patients on the deceased donor list an increased a suitable match. Long-term patient and allograft survival in this high-risk population have significantly improved over the years [38].

13.9.1.2 Current Management

Highly sensitized patients as well as ABO-incompatible kidney transplant recipients have received kidney transplants with success [39–41]. Presence of donor-specific antibodies (DSAs) has a negative impact on renal allografts [38] resulting in developing protocols devised to preemptively treat such patients prior to receiving a kidney transplant. The aim of any desensitization regimen is to achieve a negative crossmatch by eliminating donor-specific antibodies. Most protocols include high- or low-dose intravenous immunoglobulin (IVIG) at a dose of 2 mg/kg [42] in combination with rituximab [43] (B-cell-depleting agents). There are limited randomized controlled trial studies [44–46]; making it challenging to compare the various protocols due to heterogeneity of these studies and methods.

13.9.1.3 Plasmapheresis Management

The use of plasmapheresis and desensitization with immunosuppressive treatment in patients receiving ABO-incompatible renal transplants was suggested in 1980s and has increased in the last 30 years. The mechanism is targeted in removal of isoagglutinins and/or anti-HLA antibodies. Immunoadsorption is more specific than TPE and is mainly targeted at removal of IgG with no need for replacement fluids. Studies from Johns Hopkins Hospital report higher survival rates among desensitized adult patients compared to remaining on dialysis or awaiting a compatible allograft [41]. Mayo Clinic reported 13 patients receiving IVIG alone compared to IVIG and TPE for desensitization with higher rates of desensitization among the combined group 38% vs 80%, respectively, as well as higher ABMR rates in the IVIG group [45]. The pediatric protocols are mostly adapted from the adult data with limited studies.

Despite desensitization protocols these patients are at higher risk for antibody-mediated rejection (AMR). The incidence of AMR after desensitization treatments is approximately 30% [37]. The goal of TPE in ABO-incompatible kidney transplant is to reduce the isoagglutinin titer to less than critical threshold, which may vary depending on technique used, in general pre-kidney transplant both IgG and IgM <1:16. Prior to kidney transplant, intense TPE with 1.5× TPV can be performed daily until IgG and IgM titers reduce to 1:16. Replacement fluids include 5% albumin, plasma, or both. However, FFP must be used as replacement fluid during the minimum 3–5 days pre- and posttransplantation to prevent postoperative bleeding.

13.9.2 Allograft Rejection

13.9.2.1 Brief Description

Renal graft failure remains an important clinical problem. Data from the USRDS describe high rates of graft failure leading to ESRD, making kidney transplant failure the fourth leading cause of ESRD. The reasons leading to graft failure include cellular rejection, antibody-mediated rejection (AMR), and recurrent renal diseases as well as infections and medication toxicities. Rejection can either be a cellular rejection mediated by cytotoxic T cells or a humoral process mediated by antibodies. Both of these can present either acutely or as a more chronic process leading to decreased graft function and subsequently if remains untreated allograft loss. The differential diagnosis for rejection can be other reasons leading to graft dysfunction, and the final diagnosis is by a kidney biopsy demonstrating pathognomonic changes consistent with rejection using the Banff classification. Positive donor-specific antibodies can support findings consistent with AMR as well as staining for complement activations such as C4d [47].

13.9.2.2 Current Management

The cornerstone of cellular rejection is focused on immunosuppressive therapy with first-line high-dose steroids and if significant rejection is evident on biopsy or there is limited response to steroids subsequent treatment with anti-thymoglobulin antibodies. In a systematic review, Wan et al. identified 21 studies including 10 RCT evaluating therapies targeted in AMR with IVIG and TPE demonstrating the best outcome and are considered standard of care [48]. IVIG is known to be a modulator of immunity although the exact mechanism isn't known. Newer treatments with rituximab, bortezomib, and complement pathway inhibitor treatment have been reported in the literature, but their role isn't clear.

13.9.2.3 Plasmapheresis Management

Plasmapheresis for AMR is based on antibody removal of donor-specific antibodies involved in the pathogenesis of the rejection. Lefaucheur et al. reported a retrospective comparison of high-dose IVIG alone (12 patients) vs IVIG + rituximab + plasma exchange (12 patients) for treating AMR. The IVIG-alone group was treated between January 2000 and December 2003, whereas patients receiving combined therapy were treated from January 2004 to December 2005. The investigators reported that the combined therapy was superior to IVIG alone in providing improved graft survival at 36 months (91.7% combined to 50%) [49]. Jordan et al. reviewed their experience and current data of management of AMR and provided a protocol of treatment in severe AMR, with plasma exchange followed by IVIG and rituximab [37]. There are various protocols in different centers including plasmapheresis which usually includes daily apheresis for 3 days and subsequently alternating day treatments with cessation of therapy depending on antibody levels.

A newer modality for cellular rejection which is mediated by aberrant T lymphocytes is extracorporeal photopheresis (ECP) which is considered to be a promising immunomodulatory therapy in diseases caused by aberrant T lymphocytes. ECP has been used in patients with graft-versus-host disease and systemic scleroderma as well as in solid organ transplant rejection. The recommended TPE dose for desensitization protocol includes daily or every other day until crossmatch becomes negative. For AMR, TPE can be started posttransplantation or continued, if already started, along with immunosuppressive drugs for a minimum of 3–5 procedures. It is important to use FFP as replacement fluids to prevent post-op bleeding.

13.10 Focal Segmental Glomerulosclerosis (FSGS) Recurrence After Transplant

13.10.1 Brief Description

FSGS is a characteristic pathological finding on kidney biopsies of children or adults presenting with proteinuria or full-blown nephrotic syndrome and includes multiple entities. FSGS may be idiopathic or secondary to known genetic mutations in podocyte genes, resulting in podocyte effacement altering the glomerular basement barrier leading to extensive proteinuria and subsequently nephrotic syndrome presenting with nephrotic range proteinuria, hypoalbuminemia, and edema. Children presenting with FSGS will mostly be resistant to conservative therapy, and over 50% will progress to ESKD within 5–10 years after diagnosis; FSGS is the cause of 10% of cases of ESRD in children receiving dialysis [50]. After kidney transplantation there is a 50% rate of recurrence of FSGS [51] which can appear within hours-days after transplantation and is a challenge to treat.

Despite extensive research the specific cause for idiopathic FSGS has yet to be found. A case report published in the NEJM in 2012 described a 27-year-old with primary FSGS who recurred in a kidney transplant with extensive proteinuria within days posttransplant; at day 14 the kidney allograft was removed, and re-transplantation in a 66-year-old diabetic patient with resolution of proteinuria after transplantation suggesting a soluble factor present in the patient's serum is the cause for the disease [52]. That elusive humoral factor has yet to be found but has established the proposed mechanism for FSGS recurrence treatment with plasmapheresis.

13.10.2 Current Management

FSGS is a challenging disease to treat, and management includes both immune- and nonimmune-based treatments. Treatment of secondary FSGS is targeted at controlling the primary illness (such as SLE, HIV, etc.) as well as focused on chronic kidney disease progression improving blood pressure control and reducing proteinuria with ACE inhibitors or ARBs. Primary FSGS is treated first with immunosuppression (including steroids—most patients will be resistant), calcineurin inhibitors, and rituximab as well as anti-proteinuria and antihypertensive agents. Recurrent FSGS can lead to early graft failure, but in rare case, it can resolve spontaneously. Data of over 2000 children from the North American Pediatric Renal Transplant Collaborative Study (NAPRTCS) database between 1987 and 2001 recurrent FSGS accounted for 15% of all graft failures [53]. Given the high rate of recurrence and its leading to graft failure and no successful therapies, plasmapheresis has a significant role in recurrence management.

13.10.3 Plasmapheresis Management

Plasmapheresis in primary FSGS is not a used modality although some studies have been conducted in primary FSGS using low-density lipoprotein (LDL) apheresis with some encouraging results. The common regimen to attain remission after FSGS recurrence may defer between centers. Garcia treated 9 children with 10 TPEs and immunosuppression with a 55% of full remission [54]. A 2016 review reported the outcome of 53 kidney transplant recipients recorded in the National Israeli Kidney Transplant Registry with a 64% recurrence rate. Plasmapheresis achieved partial and complete remission in 7/18 who were treated [55].

Rationale for TPE in recurrent FSGS may be due to removal of a plasma factor or factors that increases glomerular permeability. The standard approach is a 3-day daily TPE treatments followed by additional alternating TPE treatments over another 2 weeks period. There are other approaches with a gradual taper over 9 months depending upon urine protein/creatinine ratios. Albumin is the primary replacement fluid unless TPE is performed daily.

13.11 Thrombotic Microangiopathy (TMA)

Thrombotic microangiopathy (TMA) is a complex process where the main pathological process is endothelial injury either secondary to HPC transplant, medications, infection triggered (*E. coli* STEC), immune or congenital due to mutations in genes encoding complement regulators, or ADAMTS13 deficiency [56]. The clinical spectrum includes thrombocytopenia, intravascular hemolysis secondary to microangiopathy, and multisystem involvement of the central nervous system and kidney (including renal failure, hematuria, and proteinuria). TMA is a pathological diagnosis and can be also divided into various clinical entities, for example, *TTP* thrombotic thrombocytopenic purpura and *HUS* hemolytic uremic syndrome typical or atypical. There is much overlap between the different entities, and we will briefly discuss the ones which there may be a role for plasmapheresis as part of therapy: TMA after HSCT, complement related (secondary to antibodies), and TTP.

13.12 Post Hematopoietic Stem/Progenitor Cell Transplantation (HSCT/HPCT)

13.12.1 Brief Description

TMA is increasingly recognized as a cause of acute kidney injury (AKI) after HSCT. The endothelial cell injury leads to microangiopathic hemolytic anemia, thrombocytopenia, and subsequent vessel damage leading to significant organ damage. After HSCT the kidney is a common target of involvement although other organs can have involvement such as the lung, bowel, heart, and brain (seizures and altered mental status) [57]. Children developing AKI and clinical or histological evidence of TMA have been found to have abnormalities in the alternative pathway of complement including factor H autoantibodies and deletions in factor H-related genes [58].

13.12.2 Current Management

Chapter 8 describes in-depth TMA after HSCT. We will focus here on the plasmapheresis aspect.

13.12.3 Plasmapheresis Management

There are two approaches managing TMA after HSCT: the first includes a supportive approach with close monitoring and a trial of TPE in a selected group of patients. TPE is a relative cheap therapy with limited side effects. The second approach is the growing use/consideration of eculizumab (a targeted complement inhibitor); the basis of it is that there is a percentage of children (unclear) which may have complement dysregulation, and targeted therapy has shown efficacy in some patients. In a recent retrospective review of a single center and 18 children with transplant-associated TMA, it was seen that early initiation of TPE might be beneficial even in those with multiorgan failure [59]. Another retrospective study by Jodele et al. of 10 pediatric patients receiving plasmapheresis suggests that early initiation may improve outcome in 9/10 children who received TPE demonstrated normalization of their abnormal laboratory findings [60]; the 5 children who gained renal recovery started TPE at a median of 17 days (range 4–24 days) compared with the remainders who started TPE after a median of 32 days (range 17–73 days); all these patients died. Deciding which approach is better is not completely answered in the literature. Complement testing can take a while to return, and therapy may need to be initiated earlier; it is an expensive modality as well as encompasses the additional risk of infections. A recent review by Bohl [61] tried to address this question and compared 24 patients treated with conventional therapy in an earlier era and 15 patients who received eculizumab. The conventional therapy group was treated predominantly with defibrotide alone or in combination with plasmapheresis or rituximab. Despite an initial response rate of 61%, only 4 patients (16%) were long-term survivors, 2 of whom had a low-risk thrombotic microangiopathy without multiorgan damage. The overall response rate in the eculizumab group was significantly higher, at 93%. In addition, eculizumab treatment was discontinued in five patients (33%), with persistent recovery.

13.13 Complement Mediated (Complement Factor Autoantibodies)

13.13.1 Brief Description

Growing knowledge of atypical HUS has found multiple complement factor mutations leading to hyperactive complement pathway resulting in TMA. Factors involved include membrane cofactor protein, factor I, factor B, and factor H. Autoantibodies directed against those factors can lead to an acquired complement dysregulation with a similar form of TMA. The clinical presentation can include intravascular hemolysis, thrombocytopenia, and acute kidney injury with hematuria, proteinuria, and disproportionate hypertension which may be refractory to treatment.

13.13.2 Current Management

Suspected complement-mediated TMA will be treated with complement pathway inhibition; currently the mainstay of treatment is eculizumab. This is a monoclonal antibody targeted against terminal complement factor 5. Inhibition of this factor inhibits formation of the membrane attack complex and inhibits complement cascade activation.

13.13.3 Plasmapheresis Management

The rationale for using plasmapheresis is in the cases that the cause of HUS is the presence of complement autoantibodies such as factor H antibodies which can be removed during TPE.

Eculizumab has growing evidence and currently is considered first-line therapy, but due to a high cost and limited availability in some areas, TPE can be considered. No RCT have been done in children or adults.

13.14 Thrombotic Thrombocytopenic Purpura (TTP) Secondary to ADAMTS13 Deficiency

13.14.1 Brief Description

Thrombotic thrombocytopenic purpura is a rare clinical entity on the spectrum of TMA which presents with five hallmark features: thrombocytopenia, hemolytic anemia, neurological manifestations, acute kidney injury, and fever. The cause for the disease is deficient activity of ADAMTS13 enzyme, which cleaves von Willebrand factor multimers and prevents microthrombosis. The lack of ADAMTS13 enzyme activity either congenital or secondary to an antibody leads to TTP. Given the rare pediatric cases, most reports are case reports with few larger studies. In a population-based registry from Oklahoma, the pediatric population has an incidence rate of 3% compared to the adult rate (0.09 per 100,000 children) more common among females with significant multisystem involvement [62].

Acquired TTP is diagnosed in the setting of abrupt thrombocytopenia and Coombs-negative microangiopathic hemolytic anemia with normal PT/ INR and PTT and is suggested to be secondary to IGG autoantibodies directed against ADAMTS13 [63]. Mortality is high among patients with TTP with over 90% mortality with no intervention leading to aggressive therapy which has demonstrated to reduce mortality especially TPE which is discussed here [1, 64].

13.14.2 Current Management

The removal of the offending antibody and the simultaneous administration of ADAMTS13 protein in plasma is the mainstay treatment in TTP.

There have been studies which addressed concomitant steroid therapy with TPE in 54 patients in each arm demonstrating no survival benefit 90% vs 93% but possible increased remission rates.

IF TPE is not available, simple transfusion with plasma or cryo which contain ADAMTS13 is appropriate [65].

13.14.3 Plasmapheresis Management

TPE has effectively decreased overall mortality of TTP from fatal to below 10%. It is thought to remove inhibitors of ADAMTS13, von Willebrand factor (vWF) cleaving protease and simultaneously replenishing the protease with plasma replacement. The treatment is done daily with 1–1.5× TPV with replacement of plasma (i.e., FFP or thawed plasma) or plasma cryoprecipitate reduced (i.e., cryosupernatant or plasma cryoprecipitate removed) until platelets/LDH normalize for at least 2–3 consecutive days.

13.15 Sepsis with Multiorgan Failure Including AKI

Septic shock is a life-threatening clinical condition secondary to a dysregulated inflammatory state in response to an infection with elevated proinflammatory cytokine levels, toxins, and procoagluble factors which are associated with high rates of multiorgan failure such as acute kidney injury [66]. Septic shock is the 10th most common cause of death in the USA and accounts for 2–3% of all hospital admissions. Mortality rates of sepsis-associated shock in the pediatric population are reported to be as high as 28–88% depending on extent and number of organs involved [67]. Various extracorporeal therapies have shown some positive results as adjunctive therapeutic intervention in addition to traditional antimicrobials, pressors, and fluid management therapies in an effort to remove the inflammatory mediators and improve poor organ perfusion caused by the hypotension state and microvascular thrombosis [68, 69].

13.15.1 Current Management/Treatment

Guidelines for septic shock management have emerged from well-based studies that early resuscitation and shortening of hypotension state can decrease organ damage and mortality. The treatment is focused on antimicrobial agents as well as treatment of infection source as well as hemodynamic stabilization with fluid resuscitation and pressors. Additional treatments may include steroids (to treat secondary adrenal insufficiency), antithrombin, and nutritional support.

13.15.2 Plasmapheresis Management

The rationale behind utilizing TPE includes improving organ function and hemodynamic state by removing inflammatory cytokines as well ant fibrinolytic factors and supplementing with plasma which contains coagulant, natural anticoagulants, as well as ADAMTS13 in order to restore hemostasis. Various observational studies demonstrating the benefit of TPE in sepsis report a survival of 60–87% compared to those reported previously where a survival rate of 20–40% was seen. Many case series have suggested that early treatment would have an advantage over delayed initiation of therapy and may lead to hemodynamic stabilization.

An improvement in 28-day mortality was seen in a retrospective cohort of 42 patients after controlling for illness severity. The suggestion of efficacy of TPE in sepsis in prospective randomized studies is conflicting as against that noted in observational studies. Among the four RCTs that have been published involving 106 patients, the largest is that of Busund et al. who instituted a single TPE in 69 patients followed by another session the next day if the patient failed to improve [70]. It was noted that there was 33% mortality in treatment group and 53.8% mortality in the control arm at 28 days follow-up ($p < 0.05$). The significance of the effect of TPE became nonsignificant once the other contributing factors were controlled. Another study involving 22 adults and 8 children to study the effect of continuous plasma filtration found no difference in mortality, but reduction of some acute phase reactants such as C3, CRP, haptoglobin, and a1-antitrypsin was achieved. In another RCT involving 48 adults and children, there was no significant difference that was noted in 28-day mortality when plasma filtration was compared to standard therapy, but the study closed early due to poor enrolment [71].

A recent study evaluated TPE in thrombocytopenia-associated multiple organ failure (TAMOF); this study demonstrated decreased ADAMTS13 activity which correlates with platelet counts, and vWF antigen and children with TAMOF syndrome may have vWF-mediated thrombotic microangiopathy. In a randomized trial [72], children with severe TAMOF (platelet counts < 100,000/mm^3 and >3 organ failure) were randomized to TPE or standard therapy. Five patients received TPE and five patients received standard therapy. TPE ($n = 5$, median 12 days, 4–28 days) restored ADAMTS13 activity and organ function, compared to standard therapy ($n = 5, p < 0.05$). Similar to adult experience, TPE can replenish ADAMTS13 activity and reverse organ failure. Given the multiorgan failure and high rates of AKI, there have been developed techniques of tandem use of CRRT, plasmapheresis, and/or extracorporeal membrane oxygenation (ECMO).

Tandem plasmapheresis and continuous renal replacement therapy (*CRRT*) simultaneous use of continuous veno-venous hemodiafiltration (CVVHDF), a subtype of CRRT, and plasmapheresis in critically ill patients is a feasible process. The patient is connected to the CRRT machine through a central hemodialysis catheter with blood removed from the access line (A) and returned to the patient through the return line (R); blood from the A line of the hemodialysis catheter is directed by a stopcock to both the plasmapheresis machine and CRRT machine. Blood is returned from both CRRT and plasmapheresis machines via the return line stopcocks. Anticoagulation (usually with citrate) is given using a pump, and ionized calcium levels are closely monitored both in the CVVHDF circulation, plasmapheresis circuit, and the patient. Ten percent calcium gluconate must be infused intravenously to prevent hypocalcemia due to citrate toxicity. When TPE and CRRT are performed simultaneously through the ECMO line, additional anticoagulant is not needed since patient is already heparinized for the ECMO. Although the volume of calcium replacement is less than required with TPE using citrate anticoagulant, supplemental calcium must be administered when FFP is used as replacement solution.

13.16 Adverse Effects of TPE

In a retrospective review of 186 children receiving a total of 1632 apheresis in Canada, adverse reactions were reported in 55% of procedures in 82% of patients [11]. This incidence of pediatric adverse effects is much higher than the 4.3–28% of procedures in approximately 40% of adult patients reported in the literature.

The most frequent complications which reported included hypotension (48% of patients), hypocalcemia (28.5%), allergic reactions (5.9%), catheter-related thrombosis (12.4%), catheter-related infection (16.1%), and severe anemia (17.2%). There were two deaths (1% of patients) in this cohort [73]. Most of these adverse reactions could be prevented or at least minimized by careful planning of the procedure with emphasis on maintenance of isovolemia and critical circulating red cell mass with blood prime, prophylactic calcium infusion, and meticulous management of central venous devices. In general, apheresis procedures can be performed relatively safely in critically ill patients. Adverse reactions during therapeutic apheresis procedures may often be related to the type of anticoagulant, volume shifts, transfused blood components, underlying disease, or other physiologic disturbances.

Of those adverse effects, three types of complications are discussed because they appear to be more common and serious in children than in adults, and some are difficult to recognize at an early stage. These are hypotension, hypocalcemia, and iron deficiency anemia as a result of long-term apheresis due to chronic iatrogenic blood loss.

Hypotension Hypotension may result from various factors during the TPE, primarily secondary to hypovolemia, hypocalcemia, or vasovagal reaction. Minor symptoms of hypovolemia without changes in vital signs may get resolved if the patients head is lowered below the level of legs and trunk. The procedure should however be halted temporarily, if in case significant hypotension sets in, until the vitals have returned to normal. Hypotension should be treated by administration of normal saline bolus or colloid solution. Hypotension can be prevented in pediatric patients by careful management of intravascular volume shift. Symptomatic hypotension may occur when the extracorporeal volume is greater than 15% of TBV. When children manifest hypotension during apheresis, it is often difficult to differentiate hypotension secondary to hypovolemia, hypocalcemia, or vasovagal reaction.

Citrate Toxicity Citrate-induced hypocalcemia is often manifested as perioral tingling or numbness and parenthesis in adults; however, children rarely report these symptoms. More commonly, children experience nausea and vomiting as the first sign of citrate toxicity. Hypotension is also common with citrate toxicity. Severe hypocalcemia may be associated with frank tetany, electrocardiogram abnormalities, dysrhythmias, and decreased cardiac output. Serum ionized calcium levels should be measured before treating patients and during the procedure and with suspected reactions. Symptoms of hypocalcemia can be treated or prevented by slowing the reinfusion rate, decreasing the amount of citrate infusion by reducing the drawing flow rate, pausing the procedure, administering calcium, or using a combination of these maneuvers. Oral calcium in the form of calcium carbonate [e.g., Tums (GlaxoSmithKline, Brentford, UK) has been shown to reduce the severity of paresthesias but not the occurrence of more severe symptoms. Intravenous calcium supplementation using 10% calcium gluconate may be necessary for immediate correction of low serum ionized calcium level and severe citrate reactions. In addition, the risk of citrate toxicity potentiates with the use of a large volume of citrate blood, such as FFP, as replacement solution.

Vasovagal Reactions When children present with pallor, diaphoresis, and hypotension, vasovagal reactions must be ruled out. Vasovagal reactions are characterized by bradycardia, hypotension, diaphoresis, pallor, nausea, and apprehension. Hypotension may otherwise be caused by hypovolemia, but the two reactions can be distinguished by the pulse rate: bradycardia typically occurs in vasovagal reactions, while tachycardia occurs with hypovolemia. Vasovagal reactions are treated by pausing the procedure and placing the patient in the Trendelenburg position and distracting the child's attention from the procedure; these maneuvers usually allow resumption of the procedure.

Iron Deficiency Anemia At the end of each procedure, the contents of centrifuge need to be rinsed back to the patient. During this small amount of RBCs are left in the disposable set, known as residual RBC volume. Therefore, a long-term complication of therapeutic apheresis is chronic blood loss with repeated procedures causing iron deficiency anemia. These losses may be significant in infants and small children who require long-term apheresis; however, it may not be significant in older children requiring fewer procedures. It is advisable to monitor the patient's hematocrit levels and serum ferritin levels regularly and supplement with oral iron in the form of ferrous sulfate at 3–4 mg/kg/day when a fall in the hematocrit level greater than 5% from the baseline level.

13.17 Conclusions and Future Directions

TPE is a growing modality used in the treatment of various diseases with kidney involvement leading to improved morbidity rates and decreased mortality. It does encompass risks such as central venous line associated risks such as infections, thrombosis, and bleeding as well as removal of essential factors from the plasma which are needed for homeostasis. It is important to weigh the benefits and risks of TPE prior to initiation and tailor the treatment depending on specific targeted endpoints.

Key Learning Points

1. Apheresis is a useful and lifesaving modality in children with kidney disease.
2. TPE should be considered early in the course of the diseases where it is indicated.
3. There are various technical considerations in children which should be addressed prior to initiation.

References

1. Schwartz J, Padmanabhan A, Aqui N, et al. Guidelines on the use of therapeutic apheresis in clinical practice-evidence-based approach from the writing committee of the American society for apheresis: the seventh special issue. J Clin Apher. 2016;31(3):149–62.
2. Galacki DM. An overview of therapeutic apheresis in pediatrics. J Clin Apher. 1997;12(1):1–3.

3. Friedman D, Kim H. Apheresis (chapter 38). In: Warady B, Alexander R, Fine RN, Schaefer F, editors. Pediatric dialysis. Dordrecht: Kluwer Academic Publishers; 2004. p. 629–48.
4. Wong EC, Balogun RA. Therapeutic apheresis in pediatrics: technique adjustments, indications and nonindications, a plasma exchange focus. J Clin Apher. 2012;27(3):132–7.
5. Kim H. Therapeutic apheresis in pediatric patients. In: McLeod B, Szczepiorkowski Z, Weinstein R, Winters J, editors. Apheresis: principles and practice. 3rd ed. Bethesda: AABB Press; 2010. p. 445–64.
6. Kim H. Pediatric apheresis. In: Crookston K, editor. Therapeutic apheresis. A physician's handbook. 6th ed. Bethesda: AABB Press; 2017. p. 231–71.
7. Kim HC. Red cell exchange: special focus on sickle cell disease. Hematology Am Soc Hematol Educ Program. 2014;2014(1):450–6.
8. Eguiguren JM, Schell MJ, Crist WM, Kunkel K, Rivera GK. Complications and outcome in childhood acute lymphoblastic leukemia with hyperleukocytosis. Blood. 1992;79(4):871–5.
9. Ganzel C, Becker J, Mintz PD, Lazarus HM, Rowe JM. Hyperleukocytosis, leukostasis and leukapheresis: practice management. Blood Rev. 2012;26(3):117–22.
10. Inaba H, Fan Y, Pounds S, et al. Clinical and biologic features and treatment outcome of children with newly diagnosed acute myeloid leukemia and hyperleukocytosis. Cancer. 2008;113(3):522–9.
11. Giles FJ, Shen Y, Kantarjian HM, et al. Leukapheresis reduces early mortality in patients with acute myeloid leukemia with high white cell counts but does not improve long- term survival. Leuk Lymphoma. 2001;42(1-2):67–73.
12. Stegmayr B, Ptak J, Wikstrom B, et al. World apheresis registry 2003-2007 data. Transfus Apher Sci. 2008;39(3):247–54.
13. De Silvestro G, Tison T, Vicarioto M, Bagatella P, Stefanutti C, Marson P. The Italian registry of pediatric therapeutic apheresis: a report on activity during 2005. J Clin Apher. 2009;24(1):1–5.
14. Delaney M, Capocelli KE, Eder AF, et al. An international survey of pediatric apheresis practice. J Clin Apher. 2014;29(2):120–6.
15. Goto H, Matsuo H, Nakane S, et al. Plasmapheresis affects T helper type-1/T helper type-2 balance of circulating peripheral lymphocytes. Ther Apher. 2001;5(6):494–6.
16. Mohammad AJ, Jacobsson LT, Westman KW, Sturfelt G, Segelmark M. Incidence and survival rates in wegener's granulomatosis, microscopic polyangiitis, churg-strauss syndrome and polyarteritis nodosa. Rheumatology (Oxford). 2009;48(12):1560–5.
17. Watts RA, Al-Taiar A, Scott DG, Macgregor AJ. Prevalence and incidence of wegener's granulomatosis in the UK general practice research database. Arthritis Rheum. 2009;61(10):1412–6.
18. Kamesh L, Harper L, Savage CO. ANCA-positive vasculitis. J Am Soc Nephrol. 2002;13(7):1953–60.
19. Kouri AM, Andreoli SP. Clinical presentation and outcome of pediatric ANCA-associated glomerulonephritis. Pediatr Nephrol. 2017;32(3):449–55.
20. Stone JH, Merkel PA, Spiera R, et al. Rituximab versus cyclophosphamide for ANCA-associated vasculitis. N Engl J Med. 2010;363(3):221–32.
21. Walsh M, Catapano F, Szpirt W, et al. Plasma exchange for renal vasculitis and idiopathic rapidly progressive glomerulonephritis: a meta-analysis. Am J Kidney Dis. 2011;57(4):566–74.
22. Jayne DR, Gaskin G, Rasmussen N, et al. Randomized trial of plasma exchange or high-dosage methylprednisolone as adjunctive therapy for severe renal vasculitis. J Am Soc Nephrol. 2007;18(7):2180–8.
23. McAdoo SP, Pusey CD. Anti-glomerular basement membrane disease. Clin J Am Soc Nephrol. 2017;12(7):1162–72.
24. Lerner RA, Glassock RJ, Dixon FJ. The role of anti-glomerular basement membrane antibody in the pathogenesis of human glomerulonephritis. J Exp Med. 1967;126(6):989–1004.
25. Clark WF, Huang SS, Walsh MW, Farah M, Hildebrand AM, Sontrop JM. Plasmapheresis for the treatment of kidney diseases. Kidney Int. 2016;90(5):974–84.
26. Levy JB, Turner AN, Rees AJ, Pusey CD. Long-term outcome of anti-glomerular basement membrane antibody disease treated with plasma exchange and immunosuppression. Ann Intern Med. 2001;134(11):1033–42.
27. Bayat A, Kamperis K, Herlin T. Characteristics and outcome of goodpasture's disease in children. Clin Rheumatol. 2012;31(12):1745–51.

28. van Daalen EE, Jennette JC, McAdoo SP, et al. Predicting outcome in patients with anti-GBM glomerulonephritis. Clin J Am Soc Nephrol. 2018;13(1):63–72.
29. Hellmark T, Johansson C, Wieslander J. Characterization of anti-GBM antibodies involved in goodpasture's syndrome. Kidney Int. 1994;46(3):823–9.
30. Hellmark T, Segelmark M. Diagnosis and classification of goodpasture's disease (anti-GBM). J Autoimmun. 2014;48–49:108–12.
31. Williamson SR, Phillips CL, Andreoli SP, Nailescu C. A 25-year experience with pediatric anti-glomerular basement membrane disease. Pediatr Nephrol. 2011;26(1):85–91.
32. Johnson JP, Moore J Jr, Austin HA 3rd, Balow JE, Antonovych TT, Wilson CB. Therapy of anti-glomerular basement membrane antibody disease: analysis of prognostic significance of clinical, pathologic and treatment factors. Medicine (Baltimore). 1985;64(4):219–27.
33. Zhang YY, Tang Z, Chen DM, Gong DH, Ji DX, Liu ZH. Comparison of double filtration plasmapheresis with immunoadsorption therapy in patients with anti-glomerular basement membrane nephritis. BMC Nephrol. 2014;15:128.
34. Tonelli M, Wiebe N, Knoll G, et al. Systematic review: kidney transplantation compared with dialysis in clinically relevant outcomes. Am J Transplant. 2011;11(10):2093–109.
35. Gillen DL, Stehman-Breen CO, Smith JM, et al. Survival advantage of pediatric recipients of a first kidney transplant among children awaiting kidney transplantation. Am J Transplant. 2008;8(12):2600–6.
36. Saran R, Li Y, Robinson B, et al. US renal data system 2015 annual data report: epidemiology of kidney disease in the United States. Am J Kidney Dis. 2016;67(3 Suppl 1):Svii, S1–305.
37. Jordan SC, Vo AA, Tyan D, Nast CC, Toyoda M. Current approaches to treatment of antibody-mediated rejection. Pediatr Transplant. 2005;9(3):408–15.
38. Mohan S, Palanisamy A, Tsapepas D, et al. Donor-specific antibodies adversely affect kidney allograft outcomes. J Am Soc Nephrol. 2012;23(12):2061–71.
39. Fuchinoue S, Ishii Y, Sawada T, et al. The 5-year outcome of ABO-incompatible kidney transplantation with rituximab induction. Transplantation. 2011;91(8):853–7.
40. Genberg H, Kumlien G, Wennberg L, Berg U, Tyden G. ABO-incompatible kidney transplantation using antigen-specific immunoadsorption and rituximab: a 3-year follow-up. Transplantation. 2008;85(12):1745–54.
41. Montgomery RA, Lonze BE, King KE, et al. Desensitization in HLA-incompatible kidney recipients and survival. N Engl J Med. 2011;365(4):318–26.
42. Jordan SC, Tyan D, Stablein D, et al. Evaluation of intravenous immunoglobulin as an agent to lower allosensitization and improve transplantation in highly sensitized adult patients with end-stage renal disease: report of the NIH IG02 trial. J Am Soc Nephrol. 2004;15(12):3256–62.
43. Ejaz NS, Shields AR, Alloway RR, et al. Randomized controlled pilot study of B cell-targeted induction therapy in HLA sensitized kidney transplant recipients. Am J Transplant. 2013;13(12):3142–54.
44. Schweitzer EJ, Wilson JS, Fernandez-Vina M, et al. A high panel-reactive antibody rescue protocol for cross-match-positive live donor kidney transplants. Transplantation. 2000;70(10):1531–6.
45. Stegall MD, Gloor J, Winters JL, Moore SB, Degoey S. A comparison of plasmapheresis versus high-dose IVIG desensitization in renal allograft recipients with high levels of donor specific alloantibody. Am J Transplant. 2006;6(2):346–51.
46. Adamusiak AM, Stojanovic J, Shaw O, et al. Desensitization protocol enabling pediatric crossmatch-positive renal transplantation: successful HLA-antibody-incompatible renal transplantation of two highly sensitized children. Pediatr Nephrol. 2017;32(2):359–64.
47. Velidedeoglu E, Cavaille-Coll MW, Bala S, Belen OA, Wang Y, Albrecht R. Summary of 2017 FDA public workshop: antibody mediated rejection in kidney transplantation. Transplantation. 2018;102(6):e257–64.
48. Wan SS, Ying TD, Wyburn K, Roberts DM, Wyld M, Chadban SJ. The treatment of antibody-mediated rejection in kidney transplantation: an updated systematic review and meta-analysis. Transplantation. 2018;102(4):557–68.

49. Lefaucheur C, Nochy D, Andrade J, et al. Comparison of combination plasmapheresis/IVIg/anti-CD20 versus high-dose IVIg in the treatment of antibody-mediated rejection. Am J Transplant. 2009;9(5):1099–107.
50. Kiffel J, Rahimzada Y, Trachtman H. Focal segmental glomerulosclerosis and chronic kidney disease in pediatric patients. Adv Chronic Kidney Dis. 2011;18(5):332–8.
51. Trachtman R, Sran SS, Trachtman H. Recurrent focal segmental glomerulosclerosis after kidney transplantation. Pediatr Nephrol. 2015;30(10):1793–802.
52. Gallon L, Leventhal J, Skaro A, Kanwar Y, Alvarado A. Resolution of recurrent focal segmental glomerulosclerosis after retransplantation. N Engl J Med. 2012;366(17):1648–9.
53. Baum MA, Ho M, Stablein D, Alexander SR, North American Pediatric Renal Transplant Cooperative Study. Outcome of renal transplantation in adolescents with focal segmental glomerulosclerosis. Pediatr Transplant. 2002;6(6):488–92.
54. Garcia CD, Bittencourt VB, Tumelero A, Antonello JS, Malheiros D, Garcia VD. Plasmapheresis for recurrent posttransplant focal segmental glomerulosclerosis. Transplant Proc. 2006;38(6):1904–5.
55. Cleper R, Krause I, Bar Nathan N, et al. Focal segmental glomerulosclerosis in pediatric kidney transplantation: 30 years' experience. Clin Transpl. 2016;30(10):1324–31.
56. George JN, Nester CM. Syndromes of thrombotic microangiopathy. N Engl J Med. 2014;371(19):1847–8.
57. Jodele S, Laskin BL, Dandoy CE, et al. A new paradigm: diagnosis and management of HSCT-associated thrombotic microangiopathy as multi-system endothelial injury. Blood Rev. 2015;29(3):191–204.
58. Jodele S, Licht C, Goebel J, et al. Abnormalities in the alternative pathway of complement in children with hematopoietic stem cell transplant-associated thrombotic microangiopathy. Blood. 2013;122(12):2003–7.
59. Christidou F, Athanasiadou A, Kalogiannidis P, et al. Therapeutic plasma exchange in patients with grade 2-3 hematopoietic stem cell transplantation-associated thrombotic thrombocytopenic purpura: a ten-year experience. Ther Apher Dial. 2003;7(2):259–62.
60. Jodele S, Laskin BL, Goebel J, et al. Does early initiation of therapeutic plasma exchange improve outcome in pediatric stem cell transplant-associated thrombotic microangiopathy? Transfusion. 2013;53(3):661–7.
61. Bohl SR, Kuchenbauer F, von Harsdorf S, et al. Thrombotic microangiopathy after allogeneic stem cell transplantation: a comparison of eculizumab therapy and conventional therapy. Biol Blood Marrow Transplant. 2017;23(12):2172–7.
62. Reese JA, Muthurajah DS, Kremer Hovinga JA, Vesely SK, Terrell DR, George JN. Children and adults with thrombotic thrombocytopenic purpura associated with severe, acquired Adamts13 deficiency: comparison of incidence, demographic and clinical features. Pediatr Blood Cancer. 2013;60(10):1676–82.
63. Tsai HM, Lian EC. Antibodies to von willebrand factor-cleaving protease in acute thrombotic thrombocytopenic purpura. N Engl J Med. 1998;339(22):1585–94.
64. Sarode R, Bandarenko N, Brecher ME, et al. Thrombotic thrombocytopenic purpura: 2012 American society for apheresis (ASFA) consensus conference on classification, diagnosis, management, and future research. J Clin Apher. 2014;29(3):148–67.
65. Bell WR, Braine HG, Ness PM, Kickler TS. Improved survival in thrombotic thrombocytopenic purpura-hemolytic uremic syndrome. Clinical experience in 108 patients. N Engl J Med. 1991;325(6):398–403.
66. Dellinger RP, Levy MM, Rhodes A, et al. Surviving sepsis campaign: international guidelines for management of severe sepsis and septic shock, 2012. Intensive Care Med. 2013;39(2):165–228.
67. Wilkinson JD, Pollack MM, Glass NL, Kanter RK, Katz RW, Steinhart CM. Mortality associated with multiple organ system failure and sepsis in pediatric intensive care unit. J Pediatr. 1987;111(3):324–8.
68. Stegmayr B, Ramlow W, Balogun RA. Beyond dialysis: current and emerging blood purification techniques. Semin Dial. 2012;25(2):207–13.

69. Hamishehkar H, Beigmohammadi MT, Abdollahi M, et al. Pro-inflammatory cytokine profile of critically ill septic patients following therapeutic plasma exchange. Transfus Apher Sci. 2013;48(1):75–8.
70. Busund R, Koukline V, Utrobin U, Nedashkovsky E. Plasmapheresis in severe sepsis and septic shock: a prospective, randomised, controlled trial. Intensive Care Med. 2002;28(10):1434–9.
71. Reeves JH, Butt WW, Shann F, et al. Continuous plasmafiltration in sepsis syndrome. Plasma filtration in sepsis study group. Crit Care Med. 1999;27(10):2096–104.
72. Nguyen TC, Han YY, Kiss JE, et al. Intensive plasma exchange increases a disintegrin and metalloprotease with thrombospondin motifs-13 activity and reverses organ dysfunction in children with thrombocytopenia-associated multiple organ failure. Crit Care Med. 2008;36(10):2878–87.
73. Michon B, Moghrabi A, Winikoff R, et al. Complications of apheresis in children. Transfusion. 2007;47(10):1837–42.

Neonatal Acute Kidney Injury

14

Indrani Bhattacharjee, Marissa J. DeFreitas, Maroun Mhanna, and Carolyn Abitbol

14.1 Case Presentation

Twin girls were born at 29 weeks' gestation of a 38-year-old primigravida after in vitro fertilization. The pregnancy was uneventful until the mother developed severe hypertension (preeclampsia) with rapid deterioration in clinical status requiring emergency C-section. Twin A weighed 920 g and was limp at birth requiring stimulation, suction, and intubation. Apgar scores were 2, 4, and 8 at 1, 5, and 10 min of life, respectively. Twin B weighed 900 g and was more vigorous at birth with Apgar score of 6, 8, and 8. She was suctioned and placed on high flow oxygen and continuous positive airway pressure. The blood pressures in both infants were initially at mean arterial pressures (MAP) around 50 mmHg, but Twin A suddenly became hypotensive requiring vasopressor support. Urine output fell below 0.5 ml/kg/h for 6 h but responded well to fluid resuscitation and improvement in MAP. Both

I. Bhattacharjee
Neonatology, Case Western Reserve University, Neonatal Perinatal Medicine, MetroHealth Medical Center/Cleveland Clinic Foundation, Cleveland, OH, USA
e-mail: ibhattacharjee@metrohealth.org

M. J. DeFreitas
Clinical Pediatrics, Department of Pediatrics/Division of Pediatric Nephrology, Holtz Children's Hospital/Jackson Memorial Hospital, Miami, FL, USA
e-mail: mdefreitas@med.miami.edu

M. Mhanna
Pediatrics, Case Western Reserve University, Pediatric Critical Care and Neonatal Perinatal Medicine, MetroHealth Medical Center, Cleveland, OH, USA

C. Abitbol (✉)
Pediatrics, Pediatric Dialysis, University of Miami/Holtz Children's Hospital, Miami, FL, USA
e-mail: cabitbol@med.miami.edu

S. K. Sethi et al. (eds.), *Critical Care Pediatric Nephrology and Dialysis: A Practical Handbook*, https://doi.org/10.1007/978-981-13-2276-1_14

infants were given ampicillin and gentamycin for sepsis precautions. The initial serum creatinine (SCr) was 0.8 mg/dL (70 mM/L) in both infants. However, Twin A developed signs of sepsis and abdominal distension during the first week of life which progressed to necrotizing enterocolitis (NEC). It was treated with abdominal drains without resection. Renal function was monitored in both infants, and the progression of SCr rise and decline is pictured on the graph. Twin A's peak SCr was 1.2 mg/dL (106 mM/L), while Twin B peaked at 0.9 mg/dL (79 mM/L). The nadir at 14 days was 0.7 mg/dL (62 mM/L) for Twin A and 0.3 mg/dL (26 mM/L) for Twin B.

1. Which, if either, twin developed neonatal acute kidney injury (nAKI)?
2. By what criteria was it diagnosed?
3. Which, if either, twin needs long-term follow-up and for how long?

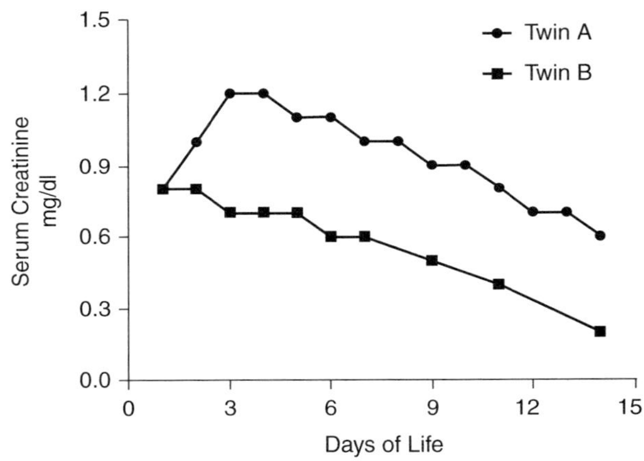

14.2 Introduction

Newborns are uniquely vulnerable to *neonatal* acute kidney injury (nAKI) due to their physiologic and developmental immaturity and their required adaptations during the transition from the intra- to extrauterine environment. The incidence of reported nAKI has varied from 16% to 40% depending on the cohort studied and the definitions applied [1–3]. The World Health Organization has recognized an urgency regarding the early identification and treatment of noncommunicable diseases including chronic kidney disease (CKD) arising from the developmental programming of infants born either preterm or small for gestational age who survive their course in the neonatal intensive care unit (NICU) [4]. With this as the impetus, the National Institutes of Health convened a workshop in April 2013 dedicated to promoting the collaboration between nephrologists and neonatologists in the study of nAKI [5, 6]. From this workshop emerged the *Neonatal Kidney Collaborative*

(NKC), an international collaboration of 24 centers of neonatologists and nephrologists [7]. The inaugural study was entitled the *AWAKEN* (Assessment of Worldwide Acute Kidney Injury Epidemiology in Neonates), a retrospective observational study of neonates across all gestational ages [7]. To date, this is the single largest cohort of neonates studied for the development of early and late nAKI. Initial reports provide important data on the incidence of nAKI, associated risks, and potential early interventions to modify the course and consequences of the disease in this vulnerable population [8, 9]. Figure 14.1 shows the distribution of nAKI in the AWAKEN population across gestational ages [8]. However, the *AWAKEN* study used an adapted SCr-based definition for nAKI that has not yet been validated. Hence, much more needs to be studied as we move forward in refining the scientific and clinical approaches to the diagnosis, management, and follow-up of infants affected by *nAKI*.

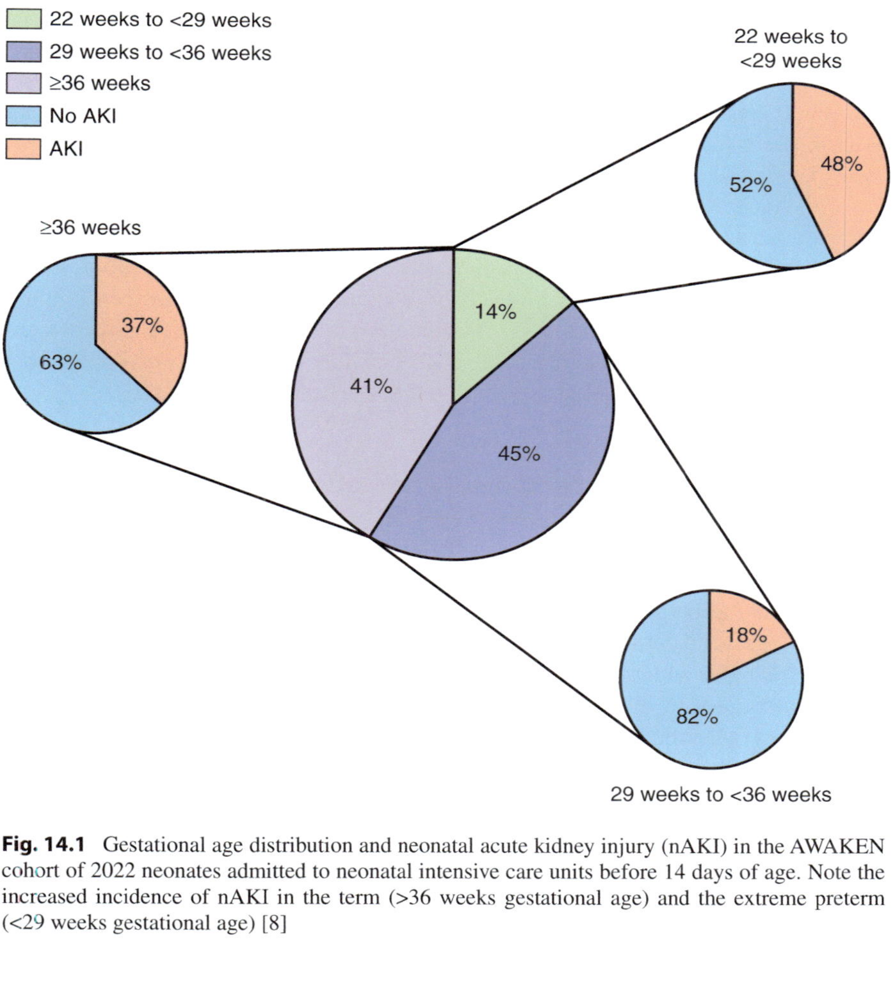

Fig. 14.1 Gestational age distribution and neonatal acute kidney injury (nAKI) in the AWAKEN cohort of 2022 neonates admitted to neonatal intensive care units before 14 days of age. Note the increased incidence of nAKI in the term (>36 weeks gestational age) and the extreme preterm (<29 weeks gestational age) [8]

14.3 Unique Developmental Physiology

The normal adaptation of the human kidneys to extrauterine life renders them vulnerable and at risk of injury in the neonatal period. Certain populations of infants, such as those born with growth restriction, preterm, and/or congenital anomalies of the kidney and urinary tract (CAKUT), are placed at the greatest risk of kidney injury due to a decreased nephron endowment and, therefore, a limited number of nephrons able to sustain the ischemic and nephrotoxic insults commonly endured in this group [10, 11]. During fetal life, the kidneys are mostly responsible for the production of amniotic fluid, while the placenta functions to maintain fluid and electrolyte homeostasis. After birth, this demand shifts, and the kidneys, which have been developing rapidly during the last trimester, begin to assume their destined functional responsibilities [11, 12].

14.3.1 Congenital Nephron Endowment

Nephrogenesis is complete by around 36 weeks' gestation, with a rapid succession of nephron generations from the corticomedullary junction extending peripherally up to the nephrogenic zone. After birth, tubular and vascular growth and interstitial tissue expansion account for progressive renal growth, and no new nephrons are formed [10–12]. Autopsy studies of postnatal nephrogenesis in preterm infants have found that extrauterine nephrogenesis was active but resulted in morphologically abnormal and nonfunctioning glomeruli [13, 14]. There is a wide normal distribution in the congenital nephron endowment, with a tenfold variance in nephron numbers ranging from approximately 200,000 to over 2 million per kidney. Epigenetic and environmental influences play a prominent role in an individual's final nephron endowment accounting for the wide normal distribution that has been described [10–15].

14.3.2 Postnatal Renal Functional Adaptation

In order to adapt to extrauterine life, renal blood flow (RBF) increases due to a decrease in renal vascular resistance (RVR). However, neonatal kidneys still only receive about 5–10% of cardiac output as compared to 20–25% in adult life. The decrease in RVR is mediated by several competing neurohumoral factors such as rising levels of the vasodilator nitric oxide and falling levels of the vasoconstrictors, angiotensin II which ultimately culminates in dilation of the renal vascular bed [10–12]. At birth, RBF is concentrated in the inner cortex and medulla with the increase in flow during maturation being directed to the outer cortical regions which places the outer cortex at higher risk of ischemic insult in the perinatal period. In addition, both the glomerular filtration rate (GFR) and renal plasma flow (RPF) are initially low due to the low renal perfusion pressure, high blood viscosity, and increased efferent arteriolar tone [11, 12]. With increasing RBF, the GFR also rises from 5 to 40 mL/min/1.73 m^2 during the first week of life to 65 mL/min/1.73 m^2 by 2 months of age and reaching adult levels of 110–120 mL/min/1.73 m^2 by 2 years of age [12]. In addition, the filtration fraction

(FF) = [GFR/RPF] gradually declines from 50% to a mature 20% once the glomerular capillary resistance decreases [11, 12]. The urinary flow rate is positively correlated with increasing GFR during the first few days of life in both term and preterm infants. Of note, the rate of increase of GFR is less in preterm than in term infants and can continue to be discrepant during the early childhood years [10–12]. At birth, immature renal tubules result in a limited urinary concentrating ability and increased fractional excretion of sodium which gradually matures with time [11].

14.4 Definition

AKI is defined as an abrupt decline in functional status of the kidneys resulting in fluid and electrolyte disturbances and retention of waste products. The *definition* of *nAKI* is elusive primarily because traditional definitions in adults and children are based on minor increases in SCr from a low baseline. This cannot be applied to neonates who are transitioning from an *elevated* SCr that may normally have an early rise and then decline depending on gestational age [15–17]. Since maternal SCr readily crosses the placenta, neonatal SCr levels reflect the *burden* of maternal SCr for the first few days after birth [18] (Fig. 14.2). Full developmental adaptation to a mature GFR of 110–120 mL/min/1.73 m^2 will not occur until 2 years of age [12, 19] (Tables 14.1 and 14.2, Fig. 14.3). As such, SCr is a suboptimal biomarker for diagnosing nAKI [12, 15–20]. Other non-traditional markers

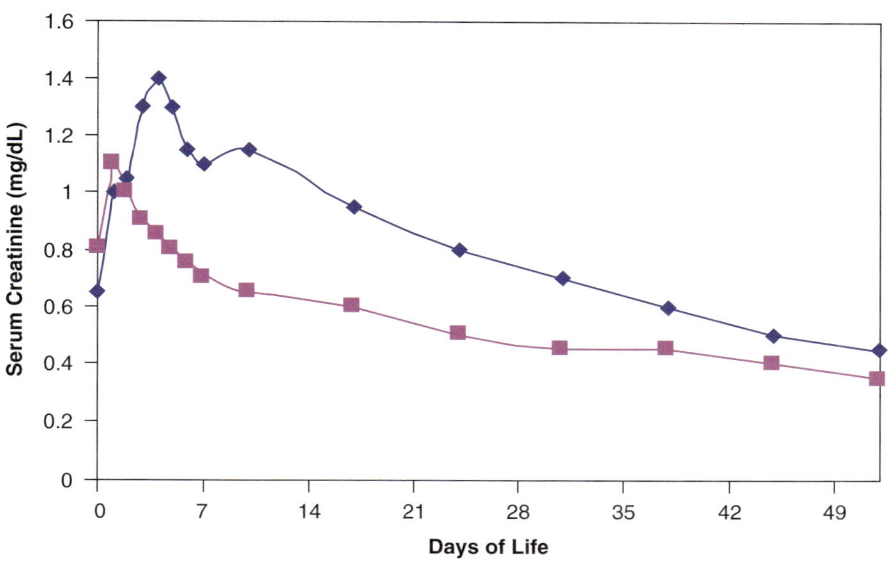

Fig. 14.2 Change in creatinine levels during the first week in preterm neonates. Note the positive change (rise) in SCr during the first 2 days of life followed by a steady decline during subsequent days which is associated with gestational age. Mean serum creatinine trends in premature infants <27 weeks' gestation (blue diamonds) and 31–32 weeks' gestation (pink squares) [16]

Table 14.1 Table of reference values and estimating equations adapted from references [17–19]

	Preterm	Term	3 MOS	6 MOS	12 MOS	24 MOS	36 MOS
SCr mg/dl	0.7 ± 0.3	0.5 ± 0.1	0.4 ± 0.2	0.3 ± 0.2	0.3 ± 0.1	0.3 ± 0.2	0.3 ± 0.2
ScysC mg/L	1.4 ± 0.2	1.3 ± 0.2	1.2 ± 0.3	1.0 ± 0.2	0.9 ± 0.2	0.7 ± 0.1	0.7 ± 0.1
GFR_{INULIN} ml/min/1.73 m^2	44 ± 9	55 ± 8	60 ± 17	87 ± 22	96 ± 12	105 ± 17	111 ± 19
$eGFR_{cr}$ ml/min/1.73 m^2	24 ± 7	46 ± 10	63 ± 8	92 ± 10	105 ± 12	120 ± 17	113 ± 10
$eGFR_{cysC}$ ml/min/1.73 m^2	46 ± 10	54 ± 8	61 ± 10	78 ± 8	92 ± 12	112 ± 10	112 ± 8
$eGFR_{TKV/cysC}$ ml/min/1.73 m^2	54 ± 8	58 ± 9	63 ± 17	75 ± 6	84 ± 20	107 ± 16	107 ± 16

None of the estimating equations have been validated in neonates

Table 14.2 Estimating equations for glomerular filtration rate in infants and children

eGFR equations (mL/min/1.73 m^2)
Creatinine and length
$eGFR_{cr} = 0.413 \times \text{Length (cm)}/SCr$
Cystatin C alone
$eGFR_{CysC} = 70.69 \times (CysC)^{-0.931}$
Total kidney volume and cystatin C
$eGFR_{TKVCysC} = [(TKV/BSA)/CysC]/1.73$
Combined equations
$eGFR = 3.98 \times (\text{Length (cm)}/Cr)^{0.456}\,(1.8/CysC)^{0.418}\,(30/BUN)^{0.079}$

SCr serum creatinine, *mg/dl* milligrams/deciliter, *CysC* serum cystatin C, *mg/L* milligrams/liter, *TKV* total kidney volume measured by ultrasound and calculated from the equation of an ellipsoid in milliliters (ml), *BSA* body surface area in square meters (m^2), GFR_{INULIN} glomerular filtration rate measured by inulin, *ml/min/1.73 m^2* milliliters/minute/1.73 meters^2, $eGFR_{cr}$ estimated GFR by creatinine, $eGFR_{CysC}$ estimated GFR by cystatin C, $eGFR_{TKV/CysC}$ estimated GFR from TKV

such as cystatin C (CysC) and beta-trace protein (BTP) have been included in estimating equations for neonatal GFR derived from clearances measured by inulin as well as iothalamate and iohexol [12, 17–19]. Ultimately, the definition of nAKI may include a combination of these alternative markers. Additionally, total kidney volume referenced to body surface area (TKV/BSA) is an important determinant of neonatal kidney function and has been incorporated into a GFR estimating equation with CysC in neonates [17–19]. This adds impetus to routinely perform renal ultrasounds on neonates to use TKV/BSA as an indirect measure of nephron endowment and baseline GFR which can be incorporated into long-term follow-up [12, 17–20]. Tables 14.1 and 14.2 and Fig. 14.3 show the progression of normal GFR from birth to 3 years of age according to SCr and CysC. Reference values are derived from the literature [12, 17–21]. The *Treiber* equation incorporating total kidney volume (TKV) referenced to body surface area (BSA) and

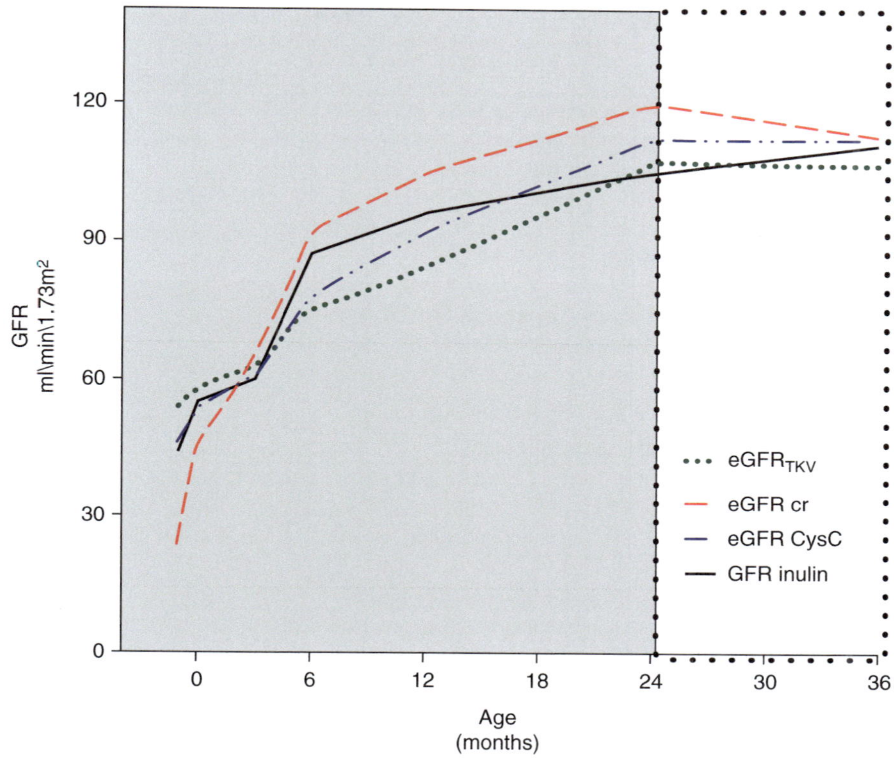

Fig. 14.3 Progression of renal function from birth as measured by inulin clearance compared to estimated glomerular filtration rates from biomarkers. Plot and comparison of the estimated glomerular filtration rates (eGFR) derived from two endogenous markers: creatinine (cr), cystatin C (CysC), and total kidney volume/body surface area (TKV/BSA) in colors against the measured inulin clearance from preterm birth through the first 36 months of life. At birth, especially in the preterm infant, eGFRcr markedly underestimates GFR-inulin, whereas GFR CysC and GFR TKV closely approximates measured or "true" GFR. After 6 months, GFRcr overestimates, and GFR CysC and GFR TKV underestimate "true" GFR. It is not until 3 years of age that all the eGFR seem to accurately assess GFR (adapted from reference [18]).

factored by CysC incorporates the important role of nephron mass on kidney function [18, 19].

With the inception of the NKC in 2014, a consensus agreement led to the adoption of the SCr-based KDIGO (Kidney Diseases: Improving Global Outcomes) definition for adults and children to be applied to neonates [3, 6–8]. This was modified empirically for the purpose of research conformity to be used in the AWAKEN trial (Table 14.3) [3, 6–8]. For the purposes of this chapter and universal applicability, we have provided an abbreviated SCr-based definition which incorporates the main components of neonatal physiologic adaptations and will earmark the great majority of neonates who experience AKI. It is derived from prior experiences in different *neonatal* cohorts and includes a rise in SCr ≥0.3 mg/

Table 14.3 Neonatal AKI KDIGO (Kidney Diseases: Improving Global Outcomes) definition [7–9]

Stage	Serum creatinine	Urine output over 24 h
0	No change in serum creatinine or rise <0.3 mg/dL	>1 mL/kg/h
1 (*risk*)	SCr rise ≥ 0.3 mg/dL within 48 h or SCr rise ≥ 1.5–1.9 × reference SCr[a] within 7 days	>0.5 and ≤0.5 mL/kg/h
2 (*injury*)	SCr rise ≥ 2–2.9 × reference SCr[a]	>0.3 and ≤0.5 mL/kg/h
3 (*failure*)	SCr rise ≥ 3 × reference SCr[a] or SCr ≥ 2.5 mg/dL[b] or receipt of dialysis	≤0.3 mL/kg/h

SCr serum creatinine
[a]Reference SCr is defined as the lowest previous SCr value
[b]SCr value of 2.5 mg/dL represents a clearance <10 mL/min/1.73m^2

Table 14.4 Short definition of neonatal acute kidney injury

Short definition of neonatal acute kidney injury	
SCr rise	Rise in SCr ≥ 0.3 mg/dL (27 mM/L)[a]
Peak SCr	Peak SCr ≥ 1.5 mg/dL (132 mM/L)[b]
Nadir SCr	Nadir SCr ≥ 0.5 mg/dL (44 mM/L)[c]

SCr serum creatinine
[a]Reference SCr is defined as the lowest previous SCr value
[b]Peak SCr is the highest SCr from baseline
[c]Nadir SCr is the lowest SCr at discharge or 30 days of age

dL (26 mM/L), a “critical” SCr ≥1.5 mg/dL (132 mM/L), and a “nadir” SCr ≥0.5 mg/dL (44 mM/L) [2, 21–23]. This may be applied during the birth hospitalization and at the time of discharge. It will capture all the stages of nAKI included in the KDIGO definition except for periods of oliguria. Ultimately, it is anticipated that the NKC will develop a prospective multicenter trial to study and validate a unique definition of *nAKI*.

Importantly, the development and application of novel biomarkers of kidney injury will allow early diagnosis of nAKI [24]. These biomarkers include CysC, neutrophil gelatinase-associated lipocalin (NGAL), kidney injury molecule 1 (KIM1), and others currently under investigation [24]. Theoretically, by detecting kidney damage early, these biomarkers may allow preventive or early interventions in neonates with impending or progressive nAKI. As promising data emerge in support of these biomarkers, more refined and early definitions of nAKI will be forthcoming (Table 14.4).

14.5 Etiologies

Neonatal AKI may occur during the prenatal, perinatal, or postnatal period and has traditionally been classified as prerenal, intrinsic, or postrenal in etiology [16, 25, 26]. Prerenal injury occurs following a decrease in effective systemic blood flow to the kidneys. Intrinsic renal injury results from injury to the renal parenchyma or

Table 14.5 Etiologies of neonatal acute kidney injury

Etiologies of neonatal AKI		
Prerenal (85%) (*Risk*)	Intrinsic (12%) (*Injury ↔ failure*)	Postrenal (obstructive) (3%) (*Failure ↔ injury*)
Volume contraction – Decreased placental perfusion – Increased insensible water losses – Increased gastrointestinal losses Hemorrhage – Fetomaternal hemorrhage – Twin-twin transfusion – Disseminated intravascular coagulation – Induced coagulopathy Hypoxia ischemia Sepsis Cardiac conditions – History of patent ductus arteriosus – Asphyxia-related cardiomyopathy – Obstructive cardiac lesions (hypoplastic left heart, coarctation of the aorta) Polycythemia	*Acute tubular necrosis* – Drug induced – Hypoxia – Contrast nephropathy – Prolonged hypoperfusion *Drugs* – Aminoglycosides – Vancomycin – Angiotensin-converting enzyme inhibitors – Acyclovir – Intravenous immunoglobulin – Albumin *Vascular* – Renal venous thrombosis – Renal artery thrombosis *Cystic renal diseases* – Multicystic dysplastic kidney – Polycystic kidney disease	*CAKUT (often with dysplasia)* *Obstructive uropathy* – Posterior urethral valves – Urethral stenosis/atresia – Ureteral pelvic or vesical junction abnormalities – Ureterocele(s) – Urogenital sinus anomaly – Calculi *Fungal balls* *Urate nephropathy*

tubules, and postrenal injury results from an obstruction to urinary flow. The distinction among the three forms is often ambiguous since the etiology of nAKI may be multifactorial progressing across stages and involving genetic and developmental alterations in function and structure. Table 14.5 summarizes the of nAKI according to these three designations. A brief synopsis of these etiologies follows.

14.5.1 Prerenal AKI

Prerenal AKI is the most common type of renal injury seen in the neonatal population. It accounts for 85% of all cases of nAKI. This phase is arguably the most urgent and actually represents the "risk" or "impending" and potentially *reversible* stage of nAKI [16, 25, 26]. Therefore, the clinical focus should be on identification, prevention, and expeditious medical intervention.

14.5.1.1 Systemic Hypoperfusion

Intravascular volume depletion is an important contributor to prerenal AKI in newborns and can result from a myriad of conditions ranging from inadequate placental transfusion to gastrointestinal and excessive insensible fluid losses in preterm infants. A relative volume contraction may occur following an increase in capillary permeability, termed "capillary leak," secondary to a cytokine-induced injury. Cytokine release is seen in inflammatory conditions such as sepsis or NEC [25–27].

14.5.1.2 Congestive Heart Failure

In conditions of hemodynamic instability such as significant patent ductus arteriosus (PDA), there may be a decrease in effective circulating blood volume, leading to a relative intravascular volume contraction and a decrease in end-organ perfusion. Other related conditions in newborn infants include myocardial injuries secondary to sepsis, myocardial ischemia secondary to hypoxic ischemic injury, and postcardiac surgery [16, 25–28]. At least 25% of infants born with obstructive cardiac conditions such as hypoplastic left heart syndrome develop nAKI [25–28].

14.5.1.3 Hypoxic Ischemic Injury

Hypoxic ischemic injury in newborn infants may result in AKI via several mechanisms bridging both prerenal and intrinsic renal injuries [16, 25–29]. Initially, systemic hypoperfusion secondary to both hypovolemia and cardiac failure results in a decrease in cardiac output leading to prerenal AKI. However, the final consequence of these two mechanisms leads to an intrinsic renal injury. Other contributing factors include a prolonged renal ischemia and tubular injury secondary to inflammatory cytokines [16, 25–28]. Vascular compromise such as renal venous thrombosis may also be a spectrum of kidney disease seen in hypoxic/ischemic renal injury.

14.5.2 Intrinsic AKI

An intrinsic renal cause is the second most common cause of *nAKI* with an incidence of 11–12% [16, 25–28]. The most common cause of intrinsic *nAKI* is acute tubular necrosis [16, 25]. Predisposing conditions to tubular injury in newborn infants include perinatal asphyxia, systemic sepsis, postcardiac surgery, prolonged prerenal injury, and nephrotoxic medication exposure. Intrinsic *nAKI* can be secondary to a vascular compromise as seen in bilateral renal venous thrombosis or renal artery thrombosis secondary to an umbilical vascular catheter with thrombotic clot embolization or extension [16, 28, 29]. Cystic renal diseases like autosomal recessive polycystic kidney disease or cystic renal dysplasia are also important causes of intrinsic AKI in newborns.

14.5.2.1 Drug Induced

Renal injury secondary to drugs could be either due to alterations in renal blood flow by drugs such as nonselective cyclooxygenase (COX) inhibitors, angiotensin-converting enzyme (ACE) inhibitors, or angiotensin 1 (AT1) receptor antagonists. NSAIDs such as indomethacin or ibuprofen interfere with renal regulation by prostaglandins. ACE inhibitors/AT1 receptor antagonists interfere with tubular regulation of sodium. Different medications are known to have different mechanisms of injury. For instance, aminoglycosides have a direct toxic effect on the tubular epithelium, and vancomycin has an oxidative injury on the proximal tubular cells. Amphotericin B directly damages renal tubules and constricts peritubular capillaries [16, 30, 31]. Acyclovir-induced toxicity is due to deposition of crystals in the tubules [16, 30, 31].

14.5.3 Postrenal AKI

Obstructive kidney injury is the least common variant of kidney injury in newborn infants accounting for 3% of all nAKI [16, 25–30]. Many of these conditions are associated with various degrees of renal dysplasia and, hence, are synonymous with *intrinsic renal* disease that leads to CKD despite early relief of obstruction.

14.6 Assessment and Management

The evaluation of nAKI should include an in-depth clinical assessment with supporting imaging and laboratory investigations to best classify the etiology of the AKI and risk for ongoing injury. Figure 14.4 outlines key steps to guide practitioners in their evaluation and management of nAKI. Once intrinsic injury has occurred, urinalysis results show granular casts and variable degrees of proteinuria. Urine osmolality and urinary sodium concentrations are affected, as the solute concentrating capacity of tubules is compromised. These changes are summarized in Table 14.6. The diagnostic utility of these urine indices is limited in preterm infants due to physiologic tubular immaturity.

Once the neonate has been evaluated fully and appropriate interventions undergone to address the AKI episode, repeat renal assessments during the NICU course are warranted as the risk for recurrent AKI and/or future risk of CKD will need to be followed. In particular, trends in renal function as assessed by eGFR by creatinine and CysC should be followed as this varies in early postnatal life as the kidneys adapt and respond to injury. Although not validated in neonates, combined (SCr + CysC) eGFR formulae have most accurately matched historical inulin clearances [18, 19]. A discharge SCr and CysC are also important to guide practitioners to trend renal function progression in early childhood until full renal maturation is achieved.

The management of nAKI should be directed at risk stratification and prevention, restoration of fluid and electrolyte balance, maintenance of hemodynamic stability, provision of adequate nutrition, avoidance of nephrotoxic exposures, and establishment of long-term follow-up (Fig. 14.4). Importantly, once nAKI is diagnosed and treated, ongoing preventive strategies should be undertaken to avoid recurrent AKI episodes. Conservative management should be the mainstay with renal replacement therapy reserved for the most critically ill patients. Dialytic interventions require skilled technical adaptations and resources. Formal renal consultation is recommended as it secures long-term follow-up of these neonates for CKD. Key considerations for correction of electrolyte abnormalities as well as available RRT options are outlined below.

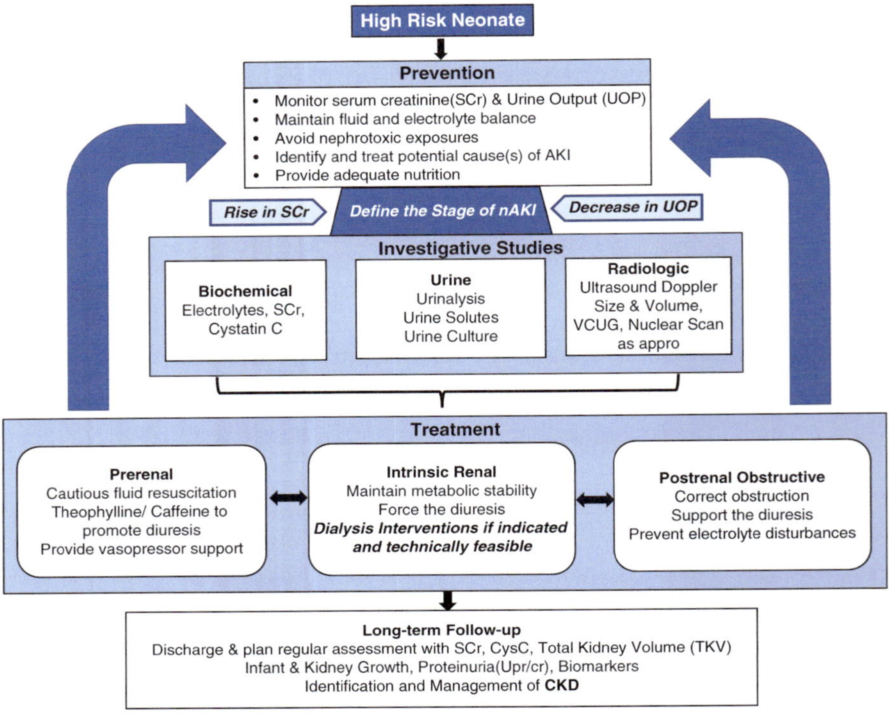

Fig. 14.4 Algorithm for the assessment and treatment of neonatal acute kidney injury (nAKI)

Table 14.6 Urinary indices in prerenal and intrinsic nAKI[a]

Parameter	Prerenal AKI	Intrinsic AKI
Urine-specific gravity	>1.020	<1.010
Urine osmolality (mOsm/L)	>400	<300
Urine/plasma osmolality ratio	>1.3	<1.0
Urinary Na (mEq/L)	<10–50	30–90
FeNa (%)	<1%	>3%
Renal failure index	<3.0	>3.0
FeUN (%)	<35%	>50%
Urine Pr/Cr (mg/mg)	<0.3	>0.6
Urine Alb/Cr (mcg/mg)	<100	>100

Fractional excretion of solute (X)%: FeX = (urine [X] × plasma [Cr])/(urine[Cr] × plasma [X]) × 100

Renal failure index (RFI): urine [Na]/(urine [Cr]/plasma [Cr])

Cr creatinine, *UN* urea nitrogen, *Na* sodium, *FeNa* fractional excretion of sodium, *FeUN* fractional excretion urea nitrogen, *Pr/Cr* protein/creatinine ratio, *Alb/Cr* albumin/creatinine ratio

[a]All of these indices are based on small sample sizes and should be used for understanding the physiologic dynamic during renal stress to support a diagnosis which is a clinical determination

14.6.1 Restore Fluid and Electrolyte Balance [15, 31]

- Correct hyponatremia *slowly* avoiding hypertonic saline. Calculate correction by 5 mEq/kg.
- Correct hypernatremia *slowly* and with enteral free water if possible.
- Correct hyperkalemia (>7.0 mM/L) *expeditiously but cautiously; then, prevent recurrence.*
  - Albuterol (beta-adrenergic agonists) by inhalation (0.4 mg in 2 mL of saline).
  - Glucose and insulin (Dextrose 10% at 5 mL/kg with regular insulin 0.1 units/kg) over 30 min.
  - Force a diuresis with theophylline (3–5 mg/kg) and furosemide (1–2 mg/kg).
  - Discontinue all potassium-containing intravenous/enteral sources.
  - Correct acidosis slowly with isotonic sodium bicarbonate solution (do not exceed 2% solution).
  - Sodium polystyrene sulfonate (SPS) (Kayexalate) preferably by pretreating the formula and avoid giving directly to the infant.
- Provide adequate nutrition with special attention to adequate provision of protein (2–4 g/kg/day).
- Avoid nephrotoxic medications.

14.6.2 Renal Replacement Therapies [15, 29, 31–33]

Renal replacement therapy (RRT) in neonates is rarely required unless there is total anuria without the possibility of reversal as in bilateral renal aplasia/dysplasia or autosomal recessive polycystic kidney disease. With rare exceptions, the natural course of neonatal kidney disease is toward the improvement in function as adaptive developmental mechanisms come into play. Even with marked elevations in SCr and metabolic disturbances, careful medical management with initiation and support of a diuresis will allow the infant to reach a "nadir SCr" and a conservative plateau in renal function that may allow a safe bridge of months or years without RRT. There are multiple reasons to avoid RRT, especially related to conserving peritoneal and vascular access for future dialysis. Those individuals requiring RRT at <1 year of age have a marked decrease in longevity, particularly those on hemodialysis. Much of this is related to loss of peritoneal and vascular access at a young age. Comorbidities also impact on the quality of life and the prognosis of infants who are initiated on RRT. Such comorbidities include pulmonary hypoplasia, other congenital anomalies including the heart and nervous system, and any disruption of the abdominal cavity such as NEC. Available resources include not only financial support but also the institutional/local availability of medical expertise and technical equipment and supplies. Despite the USA being an affluent nation, specialized equipment for the RRT of infants and small children is not FDA approved, and special adaptations need to be made to accommodate the larger machines to the small size and needs of infants. Finally, when considering the initiation of RRT in a neonate, it is imperative that ethical issues be considered for each individual infant, family, and treatment team. There are no clear choices, and it is important to include ethical discussions regarding prognosis, longevity, and quality of life. Ultimately, the treatment plan should reflect a focus in the best interest of the individual child.

The modality of choice for RRT depends on the immediate goals relative to fluid removal and metabolic and drug clearances. If feasible, the modality of choice is peritoneal dialysis since it avoids vascular access, is relatively inexpensive and safe, and can be performed manually until the infant is large enough for an automated cycling machine. If an extracorporeal modality is chosen, a blood prime of the circuit is usually required since no more than 10% of the blood volume (80–85 mL/kg) can be safely used to fill the circuit. Moreover, the preferred membrane is a polysulfone membrane since the AN69 membrane causes a "bradykinin release" syndrome with a blood prime that results in hemodynamic collapse when the acid blood reacts to the banked blood. In the USA, Dr. David Askenazi has adapted the Aquadex™, a small machine for aquapheresis, as an extracorporeal system for continuous veno-venous ultrafiltration in infants [33]. A comparison chart of available dialysis modalities with their characteristics and availability is shown in Table 14.7.

Key Points

- There is to date no validated definition of *neonatal acute kidney injury* (nAKI).
- Serum creatinine-based definitions of nAKI will vary with gestational and postnatal age.

Table 14.7 Dialysis modalities for infants and small children

Modality	Efficiency	Fluid removal	Extracorporeal volume (mL)	Availability
Peritoneal dialysis				
• Manual	+/–	+/–	0	Often
• Continuous cycling peritoneal dialysis	+/–	+/–	0	Often
• Continuous flow peritoneal dialysis	+/–	+/–	0	Rarely
Intermittent hemodialysis	+	+	120–150	Often
Continuous renal replacement therapy	+	+		
• PRISMAFLEX™				
– HF1000	+	+	175	Often
– M60[a]	+	+	125	Often
– HF20	+	+	45	Europe
• Aquadex™ adapted	+/–	+	35	Rarely
• CARPEDIEM™ (cardiac and renal pediatric dialysis emergency)	+	+	10	Europe
• NIDUS™ (Newcastle infant dialysis ultrafiltration system)	+	+	6.5	United Kingdom

[a]AN69 membrane causes bradykinin release syndrome

- Early recognition and reversal of stage 1 (Prerenal) AKI requires risk assessment and frequent monitoring of renal function and injury.
- Prevention should include avoidance of nephrotoxic exposures and early intervention for reversal of cause, i.e., relieve obstruction, treat sepsis, and support blood pressure.
- Management should be directed at conservative fluid resuscitation, maintenance of diuresis, electrolyte balance, and nutritional support.
- Dialytic interventions require specialized technical adaptations of treatment modalities and consideration of comorbidities.
- Long-term follow-up is essential to recognize and treat chronic kidney disease, a likely sequela of nAKI.

References

1. Koralkar R, Ambalavanan N, Levitan EB, McGwin G, Goldstein S, Askenazi D. Acute kidney injury reduces survival in very low birth weight infants. Pediatr Res. 2011;69:354–8.
2. Carmody JB, Swanson JR, Rhone ET, Charlton JR. Recognition and reporting of AKI in very low birth weight infants. Clin J Am Soc Nephrol. 2014;9:2036–43.
3. Selewski DT, Charlton JR, Jetton JG, Guillet R, Mhanna MJ, Askenazi DJ, Kent AL. Neonatal acute kidney injury. Pediatrics. 2015;136(2):e463–73.
4. Luyckx VA, Bertram LF, Brenner BM, Fall C, Hoy WE, Ozanne SE, Vikse BE. Effect of fetal and child health on kidney development and long-term risk of hypertension and kidney disease. Lancet. 2013;382(9888):273–83.
5. Askenazi DJ, Morgan C, Goldstein SL, Selewski DT, Moxey-Mims MM, Kimmel PL, Star RA, Higgins R, Laughon M. Strategies to improve the understanding of long-term renal consequences after neonatal acute kidney injury. Pediatr Res. 2016;79(3):502–8.
6. Zappitelli M, Ambalavanan N, Askenazi DJ, Moxey-Mims MM, Kimmel PL, Star RA, Abitbol CL, Brophy PD, Hidalgo G, Hanna M, Morgan CM, Raju TNK, Ray P, Reyes-Bou Z, Roushdi A, Goldstein SL. Developing a neonatal acute kidney injury research definition: a report from the NIDDK neonatal AKI workshop. Pediatr Res. 2017;82(4):569–73.
7. Jetton JG, Guillet R, Askenazi DJ, Dill L, Jacobs J, Kent AL, Selewski DT, Abitbol CL, Kaskel FJ, Mhanna MJ, Ambalavanan N, Charlton JR, The Neonatal Kidney Collaborative. Assessment of worldwide acute kidney injury epidemiology in neonates: design of a retrospective cohort study. Front Pediatr. 2016;4:68.
8. Jetton JG, Boohaker LJ, Sethi SK, Wazir S, Rohatgi S, Soranno D, Chishti AS, Woroniecki R, Mammen C, Swanson SR, Sridhar S, Wong CS, Kupferman JC, Griffin RL, Askenazi DJ, on behalf of the Neonatal Kidney Collaborative (NKC). Incidence and outcomes of neonatal acute kidney injury (AWAKEN): a multicentre, multinational, observational cohort study. Lancet Child Adolesc Health. 2017;1:184–94.
9. Harer MW, Askenazi DJ, Boohaker LJ, Carmody JB, Griffin RL, Guillet R, Selewski DT, Swanson JR, Charlton JR, Neonatal Kidney Collaborative (NKC). Association between early caffeine citrate administration and risk of acute kidney injury in preterm neonates: results from the AWAKEN study. JAMA Pediatr. 2018;172:e180322. https://doi.org/10.1001/jamapediatrics.2018.0322.
10. Drukker A, Guignard J. Renal aspects of the term and preterm infant: a selective update. Curr Opin Pediatr. 2002;14:175–82.
11. Rosenblum S, Pal A, Reidy K. Renal development in the fetus and premature infant. Semin Fetal Neonatal Med. 2017;22(2):58–66.
12. Rodríguez MM, Gómez AH, Abitbol CL, Chandar JJ, Duara S, Zilleruelo GE. Histomorphometric analysis of postnatal glomerulogenesis in extremely preterm infants. Pediatr Dev Pathol. 2004;7(1):17–25.

13. Sutherland MR, Gubhaju L, Moore L, Kent AL, Dahlstrom JE, Horne RS, Hoy WE, Bertram JF, Black MJ. Accelerated maturation and abnormal morphology in the preterm neonatal kidney. J Am Soc Nephrol. 2011;22(7):1365–74.
14. Choker G, Gouyon JB. Diagnosis of acute renal failure in very preterm infants. Biol Neonate. 2004;86:212–6.
15. Nada A, Bonachea EM, Askenazi DJ. Acute kidney injury in the fetus and neonate. Semin Fetal Neonatal Med. 2017;22(2):90–7.
16. Kastl JT. Renal function in the fetus and neonate – the creatinine enigma. Semin Fetal Neonatal Med. 2017;22(2):83–9.
17. Mian AN, Schwartz GJ. Measurement and estimation of glomerular filtration rate in children. Adv Chronic Kidney Dis. 2017;24(6):348–56.
18. Abitbol CL, DeFreitas MJ, Strauss J. Assessment of kidney function in preterm infants: lifelong implications. Pediatr Nephrol. 2016;31(12):2213–22.
19. Treiber M, Pecovnik Balon B, Gorenjak M. A new serum cystatin C formula for estimating glomerular filtration rate in newborns. Pediatr Nephrol. 2015;30:1297–305.
20. Bruel A, Rozé JC, Quere MP, Flamant C, Boivin M, Roussey-Kesler G, Allain-Launay E. Renal outcome in children born preterm with neonatal acute renal failure: IRENEO-a prospective controlled study. Pediatr Nephrol. 2016;31(12):2365–73.
21. Abitbol CL, Bauer CR, Montané B, Chandar J, Duara S, Zilleruelo G. Long-term follow-up of extremely low birth weight infants with neonatal renal failure. Pediatr Nephrol. 2003;18(9):887–93.
22. Weintraub AS, Connors J, Carey A, Blanco V, Green RS. The spectrum of onset of acute kidney injury in premature infants less than 30 weeks gestation. J Perinatol. 2016;36(6):474–80.
23. Askenazi DJ, Koralkar R, Patil N, Halloran B, Ambalavanan N, Griffin R. Acute kidney injury urine biomarkers in very low-birth-weight infants. Clin J Am Soc Nephrol. 2016;11(9):1527–35.
24. Tóth-Heyn P, Drukker A, Guignard JP. The stressed neonatal kidney: from pathophysiology to clinical management of neonatal vasomotor nephropathy. Pediatr Nephrol Berl Ger. 2000;14(3):227–39.
25. Gouyon JB, Guignard JP. Vasomotor kidney failure in the newborn infant. Physiopathology and treatment. Arch Fr Pediatr. 1989;46(2):137–41.
26. Criss CN, Selewski DT, Sunkara B, Gish JS, Hsieh L, Mcleod JS, et al. Acute kidney injury in necrotizing enterocolitis predicts mortality. Pediatr Nephrol Berl Ger. 2018;33(3):503–10.
27. Blinder JJ, Goldstein SL, Lee V-V, Baycroft A, Fraser CD, Nelson D, et al. Congenital heart surgery in infants: effects of acute kidney injury on outcomes. J Thorac Cardiovasc Surg. 2012;143(2):368–74.
28. Polglase GR, Ong T, Hillman NH. Cardiovascular alterations and multiorgan dysfunction after birth asphyxia. Clin Perinatol. 2016;43(3):469–83.
29. Jetton JG, Askenazi DJ. Acute kidney injury in the neonate. Clin Perinatol. 2014;41(3):487–502.
30. Fanos V, Antonucci R, Zaffanello M, Mussap M. Neonatal drug induced nephrotoxicity: old and next generation biomarkers for early detection and management of neonatal drug-induced nephrotoxicity, with special emphasis on uNGAL and on metabolomics. Curr Med Chem. 2012;19(27):4595–605.
31. Jetton JG, Sorenson M. Pharmacological management of acute kidney injury and chronic kidney disease in neonates. Semin Fetal Neonatal Med. 2017;22(2):109–15.
32. Rees L. Renal replacement therapies in neonates: issues and ethics. Semin Fetal Neonatal Med. 2017;22(2):104–8.
33. Askenazi D, Ingram D, White S, Koyner JL, Arthur JM, Shaw AD, et al. Smaller circuits for smaller patients: improving renal support therapy with Aquadex. Pediatr Nephrol. 2016;31:853e60.

15 Hemolytic Uremic Syndrome

Sidharth Kumar Sethi

Case Scenario

An 8-year-old presents to the emergency with increasing pallor and cola-colored urine since last 3 days. He has no significant past history of diarrhea or dysentery or fever. He has not passed urine since the last 12 h.

On clinical examination: He is pale, and puffy with pedal edema. His blood pressure is 130/80 mm Hg in right arm. He is conscious and alert. His systemic examination is unremarkable.

His laboratory evaluation shows:

Hemoglobin: 5 g/dl

Peripheral smear: schistocytes 5% with evidence of aniso-poikilocytosis, and reticulocytosis 7%

Total leucocyte count: 11,000

Platelet count: 20,000/mm^3

Prothrombin time and APTT: normal

Blood urea: 200 mg/dl

Serum creatinine: 8 mg/dl

LDH 10,000 IU/ml

Venous blood gas: pH 7.2; bicarbonate 16 meq/L; base excess −8 mmol/L

C3 40 mg/dl; C4 20 mg/dl

He is being planned for dialysis. You have been called for planning the definitive care for the child.

S. K. Sethi (✉)
Pediatric Nephrology and Pediatric Kidney Transplantation, Kidney and Urology Institute, Medanta, The Medicity Hospital, Gurgaon, India

Secretary, Indian Society of Pediatric Nephrology, New Delhi, India

S. K. Sethi et al. (eds.), *Critical Care Pediatric Nephrology and Dialysis: A Practical Handbook*, https://doi.org/10.1007/978-981-13-2276-1_15

15.1 Introduction

There have been major advances in the understanding of pathogenesis and management of hemolytic uremic syndrome in the last decade. Since the consensus paper published in 2009 by the European Pediatric Study Group in 2009, there have been four prospective trials and multiple case reports on effective terminal blockade with Eculizumab, an international consensus on the diagnostic and therapeutic strategies for management has been published in 2015 [1–3].

15.2 Diagnosis

A classification based on etiology and pathogenesis has been proposed as follows in Fig. 15.1. This classification includes all thrombotic microangiopathies including thrombotic thrombocytopenic purpura, hemolytic uremic syndrome (HUS), and pregnancy-associated HUS. It is important to exclude Shiga toxin producing *Escherichia coli* (STEC) before defining Atypical HUS. Thrombotic thrombocytopenic purpura (TTP) either due to deficiency or antibodies to ADAM-TS 13 enzyme requires different definite therapy. Most consensus statements define aHUS as HUS without coexisting disease or infection [1–3].

Diagnosis of Hemolytic Uremic Syndrome should be suspected in the presence of all the following features:

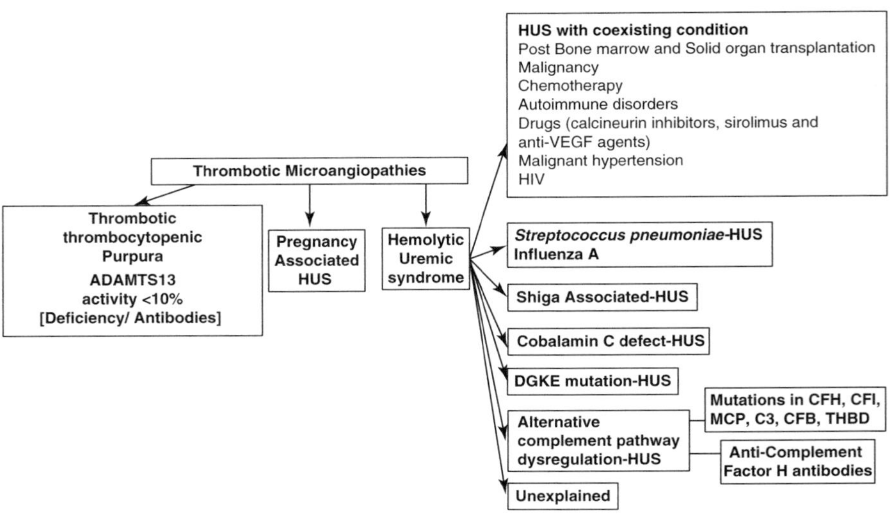

Fig. 15.1 An etiology-based classification of thrombotic microangiopathies. Adapted from Loirat et al. [3]

- Microangiopathic hemolytic anemia [hemoglobin <10 g/dl]; fragmented RBCs on peripheral smear (schistocytes >1%), and either elevated LDH or undetectable haptoglobin
- Acute kidney injury
- Thrombocytopenia [Platelets <150,000/μl]
- It is important to exclude disseminated intravascular coagulation (DIC) and thrombotic thrombocytopenic purpura (TTP), especially in setting of sepsis and malignancy as per the clinical indication

15.2.1 Infection-Associated HUS

HUS is associated with various infections including Shiga or verotoxin producing *E. coli* or *Shigella dysenteriae* type 1, invasive pneumococcal infections, and other infections including influenza A, HIV, malaria, CMV, parvovirus B19, coxsackie virus, echovirus, Epstein–Barr, salmonella, campylobacter, bartonella, dengue, and rickettsia. Hence, these infections should be borne in mind when dealing with a case of hemolytic uremic syndrome [2–4].

A probable pneumococcal HUS should be suspected especially in children more than 2 years of age, with sepsis, pneumonia, or meningitis and a positive Coombs test without disseminated intravascular coagulation. Plasma infusions/exchanges should be avoided; washed blood products and platelets should be used only if necessary.

Shiga toxin-associated *Escherichia coli* (STEC)-associated HUS should be considered in children who present with a history of bloody diarrhea in the last 2–3 weeks, or HUS occurring during a known STEC-HUS outbreak in children more than 6 months of age. All probable cases should get a rectal swab or a stool specimen as soon as possible within 6 days of diarrhea. The infection should be confirmed by any of the following: real-time PCR on fecal specimen for *stx1* and *stx2* genes; positive stool culture on MacConkey Agar (0157:H7) or other media for non-0157 serotypes and positive stool PCR; immunological tests for fecal shiga toxin, or lipopolysaccharide (LPS); elevated antibodies by ELISA to LPS of prevalent serogroups of STEC. It is important to realize that patients can have STEC-HUS in the absence of diarrhea or dysentery. Moreover, the stool excretion may be short lasting; and the referral may have been delayed and may be post-administration of antibiotics. This may hamper the yield on the stool specimens [4].

There is an association between degree of dehydration and adverse outcomes in STEC infection. Hence, it is suggested that normal hydration should be maintained in these children by early use of isotonic fluids, starting from the onset of dysentery to including the day of onset of HUS. Patients with shigella dysentery should get prompt antibiotics to reduce mortality, complications, and fecal shedding of bacteria. Ciprofloxacin has been recommended as first-line therapy by the WHO for shigellosis; second agents being cefixime and azithromycin. There is now evidence that complement is activated in acute phase of STEC infection. Hence, complement blockade with eculizumab may have a role in management of severe STEC dialysis-dependent HUS. While there is no clear benefit of routine use of eculizumab in large series from the German epidemic, few case series suggest that patients with neurological involvement may respond to timely initiation of eculizumab. Therapy with plasmapheresis or eculizumab may be considered in patients with severe neurological or cardiac manifestations, particularly STEC HUS patients with low levels of C3 or lack of recovery of renal function by 2 weeks [5–8].

15.2.2 Cobalamin [cblC] Deficiency HUS

Cobalamin deficiency-associated HUS deserves a special mention, since it may present at all ages and with different manifestations. Early recognition is important because this subset does not respond to plasma exchanges and requires specific therapy. These infants may present with failure to thrive, feeding difficulties, seizures, abnormal muscle tone, visual impairment and developmental delay, and megaloblastic anemia. Elevated blood levels of total homocysteine are characteristic of cblC deficiency. Free homocysteine levels are not required since even vitamin B12 and folate deficiency might also lead to elevated homocysteine levels. Plasma and urine methylmalonic acid (MMA) levels are usually elevated in cblC deficiency. Early treatment is recommended pending MMA levels and genetic sequencing [9].

15.2.3 Atypical HUS (aHUS)

Almost, 60–70% of children with aHUS have an identifiable mutation in the complement genes or antibodies to Factor H that leads to complement activation and thrombotic microangiopathy. Variations in six complement genes (*C3, CFH, CFI, CD46, CFB,* and *THBD*) and rearrangements of *CFHR1–5* and *CFH* are found in 19–52% of patients with aHUS. Almost all children with antibodies to complement factor H have a deficiency of complement factor H-related proteins (CFHR1 and CFHR3) due to homozygous deletions, hence MLPA should also be performed in all aHUS patients. It is important to remember that normal C3, C4, Complement Factor H and I plasma levels do not exclude a genetic defect of complement pathway, and moreover, C3 levels can be low in early phases of *Streptococcus pneumoniae* and STEC-HUS. C3 is low only in 30–40% of aHUS [10–12].

- *Recommended tests in aHUS:*
- The following are the recommended tests in all children with aHUS:
  - C3; C4; Complement Factor H; Complement Factor I; Complement Factor B
  - Anticomplement Factor H antibodies
  - MCP expression on polynuclear or mononuclear leucocytes
  - Screening for mutations using next-generation sequencing or direct sequencing Complement Factor's H; I; MCP; C3; Complement Factor B; Thrombomodulin, and DGKE

  - Screening for Complement Factor H hybrid genes and copy number variations by Multiplex ligation-dependent probe amplification (MLPA)
- *Genetic Screening*: It is recommended that all children with first episode of aHUS, especially if they do not have a causative agent, or STEC infection, or ADAMS TS 13 deficiency, or hyperhomocysteinemia or methylmalonic aciduria should get genetic screening. All children with relapsing HUS, family history, de novo or recurrent post-transplant HUS should get a genetic evaluation. Genetic characterization confirms the diagnosis, helps in management, tells about the prognosis, helps in genetic counselling of the family, and helps in taking decisions regarding kidney transplantation and strategies required during transplant in these children [10–12].

15.3 Treatment Options

- *Plasma therapies*: European Pediatric Study Group for HUS published a guideline suggesting early (within 24 h of onset) intensive plasmapheresis [2]. However, later audits showed catheter-related complications and risk of sensitization [2, 3]. Moreover, early plasmapheresis though may lead to early renal and hematological remission, these children have a poor long-term outcome in terms of proportion reaching end-stage renal disease (48% children and 67% adults reaching end-stage disease at 3 years after onset) [4]. The benefit of plasma therapy in children with DGKE mutations is uncertain.
- However in areas where Eculizumab is not available, or not affordable, the 2009 guidelines may be followed as follows:
  - Initiation of plasmapheresis 1.5 plasma volume (60–75 ml/kg) per session initiated within 24 h of diagnosis. Replace the fresh frozen plasma or Octoplas.
  - Plasmapheresis should be done daily for 5 days, then five times a week for 2 weeks, and then three times a week for another 2 weeks.
- *Eculizumab*: Eculizumab is a monoclonal humanized anti-C5 antibody. It prevents the cleavage of C5 and blocks the pro-inflammatory C5a and pro-thrombotic complement activation of C5b-9. It has been approved for aHUS in the European Union and the USA. It has been following excellent results of four prospective, open-label, single arm trials done by the Alexion Pharmaceuticals. The four trials included adults/adolescents with progressive thrombotic microangiopathy despite plasma exchanges and plasma infusion, adults/adolescents with long disease duration and chronic kidney disease under long-term plasma exchanges and plasma infusions, children with early initiation, and adults with early initiation.

Recommended dosing duration is indicated in Table 15.1.

For children who present with clinical diagnosis of aHUS, eculizumab should be initiated without any delay within 24–48 h of onset. It also avoids the needs of central venous double-lumen catheter and plasma-related complications. In the absence

Table 15.1 Recommended eculizumab dosing regimen for patients with atypical HUS (aHUS)

Patient body weight	Induction regimen	Maintenance regimen
40 kg and over	900 mg weekly × 4 doses	1200 mg at week 5; then 1200 mg every 2 weeks
30 kg to less than 40 kg	600 mg weekly × 2 doses	900 mg at week 3; then 900 mg every 2 weeks
20 kg to less than 30 kg	600 mg weekly × 2 doses	600 mg at week 3; then 600 mg every 2 weeks
10 kg to less than 20 kg	600 mg weekly × 1 dose	300 mg at week 2; then 300 mg every 2 weeks
5 kg to less than 10 kg	300 mg weekly × 1 dose	300 mg at week 2; then 300 mg every 3 weeks

of availability of eculizumab, plasma exchanges should be initiated as highlighted above. There are also reports on early switch from plasma therapy to eculizumab that may help in full renal recovery.

Confirmation of a complement mutation is not required for initiation of therapy. Anticomplement factor H antibody titer should also be sent at onset, since positive titer will require immunosuppressive therapy initiation.

It is mandatory to administer meningococcal vaccine and antibiotic prophylaxis before eculizumab therapy. Tetravalent vaccine against serotypes A, C, W135, and Y is available; however, it does not protect against serotype B. Methylpenicillin, given twice daily, remains the drug of choice for antibiotic prophylaxis. Macrolides may be given in cases of penicillin allergy. Antibiotic prophylaxis should be given during 2 weeks after the vaccination in patients receiving eculizumab. However, most of the clinicians believe in giving continuous antibiotic prophylaxis. It is important for clinicians to educate the parents regarding early recognition and treatment of meningococcal infections [10–12].

15.4 Anticomplement Factor H Antibodies aHUS

Antibodies to Factor H-related HUS appear to an important subset of patients since these patients have excellent results with a combination of plasmapheresis and immunosuppression. American Society of Apheresis assigns level I category for plasmapheresis for this subset, implying the efficacy of the plasmapheresis to remove these antibodies well. The international consensus recommends to give eculizumab along with the combination therapy since it may help in acute complement blockage, especially in severe acute injury of vital organs, e.g., heart and brain.

The anti-factor H-associated HUS is strongly associated with a polymorphism: an 84-kb homozygous deletion of the CFHR1 gene in around 90% patients. Multiplex ligation-dependent probe amplification (MLPA) or end-point PCR is useful in confirming the CFHR1 deletion. It is suggested to evaluate for copy number variation/hybrid genes in CFH and CFHR1–5 region by multiplex ligation-dependent probe amplification (MLPA) or detection of CFHR1 deletion in these patients [10–13].

The international consensus recommends the following induction regimen:

- Anti-factor H antibodies with mild or no extra renal manifestations: Two approaches can be followed:
  - Consider eculizumab, along with adding steroids and mycophenolate as immunosuppression.
  - Switch these patients to maintenance plasmapheresis with monthly cyclophosphamide pulses (total 5–6) or rituximab with steroids.
- Anti-factor H antibodies with severe extra renal manifestations: Combining eculizumab, plasmapheresis with immunosuppression of cyclophosphamide pulses or rituximab and steroids.

Plasmapheresis or eculizumab can be stopped once the titer reaches less than 1000 AU/ml. Maintenance immunosuppression is recommended to consist of prednisolone in tapering doses and mycophenolate mofetil. It can be stopped after 1 year in stable patients with hematological remission and titer less than 1000 AU/ml and normal C3. Antibodies to factor H titer should be monitored closely, at weekly intervals in the first month, and then preferably at 3–6 months thereafter during the first 12–24 months of illness [10–13].

15.5 Conclusions

With better understanding, there are now better available drugs targeting complement in these patients, with better outcomes. However, there is a lot of geographical disparity in availability and affordability of these drugs, and there is a need for more trials especially looking at newer blockers, and also safe withdrawal of treatment in these patients.

References

1. Kidney Disease Outcomes Quality Initiative. Kidney Disease Improving Global Outcomes (KDIGO) clinical practice guideline for acute kidney injury. Kidney Int Suppl. 2012;2:19–36.
2. Ariceta G, Besbas N, Johnson S, Karpman D, Landau D, Licht C, Loirat C, Pecoraro C, Taylor CM, Van de Kar N, Vandewalle J, Zimmerhackl LB, European Paediatric Study Group for HUS. Guideline for the investigation and initial therapy of diarrhea-negative hemolytic uremic syndrome. Pediatr Nephrol. 2009;24(4):687–96.
3. Loirat C, Fakhouri F, Ariceta G, Besbas N, Bitzan M, Bjerre A, Coppo R, Emma F, Johnson S, Karpman D, Landau D, Langman CB, Lapeyraque AL, Licht C, Nester C, Pecoraro C, Riedl M, van de Kar NC, Van de Walle J, Vivarelli M, Frémeaux-Bacchi V, HUS International. An international consensus approach to the management of atypical hemolytic uremic syndrome in children. Pediatr Nephrol. 2016;31(1):15–39.
4. Mody RK, Gu W, Griffin PM, Jones TF, Rounds J, Shiferaw B, Tobin-D'Angelo M, Smith G, Spina N, Hurd S, Lathrop S, Palmer A, Boothe E, Luna-Gierke RE, Hoekstra RM. Postdiarrheal

hemolytic uremic syndrome in United States children: clinical spectrum and predictors of in-hospital death. J Pediatr. 2015;166:1022–9.
5. Agger M, Scheutz F, Villumsen S, Mølbak K, Petersen AM. Antibiotic treatment of verocytotoxin-producing Escherichia coli (VTEC) infection: a systematic review and a proposal. J Antimicrob Chemother. 2015;70:2440–6.
6. Freedman SB, Xie J, Neufeld MS, Hamilton WL, Hartling L, Tarr PI, Alberta Provincial Pediatric Enteric Infection Team, Nettel-Aguirre A, Chuck A, Lee B, Johnson D, Currie G, Talbot J, Jiang J, Dickinson J, Kellner J, MacDonald J, Svenson L, Chui L, Louie M, Lavoie M, Eltorki M, Vanderkooi O, Tellier R, Ali S, Drews S, Graham T, Pang XL. Shiga toxin-producing escherichia coli infection, antibiotics, and risk of developing hemolytic uremic syndrome: a meta-analysis. Clin Infect Dis. 2016;62:1251–8.
7. Kielstein JT, Beutel G, Fleig S, Steinhoff J, Meyer TN, Hafer C, Kuhlmann U, Bramstedt J, Panzer U, Vischedyk M, Busch V, Ries W, Mitzner S, Mees S, Stracke S, Nurnberger J, Gerke P, Wiesner M, Sucke B, Abu-Tair M, Kribben A, Klause N, Schindler R, Merkel F, Schnatter S, Dorresteijn EM, Samuelsson O, Brunkhorst R, Collaborators of the DS-HUSr. Best supportive care and therapeutic plasma exchange with or without eculizumab in Shiga-toxin-producing E. coli O104:H4 induced haemolytic-uraemic syndrome: an analysis of the German STEC-HUS registry. Nephrol Dial Transplant. 2012;27:3807–15.
8. Pape L, Hartmann H, Bange FC, Suerbaum S, Bueltmann E, Ahlenstiel-Grunow T. Eculizumab in typical hemolytic uremic syndrome (HUS) with neurological involvement. Medicine (Baltimore). 2015;94:e1000.
9. Huemer M, Diodato D, Schwahn B, Schiff M, Bandeira A, Benoist JF, Burlina A, Cerone R, Couce ML, Garcia-Cazorla A, la Marca G, Pasquini E, Vilarinho L, Weisfeld-Adams JD, Kozich V, Blom H, Baumgartner MR, Dionisi-Vici C. Guidelines for diagnosis and management of the cobalamin-related remethylation disorders cblC, cblD, cblE, cblF, cblG, cblJ and MTHFR deficiency. J Inherit Metab Dis. 2017;40:21–48.
10. Johnson S, Stojanovic J, Ariceta G, Bitzan M, Besbas N, Frieling M, Karpman D, Landau D, Langman C, Licht C, Pecoraro C, Riedl M, Siomou E, van de Kar N, Walle JV, Loirat C, Taylor CM. An audit analysis of a guideline for the investigation and initial therapy of diarrhea negative (atypical) hemolytic uremic syndrome. Pediatr Nephrol. 2014;29(10):1967–78.
11. Noris M, Caprioli J, Bresin E, Mossali C, Pianetti G, Gamba S, Daina E, Fenili C, Castelletti F, Sorosina A, Piras R, Donadelli R, Maranta R, van der Meer I, Conway EM, Zipfel PF, Goodship TH, Remuzzi G. Relative role of genetic complement abnormalities in sporadic and familial aHUS and their impact on clinical phenotype. Clin J Am Soc Nephrol. 2010;5(10):1844–59.
12. Durey MA, Sinha A, Togarsimalemath SK, Bagga A. Anti-complement-factor H-associated glomerulopathies. Nat Rev Nephrol. 2016;12(9):563–78.
13. Sinha A, Gulati A, Saini S, Blanc C, Gupta A, Gurjar BS, Saini H, Kotresh ST, Ali U, Bhatia D, Ohri A, Kumar M, Agarwal I, Gulati S, Anand K, Vijayakumar M, Sinha R, Sethi S, Salmona M, George A, Bal V, Singh G, Dinda AK, Hari P, Rath S, Dragon-Durey MA, Bagga A, Indian HUS Registry. Prompt plasma exchanges and immunosuppressive treatment improves the outcomes of anti-factor H autoantibody-associated hemolytic uremic syndrome in children. Kidney Int. 2014;85(5):1151–60. https://doi.org/10.1038/ki.2013.373.

Rapidly Progressive Glomerulonephritis 16

Arvind Bagga and Shina Menon

16.1 Clinical Case

A 5-year-old girl presented to the emergency room with history of dark-colored urine for 2 days. There was history of intermittent low-grade fever and cough for the past 1 week. She had an erythematous reticular rash on the abdomen, noticed on the day of presentation. She has had decreased energy. There was no history of edema, no joint pain or swelling, and no noticeable decrease in urine output. There was no history of hemoptysis.

On examination her weight was 19.9 kg. She was afebrile and had heart rate of 107/min, blood pressure 100/48 mmHg, and respiratory rate 18/min. The erythematous, nonblanching, maculopapular rash was prominent on the chest and abdomen but also seen on the face, ears, and legs. The heart sounds were normal, with a grade 2/6 ejection systolic murmur heard best at the left lower sternal border. The lungs were clear to auscultation without any adventitious sounds. The abdomen was soft, nontender, nondistended, and had no organomegaly. Extremities were warm and well perfused without signs of edema. She had no significant neurologic deficit.

Blood levels of sodium were 130 mEq/L, potassium 5.6 mEq/L, chloride 103 mEq/L, bicarbonate 16 mEq/L, urea 120 mg/dL, creatinine 3.6 mg/dL, lactate dehydrogenase 782 U/L (normal 380–860), and albumin 3.4 g/dL. The hemoglobin level was 7.1 g/dL, hematocrit 22.6, leukocyte count 8200/cu mm with 75% neutrophils and 18% lymphocytes, and platelets 296,000/cu mm. Urinalysis showed

A. Bagga (✉)
Division of Nephrology, ICMR Advanced Center for Research in Nephrology, All India Institute of Medical Sciences, New Delhi, India

S. Menon
Division of Nephrology, Seattle Children's Hospital, University of Washington School of Medicine, Seattle, WA, USA

S. K. Sethi et al. (eds.), *Critical Care Pediatric Nephrology and Dialysis: A Practical Handbook*, https://doi.org/10.1007/978-981-13-2276-1_16

specific gravity of 1.010, pH 5.51, protein 2+, and blood 3+; there were 50–70 red cells and 3–5 leukocytes per high-power field. There were numerous granular casts and few red cell casts. Complement 3 level was 144 (normal 83–203) mg/dL and C4 10 (16–52) mg/dL. Antinuclear antibodies (ANA) were positive at a titer of 1:80; anti-double-stranded DNA was negative, and antineutrophil cytoplasmic antibodies (ANCA) were positive at 1:640, with perinuclear distribution. Antimyeloperoxidase (MPO) ANCA was 354 (normal <120) U/mL, and antiproteinase-3 (PR3) was 16 (normal <120) U/mL.

Chest CT scan showed multiple nodular opacities with surrounding halos of ground glass attenuation. Kidney biopsy showed 55 glomeruli with 50% cellular crescents and 30% fibrous, majority circumferential. There was diffuse mesangial hypercellularity and intense interstitial inflammation with lymphocytes and plasma cells, mild interstitial fibrosis, and tubular atrophy. Immunofluorescence was negative for all immunoglobulins and complement.

A diagnosis of rapidly progressive glomerulonephritis with microscopic polyangiitis was made. The patient was treated with six IV pulses of methylprednisolone, followed by oral prednisone and intravenous cyclophosphamide. In view of the pulmonary findings, she also received seven sessions of plasmapheresis.

Rapidly progressive glomerulonephritis (RPGN) is characterized by clinical features of glomerulonephritis (GN) and progressive loss of renal function. Crescentic extracapillary proliferation in the Bowman space affecting the majority of glomeruli is seen on histopathologic examination. Similar clinical phenotype may be seen in other conditions including poststreptococcal GN, renal vasculitis, immunoglobulin A (IgA) nephropathy, systemic lupus erythematosus (SLE), and C3 glomerulopathy [1, 2]. Prompt evaluation and specific therapy are necessary to prevent irreversible loss of renal function.

16.2 Definition

RPGN is a clinical syndrome characterized by an acute nephritic illness and progressive loss of renal function (more than 50% decrease in estimated glomerular filtration rate, eGFR) over days to weeks [1]. On histopathology, the characteristic feature is the presence of crescents (crescentic GN) involving more than half of the glomeruli. The presence of crescents is an indicator of severe glomerular injury, and there is a startling correlation between the severity of clinical features and the proportion of glomeruli that show crescents. The presence of circumferential crescents involving more than 80% of glomeruli is often associated with advanced acute kidney injury. On the other end, those with non-circumferential crescents in less than 50% of glomeruli tend to have an indolent course.

While the terms RPGN and crescentic GN are used interchangeably, certain conditions including hemolytic uremic syndrome (HUS), diffuse proliferative GN, and acute interstitial nephritis may present with a similar rapidly progressive course and not show any crescents on histology. Table 16.1 lists common conditions that present with RPGN in childhood.

Table 16.1 Causes of rapidly progressive glomerulonephritis (RPGN)

Immune complex GN
Postinfectious GN. Poststreptococcal nephritis, infective endocarditis, shunt nephritis, staphylococcal sepsis
Other infections. HIV, hepatitis B and C, syphilis
Systemic disease. Systemic lupus erythematosus, Henoch-Schonlein purpura, cryoglobulinemia, mixed connective tissue disorder, juvenile rheumatoid arthritis
Primary GN. IgA nephropathy, MPGN, membranous nephropathy, C1q nephropathy
Pauci-immune crescentic GN
Microscopic polyangiitis, granulomatosis with polyangiitis (Wegener's granulomatosis), renal-limited vasculitis, eosinophilic granulomatosis with polyangiitis (Churg-Strauss disease)
Idiopathic crescentic GN
Drug-induced: Penicillamine, hydralazine, propylthiouracil
Anti-glomerular basement membrane GN
Anti-GBM nephritis, Goodpasture syndrome, post-renal transplantation in Alport syndrome
Post-renal transplantation
Recurrence of IgA nephropathy, Henoch-Schonlein purpura, MPGN, systemic lupus
RPGN without crescents
Hemolytic uremic syndrome
Acute interstitial nephritis
Diffuse proliferative GN

GN glomerulonephritis, *MPGN* membranoproliferative GN, *GBM* glomerular basement membrane, *HIV* human immunodeficiency virus

16.3 Causes

Crescentic GN is classified based on histopathology and immunofluorescence staining patterns. These categories reflect different mechanisms of glomerular injury.

Immune complex GN is a heterogeneous group that includes conditions in which multiple stimuli lead to crescentic proliferative GN. On immunohistology, there are granular deposits of immunoglobulin and complement along capillary walls and in the mesangium. This can be seen secondary to infections, systemic diseases, and preexisting primary GN [1].

1. Infections: Visceral abscesses, infective endocarditis, and infected atrioventricular shunts can occasionally present with crescentic GN. It can also be seen secondary to infections with hepatitis B and C viruses, methicillin-resistant *Staphylococcus aureus*, leprosy, and syphilis [3, 4]. Occasionally, crescentic histology may also be seen in poststreptococcal GN. Although most patients with poststreptococcal GN recover completely, those with nephrotic range proteinuria, sustained hypertension, and large number of crescents may have a complicated course and an unsatisfactory outcome.
2. Systemic immune complex disease: SLE with class IV and less commonly class III nephritis can present as crescentic GN. Rarely, it may also be seen in Henoch-Schonlein purpura.

3. Primary GN: Occasionally seen in membranoproliferative GN (MPGN), IgA nephropathy, and rarely membranous nephropathy [3–5].

Pauci-immune GN is characterized by few or no immune deposits on immunofluorescence microscopy and is chiefly associated with systemic vasculitis [2]. This includes conditions like granulomatosis with polyangiitis (GPA), renal-limited vasculitis, microscopic polyangiitis (MPA) with renal manifestations, or eosinophilic granulomatosis with polyangiitis. It is characterized by antineutrophil cytoplasmic autoantibodies (ANCA) in the blood in the vast majority (80%), and the conditions are collectively classified as ANCA-associated vasculitides. Certain drugs like penicillamine, propylthiouracil, minocycline, and hydralazine can induce ANCA-positive disease [6]. A smaller subset (approximately 10–30%) of patients with pauci-immune crescentic GN do not have ANCA [7]. These patients may have a different pathophysiological basis for their disease as suggested by the presence of fewer constitutional and extrarenal symptoms and different outcomes than those who are ANCA-positive.

Anti-glomerular basement membrane (GBM) GN is rare in childhood, accounting for fewer than 10% of cases. It is characterized by linear deposition of anti-GBM antibodies that are directed against the alpha-3 chain of type IV collagen (Goodpasture antigen). These patients present with pulmonary hemorrhage and hemoptysis, due to cross-reaction of the antibodies with alveolar basement membrane components; pulmonary involvement (Goodpasture syndrome) is rare in childhood. Up to 5% of patients with Alport syndrome who undergo a kidney transplant may have anti-GBM autoantibodies and anti-GBM nephritis. This is typically seen within the first year following the transplant. However, patients with post-transplant anti-GBM nephritis do not have pulmonary hemorrhage (unlike de novo anti-GBM nephritis) because the patient's lung tissue does not contain the putative antigen. The risk of post transplantation anti-GBM nephritis is low in subjects with normal hearing, late progression to end-stage renal disease, or females with X-linked Alport syndrome.

Idiopathic RPGN includes patients with immune complex crescentic GN who do not fit into any identifiable category and those with ANCA-negative pauci-immune disease.

16.4 Epidemiology

There is insufficient data on incidence of RPGN in children. Crescentic GN has been reported in up to 5% of unselected renal biopsies in children. According to the NAPRTCS Annual Transplant Report, ~1.5–1.7% of all pediatric transplants are secondary to idiopathic crescentic GN. This figure, however, underestimates the true prevalence since other conditions, including MPGN (2.5%), SLE (1.5%), other systemic immune disorders (0.3%), GPA (0.6%), chronic GN (3.2%), and IgA nephropathy (2.4%), might also present as RPGN.

Immune complex GN accounts for ~70% of cases and is the most common pattern of crescentic GN in children [8]. Pauci-immune crescentic GN accounts for

~20–25% cases and is less frequent in children, unlike adults. Recent reports from tertiary care centers emphasize the increasing proportion of patients with pauci-immune disease [8, 9].

16.5 Clinical Features

The spectrum of presenting features in RPGN is variable. Common clinical features include macroscopic hematuria, oliguria, hypertension, and edema. It may occasionally have an insidious presentation with fatigue or edema. Some patients may have symptoms involving other organ systems including the skin (vasculitic rash), the upper respiratory tract (cough, sinusitis), the nervous system (seizures, altered sensorium), and the musculoskeletal system (joint pain, swelling). Hemoptysis and less commonly pulmonary hemorrhage may be seen in patients with anti-GBM disease. These symptoms may also be seen in GPA, SLE, and severe GN with pulmonary edema.

Detailed history and physical examination help with formulating a differential diagnosis and guide subsequent evaluation. The examination should focus on corroborating the history and screening for complications. Chief clinical features screened for include fever, malar rash, joint swelling, and oral ulcers (SLE); palpable purpura and joint pain/swelling (HSP); cough/sinus symptoms (vasculitides); bloody diarrhea and pallor (HUS); shortness of breath, rales, and S3 gallop (congestive heart failure, pulmonary hemorrhage); and hemoptysis. History is taken for change in urine color and volume, including gross hematuria (tea- or cola-colored urine) and oliguria.

16.6 Evaluation and Diagnosis

Early and accurate diagnosis is important, and delay in instituting therapy increases the risk of irreversible disease. It is important to follow a rational approach toward diagnosis and management. The diagnosis of the etiology depends on integrating clinical data with serology and renal histology. All patients should undergo the following evaluation:

1. Complete blood counts, peripheral smear for type of anemia, reticulocyte count, and erythrocyte sedimentation rate.
2. Blood levels of urea, creatinine, and electrolytes.
3. Urinalysis: proteinuria, microscopy for erythrocytes and leukocytes, and casts.
4. Complement levels (C3, C4, CH50): low total hemolytic complement (CH50) and C3 are seen in postinfectious GN, SLE, and MPGN. In addition, patients with SLE and type 1 MPGN also have low C4 due to activation of the classic complement pathway.
5. Antistreptolysin O (ASO), antinuclear antibody, anti-double-stranded DNA antibodies: ASO may be elevated in poststreptococcal GN. The latter two are seen in patients with SLE.
6. Antinuclear cytoplasmic antibodies (ANCA): ANCA is elevated in most patients with pauci-immune crescentic GN. ANCA screening can be done by indirect

immunofluorescence for the staining pattern and by enzyme-linked immunosorbent assay (ELISA) for specificity against proteinase-3 (PR3) and myeloperoxidase (MPO) [10]. A recent consensus statement on ANCA testing recommends initial testing by ELISA for PR3 ANCA and MPO ANCA in lieu of immunofluorescence [11]. Granulomatosis with polyangiitis is associated with PR3 ANCA, which produces a cytoplasmic pattern (c-ANCA). MPO ANCA, with perinuclear staining (p-ANCA), is seen in renal-limited vasculitis and drug-induced crescentic GN. Patients with microscopic polyangiitis have equal distribution of both types of ANCA. Ten percent of patients with GPA or MPA are ANCA-negative.

7. Kidney biopsy: The tissue should be sent for light microscopy, immunofluorescence, and electron microscopy.

A subset of patients needs additional evaluation based on their clinical features, including:

(a) Anti-GBM IgG antibodies: They are seen in anti-GBM nephritis or Goodpasture syndrome and correlate with disease activity.
(b) Blood levels of cryoglobulin.
(c) Hepatitis B and C serology.
(d) Chest radiograph, computed tomography (CT) scans in patients with suspected vasculitides and Goodpasture syndrome.
(e) Sinus radiograph, CT scans in patients with suspected granulomatosis with polyangiitis.

Figure 16.1 shows the classification of crescentic GN based on the clinical features, serology and histological findings.

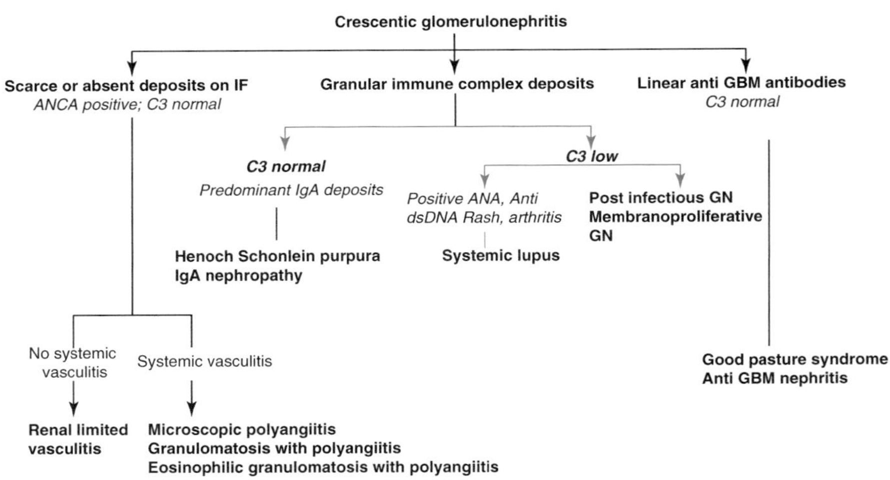

Fig. 16.1 Diagnostic evaluation of crescentic glomerulonephritis, based on renal histology and serological findings

16.6.1 Renal Histopathology

Various forms of crescentic GN present with similar histology. The defining feature is the presence of crescents, which is defined as an accumulation of two or more layers of cells that partially or completely fill the Bowman space. They may be completely cellular or show varying degrees of scarring and fibrosis. Cellular crescents demonstrate proliferation of neutrophils, macrophages, and epithelial cells (Fig. 16.2). In fibrous crescents, the cells are replaced by collagen. Fibrocellular crescents show features of both. The interstitium may show a range of changes from an acute inflammation to chronic interstitial scarring, fibrosis, and tubular atrophy. Compression of the glomerular capillary loop by the crescent can lead to ischemic changes in the tubules that derive their blood flow from that efferent arteriole.

Vasculitis is often characterized by episodic inflammation as evidenced by crescents in various stages of progression [12]. Early lesions may have segmental fibrinoid necrosis with or without an adjacent crescent. In biopsies with severe acute lesions, there may be focal or diffuse necrosis along with circumferential crescents.

The presence, location, and nature of immune deposits assist in determining the cause of crescentic GN. IgA nephropathy and HSP have mesangial deposits of IgA; postinfectious GN is characterized by granular, subepithelial deposits of IgG and C3; MPGN presents with mesangial, subendothelial, and intramembranous deposits of both IgG and C3; SLE shows "full house" capillary wall and mesangial deposits of granular IgG, IgA, IgM, C3, C4, and C1q. Patients with vasculitis, both with and without ANCA positivity, typically have few or no immune deposits in the glomeruli. Anti-GBM disease is characterized by linear staining of the GBM with IgG (rarely IgM and IgA) and C3.

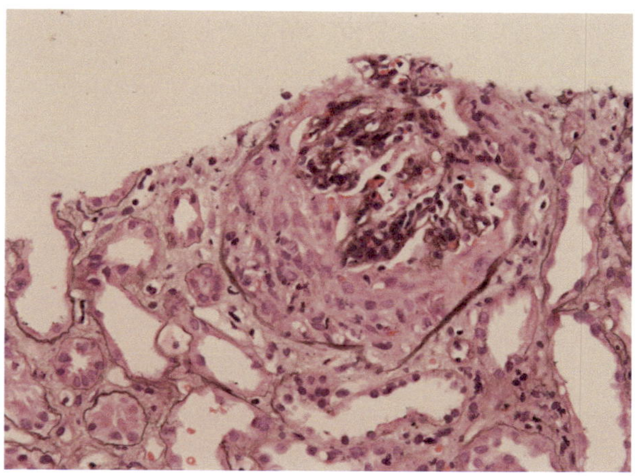

Fig. 16.2 Cellular crescent compressing the glomerular tuft. Silver methenamine stain ×800

16.7 Treatment

The heterogeneous presentation and unsatisfactory outcome associated with RPGN have given rise to a multitude of immunosuppression-based treatment regimens [13, 14]. There is limited evidence-based data, and treatment guidelines for children are derived from information from case series and prospective studies in adult patients. Supportive management includes maintenance of fluid and electrolyte balance, providing adequate nutrition, and control of infections and hypertension.

Specific treatment of RPGN comprises two phases: *induction* of remission and *maintenance* (Table 16.2). The goal of the induction phase is to control inflammation and the associated immune response. It typically includes high-dose steroids and cyclophosphamide, with additional therapy for those with life- or organ-threatening disease. Both IV and oral cyclophosphamide have been used, although IV therapy is more likely to induce remission and has a lower risk of infection and leukopenia.

Prospective studies show that B-cell depletion with multiple doses of rituximab (RTX) is an effective and safe treatment option for patients with ANCA-associated disease [15, 16]. For such patients, RTX is currently recommended as an alternative to IV cyclophosphamide for remission induction. RTX may be preferred in patients where cyclophosphamide is contraindicated or not preferred due to fertility or other concerns, or in those with relapsing disease. RTX is administered initially in 2–4

Table 16.2 Treatment of crescentic glomerulonephritis

Induction
Methylprednisolone 15–20 mg/kg (maximum 1 g) IV daily for 3–6 doses
Prednisolone 1.5–2 mg/kg/day PO for 4 weeks; taper to 0.5 mg/kg daily by 3 months; 0.5–1 mg/kg on alternate day for 3 months
Cyclophosphamide 500–750 mg/m^2 IV every 3–4 weeks for six pulses[a]
Plasma exchange (double volume) on alternate days for 2 weeks[b]
Rituximab: 375 mg/m^2 weekly for 4 weeks[c]
Maintenance
Azathioprine (1.5–2 mg/kg/d) or mycophenolate mofetil (1000–1200 mg/m^2 day) for 18–24 months
Alternate day low-dose prednisolone
Consider cyclosporine if disease activity is not controlled with azathioprine or MMF
Agents for refractory disease
Intravenous immunoglobulin, monoclonal antibodies to TNF-α, rituximab

[a]The dose of cyclophosphamide is increased to 750 mg/m^2 if no leukopenia before next dose. The dose is adjusted in patients with impaired renal function. Cyclophosphamide can be given orally at a dose of 2 mg/kg/day for 12 weeks

[b]Plasma exchange should begin early, especially if patient is dialysis dependent at presentation or if biopsy shows severe histological changes (>50% crescents). Plasma exchange is useful in anti-GBM nephritis and ANCA-associated vasculitis. It should be considered in patients with immune complex crescentic GN if there is unsatisfactory renal recovery after steroid pulses

[c]Rituximab may be used as an alternative initial treatment if cyclophosphamide is contraindicated

doses and can be repeated every 6 months for 2 years. There is limited data on the use of other agents like mycophenolate mofetil (MMF), tacrolimus, belimumab, and IVIG for induction.

Therapeutic plasmapheresis is recommended for patients with pauci-immune crescentic GN, anti-GBM GN, and life-threatening pulmonary hemorrhage and might be beneficial for patients with refractory immune complex RPGN (due to SLE or severe proliferative GN). The Kidney Disease: Improving Global Outcomes (KDIGO) Clinical Practice Guidelines recommend plasmapheresis with 60 mL/kg volume replacement [17]. For pauci-immune crescentic GN (ANCA-associated vasculitis), seven sessions of plasmapheresis over 14 days are prescribed; for anti-GBM antibody disease, daily exchanges are done for 14 days or until antibodies are undetectable [18].

After induction of remission, the maintenance phase tries to mitigate further renal damage and prevent relapses. The duration of maintenance therapy varies according to the underlying disease. Most patients with ANCA-associated disease need long-term maintenance immunosuppression due to the risk of relapses. Azathioprine is preferred over extended treatment with cyclophosphamide due to significant risks associated with the latter. MMF may be used as an alternative for maintenance therapy in patients who have ANCA vasculitis and who are intolerant of azathioprine.

Most experts recommend 18–24 months of maintenance immunosuppression following successful induction of remission; therapy may then be discontinued at physician's discretion according to patient characteristics, treatment tolerance, and relapse risk. Patients with PR3 ANCA disease are more likely to relapse and often receive longer (36–60 months) therapy.

Patients who continue to be in remission for at least 1 year on maintenance therapy should be considered for tapering corticosteroid therapy. Following steroid withdrawal, other immunosuppression may be tapered after 9–12 months. There is data from adult patients on the increased risk of infections in patients treated with immunosuppression for ANCA-associated vasculitis. Most infections involve the respiratory tract and can increase the morbidity and mortality of these patients. While there are no standard protocols for prophylaxis, some centers use cotrimoxazole, especially for patients with granulomatosis with polyangiitis as an adjuvant to immunosuppressive therapy. Therapy with cotrimoxazole is often continued until patients are on very low-dose steroids.

Patients with SLE, HSP, or IgA nephropathy presenting as RPGN are treated according to existing recommendations for those specific conditions. Most patients with poststreptococcal GN who present with extensive crescents tend to recover spontaneously. The role of intensive immunosuppression in these patients is unclear. Short courses of steroids (up to 6 months) and cyclophosphamide (3–6 months) may be used in those presenting with severe AKI and extensive crescents.

RPGN secondary to infections usually responds to treatment of the underlying infection. Patients who present with idiopathic crescentic GN should be managed similar to those with pauci-immune disease or ANCA-associated disease.

16.8 Outcome

Recent years have seen significant improvement in the renal outcomes with almost 60–70% of patients showing normal renal function in the long term. Spontaneous improvement is often seen in patients with poststreptococcal crescentic GN. Patients with pauci-immune crescentic GN, MPGN, and idiopathic RPGN generally have a less favorable outcome than those with HSP or SLE. ESRD may occur in up to 25% patients with ANCA-associated vasculitis.

Renal outcome depends on the degree of renal failure at presentation and promptness of intervention, in addition to the underlying diagnosis and renal histology. The potential for recovery corresponds with the relative proportion of cellular or fibrous components in the crescents and the degree of tubulointerstitial scarring and fibrosis.

16.9 Post-Transplant Recurrence

Crescentic GN associated with C3 glomerulopathy, especially dense deposit disease, is associated with high risk of recurrence and graft loss. Crescentic GN associated with IgA nephropathy, Henoch-Schonlein purpura, and SLE are associated with higher risk of histological recurrence, but graft losses are uncommon (<5% cases). The risk for recurrence is ~10–15% with ANCA-positive vasculitis. KDIGO guidelines recommend that these patients should be in remission for at least 1 year prior to proceeding to renal transplant [19].

Take-Home Points

1. Rapidly progressive glomerulonephritis is an acute illness with progressive loss of renal function over days to weeks, characterized histologically by extensive crescent formation.
2. Patients often present with acute onset of macroscopic hematuria, reduced urine output, hypertension, and edema. Occasionally it may have an indolent presentation.
3. Prompt diagnosis and early treatment are essential to ensure renal recovery. Patients should undergo renal biopsy and appropriate serologic assays based on clinical features and findings on renal biopsy.
4. Treatment strategies should be individualized for patients using available guidelines.

References

1. Jennette JC. Rapidly progressive crescentic glomerulonephritis. Kidney Int. 2003;63(3):1164–77.
2. Morgan MD, Harper L, Williams J, Savage C. Anti-neutrophil cytoplasm-associated glomerulonephritis. J Am Soc Nephrol. 2006;17(5):1224–34.

3. Srivastava RN, Moudgil A, Bagga A, Vasudev AS, Bhuyan UN, Sundraem KR. Crescentic glomerulonephritis in children: a review of 43 cases. Am J Nephrol. 1992;12(3):155–61.
4. El-Husseini AA, Sheashaa HA, Sabry AA, Moustafa FE, Sobh MA. Acute postinfectious crescentic glomerulonephritis: clinicopathologic presentation and risk factors. Int Urol Nephrol. 2005;37(3):603–9.
5. Hoschek JC, Dreyer P, Dahal S, Walker PD. Rapidly progressive renal failure in childhood. Am J Kidney Dis. 2002;40(6):1342–7.
6. Hattori M, Kurayama H, Koitabashi Y, Nephrology JSP. Antineutrophil cytoplasmic autoantibody-associated glomerulonephritis in children. J Am Soc Nephrol. 2001;12(7):1493–500.
7. Chen M, Kallenberg CG, Zhao MH. ANCA-negative pauci-immune crescentic glomerulonephritis. Nat Rev Nephrol. 2009;5(6):313–8.
8. Hogg RJ. A clinico-pathologic study of crescentic glomerulonephritis in 50 children. A report of the Southwest Pediatric Nephrology Study Group. Kidney Int. 1985;27(2):450–8.
9. Sinha A, Puri K, Hari P, Dinda AK, Bagga A. Etiology and outcome of crescentic glomerulonephritis. Indian Pediatr. 2013;50(3):283–8.
10. Schmitt WH, van der Woude FJ. Clinical applications of antineutrophil cytoplasmic antibody testing. Curr Opin Rheumatol. 2004;16(1):9–17.
11. Bossuyt X, Cohen Tervaert J, Arimura Y, et al. Position paper: revised 2017 international consensus on testing of ANCAs in granulomatosis with polyangiitis and microscopic polyangiitis. Nat Rev Rheumatol. 2017;13(11):683–92.
12. Berden AE, Ferrario F, Hagen EC, et al. Histopathologic classification of ANCA-associated glomerulonephritis. J Am Soc Nephrol. 2010;21(10):1628–36.
13. Levy J, Pusey C. Crescentic glomerulonephritis. In: Davison AMA, Cameron JS, Grunfeld J-P, et al., editors. Oxford textbook of clinical nephrology, vol. 3. Oxford: Oxford University Press; 2005.
14. Jindal KK. Management of idiopathic crescentic and diffuse proliferative glomerulonephritis: evidence-based recommendations. Kidney Int Suppl. 1999;70:S33–40.
15. Geetha G, Jin Q, Scott J, et al. Comparisons of guidelines and recommendations on managing ANCA-associated vasculitis. Kidney Int Rep. 2018;3(5):1039–49.
16. Stone JH, Merkel PA, Spiera R, et al. Rituximab versus cyclophosphamide for ANCA-associated vasculitis. N Engl J Med. 2010;363(3):221–32.
17. KDIGO Group. KDIGO Clinical Practice Guideline for Glomerulonephritis. Kidney Int Suppl. 2012;2:139–274.
18. Walsh M, Catapano F, Szpirt W, et al. Plasma exchange for renal vasculitis and idiopathic rapidly progressive glomerulonephritis: a meta-analysis. Am J Kidney Dis. 2011;57(4):566–74.
19. Little MA, Hassan B, Jacques S, et al. Renal transplantation in systemic vasculitis: when is it safe? Nephrol Dial Transplant. 2009;24(10):3219–25.

17 Acute Tubulointerstitial Nephritis

Uri S. Alon

17.1 Case Report

A previously healthy 12-year-old girl was transferred from an outside facility to the pediatric intensive care unit due to right lower lobe pneumonia with deterioration in respiratory function after developing pleural effusion, necessitating drainage. She was treated with ceftriaxone with gradual improvement. However on day 5 of hospitalization, it was noted that her serum creatinine increased from baseline of 0.6–1.3 mg/dL, associated with mild hyperchloremic metabolic acidosis. Urine output continued to be appropriate. Urinalysis revealed specific gravity 1.010, protein 1+, white blood cells 2+, RBC 1+, and under microscopy WBC 5–10, RBC 1–4, and a few renal epithelial cells/HPF. No eosinophils nor casts were seen. Urine protein/creatinine ratio was 0.45 (mg/mg). Urine culture was negative. On day 6 serum creatinine increased to 1.8 mg/dL. Blood pressure was normal as was the ophthalmologic examination. She was suspected to have AKI due to acute tubulointerstitial nephritis secondary to exposure to ceftriaxone. The antibiotic was discontinued and replaced by meropenem. However on days 7 and 8, serum creatinine continued to rise, reaching 2.8 mg/dL. A kidney biopsy showed acute tubulointerstitial nephritis (Fig. 17.1). Therapy with intravenous methylprednisolone 500 mg daily for 3 days was initiated followed by oral prednisone 60 mg daily for 4 weeks with subsequent taper. After reaching a peak of 3.3 mg/dL on day 10, serum creatinine started to decline, reaching baseline on day 20. On follow-ups, 1 month and 4 months later, serum creatinine continued to be normal, and urine sediment findings showed signs of resolution.

U. S. Alon (✉)
Division of Pediatric Nephrology, Children's Mercy Hospital Kansas City, University of Missouri at Kansas City, Kansas City, MO, USA
e-mail: ualon@cmh.edu

S. K. Sethi et al. (eds.), *Critical Care Pediatric Nephrology and Dialysis: A Practical Handbook*, https://doi.org/10.1007/978-981-13-2276-1_17

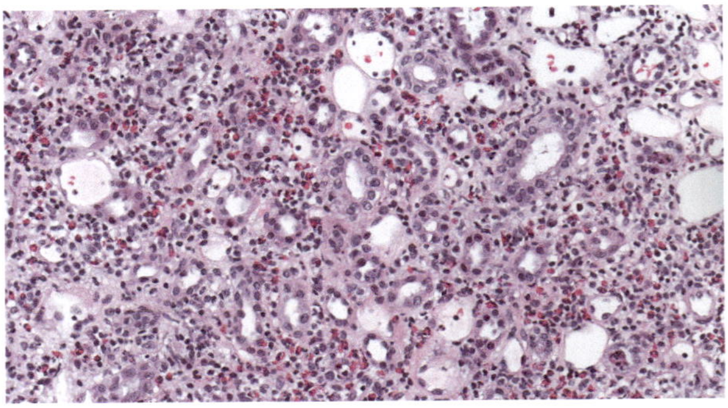

Fig. 17.1 Histopathology of acute tubulointerstitial nephritis. Acute tubulointerstitial nephritis likely secondary to ceftriaxone therapy in a 12-year-old girl. Note tubulointerstitial edema, infiltration with lymphocytes and eosinophils, and tubulitis

17.2 Introduction

The renal interstitium comprises about 80% of the renal tissue [1, 2].

Tubulointerstitial nephritis is histologically characterized by inflammation and damage to the tubulointerstitial structures with relative sparing of the glomerular and vascular elements and is divided between acute and chronic processes but should best be viewed as a continuum of manifestations of renal injury [1, 3–5]. Acute tubulointerstitial nephritis is thought to be the etiology in 10–25% of acute kidney injury (AKI) in adults and up to 7% in children [1, 6–9]. The main difficulty in reaching a more precise estimate is in establishing the diagnosis. As discussed later, acute TIN does not have any pathognomonic symptoms or signs, and definitive diagnosis can be established only by a kidney biopsy that is not routinely done [10]. Treatment is nonspecific and mostly includes removal of the underlying etiology if identified, immunosuppressive therapy, and at times concomitant renal replacement therapy. Prognosis of acute TIN is in general good, but some cases may progress to chronic kidney disease [6, 8, 10–12].

17.3 Structure and Function of the Tubulointerstitial Compartment

The tubulointerstitial compartment comprises about 80% of the renal parenchyma. The majority of tubulointerstitial volume is contributed by the tubules [2]. The interstitium is made of cells and matrix.

Two main types of cells in the interstitium are identified. Type I interstitial cells are fibroblast-like cells which are capable to produce and degrade extracellular matrix. Type II interstitial cells include dendritic antigen-presenting cells located mainly in the cortex and monocyte-derived macrophages, which are capable of phagocytosis found in all renal zones [13, 14]. The matrix is composed of a fibrillar net of basement membrane and interstitial collagens, glycoproteins, proteoglycans, and interstitial fluid [14]. The interstitium provides structural support for the nephrons and capillaries. It also plays an important role in the transport of solutes. It is the place of production of cytokines and hormones such as prostaglandins and

Table 17.1 Functional and clinical patterns of renal tubular dysfunction in tubulointerstitial nephritis

Nephron site	Functional defect	Clinical manifestations
Proximal tubule	Decreased bicarbonate, phosphate, amino acids, uric acid, and glucose reabsorption	Fanconi syndrome, hyperchloremic normal anion gap metabolic acidosis, polyuria, polydipsia, hypokalemia
Loop of Henle	Defective sodium and chloride reabsorption, decreased calcium and magnesium reabsorption	Polyuria, polydipsia, salt wasting. Calcium, magnesium, and potassium losses
Distal tubule	Defective sodium and chloride reabsorption and potassium and hydrogen ion secretion	Hyperkalemia, hyperchloremic normal anion gap metabolic acidosis, sodium and potassium losses
Collecting tubule	Defective water reabsorption	Nephrogenic diabetes insipidus

erythropoietin. Damage to different segments of the tubule results in metabolic abnormalities related to the affected segments (Table 17.1). For instance, damage to the proximal tubule may result in urinary phosphate loss, whereas damage to the collecting duct will interfere with urine concentration ability. Alteration in tubular function may at times precede decrements in glomerular filtration rate in the sequence of development of AKI [8].

17.4 Epidemiology, Pathophysiology, and Histopathology

Acute TIN accounts for 10–25% of acute kidney injury (AKI) in adults and up to 7% of children with AKI [1, 6–9]. It is important to note that in both children and adults acute TIN may be underreported, because most patients with AKI recover spontaneously after removal of the suspected offending agent, and definitive diagnosis based on a renal biopsy is not routinely established [5]. There is less reported incidence of acute TIN in children. This may reflect the more common use of nephrotoxic agents and greater prevalence of preexisting renal abnormalities in the older patients.

The hallmark of histopathology of acute inflammation is interstitial edema; infiltration with lymphocytes, macrophages, plasma cells, and eosinophils; and tubulitis with relative sparing of the glomeruli and tubules (Fig. 17.1). Rarely granulomas may be detected [15]. The similarity of the tubulointerstitial lesions in all forms of TIN is characterized by predominantly T-cell lymphocytic infiltrates. This suggests immune-mediated mechanisms of renal injury [4, 11]. Such mechanisms are likely important in either initiating tubular injury or amplifying damage induced by both immune and nonimmune causes. Studies from experimental models indicate that both cell-mediated and humoral immune mechanisms are relevant pathways for inducing renal injury [10, 11]. Specifically mechanisms include cell-mediated immunity, antibody-mediated immunity, local and extrarenal antigens, cytokines and other factors amplifying the injury, and fibrosis and atrophy [11]. Etiologies of TIN can be drug induced, infectious, idiopathic, genetic, or related to systemic inflammatory condition such as an inflammatory bowel disease or IgG4-associated immune complex multi-organ autoimmune disease [10, 11, 16–18].

A special entity of tubulointerstitial nephritis is that associated with uveitis (TINU syndrome). Patients with TINU usually have anorexia, fever, weight loss, abdominal pain, and polyuria. Eye tenderness may not be evident at presentation, as uveitis could occur later also with respect to the onset of renal disease [19, 20]. Due to the fact that uveitis might be asymptomatic, all patients with idiopathic acute tubulointerstitial nephritis require a detailed ophthalmologic examination [21]. The pathogenesis of this syndrome remains unclear, and evidence suggests roles for both humoral and cell-mediated immune mechanisms [11, 20]. In most cases, it resolves completely, either spontaneously or after steroids. In a study on 21 children with acute tubulointerstitial nephritis, TINU patients required a longer time for the renal recovery in comparison with other etiologies [22]. The uveitis in these cases often requires several steroid courses and other immunosuppressive medications like methotrexate, azathioprine, and cyclosporine A. The uveitis may relapse but carries a good long-term prognosis [11, 23].

17.5 Symptoms, Signs, and Laboratory Findings

Acute tubulointerstitial nephritis is most commonly presented to the nephrologist as acute kidney injury, although as aforementioned, in some cases it might present as tubular dysfunction involving one or more tubular segments [8, 10]. The AKI is often non-oliguric, and therefore the first suspicion of its existence may arise when a rise in serum creatinine concentration is noted. Accompanying symptoms and signs are usually nonspecific, and these patients may have malaise, elevated temperature, nausea, flank pain, arthralgia, and skin rash (Table 17.2). The latter is described as maculopapular, morbilliform, or urticarial. The patients may exhibit also signs and symptoms of the systemic disease associated with acute TIN. Edema is usually absent. The blood pressure is usually normal but at times may be elevated. Urinalysis typically shows a bland urine with minimal proteinuria, hematuria, leukocyturia, and presence of tubular cells. At times though, as is the case with NSAID etiology, the proteinuria might be massive. Studies in recent years demonstrated the possible utility of tubular proteins like alpha 1-microalbumin and beta 2-microalbumin as biomarkers of tubular injury [8, 20, 24]. Similarly, blood work is nonspecific. Serum creatinine is elevated, and patients may have hyperchloremic metabolic acidosis. The latter may result from renal failure per se and the reflection of involvement of tubular segments in acid-base homeostasis. Additional biochemical findings that can be detected based on damage to the tubules involvement are detailed in Table 17.1. Fractional excretion of sodium exceeds 1% indicating tubular injury and as aforementioned tubular proteinuria may be present.

Although the findings of eosinophilia and eosinophiluria can direct to the diagnosis of acute TIN, they are found only in a minority of patients. They are more common in those with drug-induced acute TIN [9, 18]. To test for eosinophiluria, Wright's or Hansel's stains are required [25]. However, the detection of eosinophiluria is not specific for acute tubulointerstitial nephritis, as the sensitivity for its diagnosis is estimated to be 60% with specificity of 85% and positive

Table 17.2 Clinical presentation of acute tubulointerstitial nephritis

History
Exposure to toxins
Family history
Nephrotoxin use
Symptoms
Abdominal pain
Anorexia[a]
Arthralgias
Diarrhea
Dysuria
Edema
Emesis[a]
Fatigue[a]
Fever[a]
Flank or loin pain
Headache
Lymphadenopathy
Malaise
Myalgia
Nocturia
Polydipsia
Polyuria
Rash
Sore throat[a]
Weight loss[a]
Signs
Abdominal pain
Arthritis
Costovertebral tenderness
Edema
Fever[a]
Hypertension
Lethargy
Pallor[a]
Pharyngitis
Rash (may be maculopapular, morbilliform, or urticarial)
Volume depletion

[a]A common finding in children

predictive value of only 40% [26, 27]. Eosinophiluria is more characteristic for acute tubulointerstitial nephritis when the eosinophils are seen embedded in white blood cell casts [26, 27].

Once acute tubulointerstitial nephritis is suspected a detailed history of possible offending agents and in particular recent medications should be obtained and reviewed. In case of suspected infectious etiology, the appropriate confirmatory laboratory tests should be conducted. Imaging studies of the kidneys and in particular urinary tract ultrasound show diffusely enlarged and hyperechogenic kidneys consistent with medical parenchymal disease. Additional imaging studies are usually not indicated, and computed tomography with contrast should be avoided.

In many cases the diagnosis is suspected based on the composition of the above findings combined with exclusion of other etiologies of AKI.

In mild cases and in those with spontaneous resolution of the disease, no further evaluation is required. In more complex conditions, definitive diagnosis can be established only by examination of renal histology, which has characteristic findings as described above (Fig. 17.1).

17.6 Treatment

In cases in which the offending agent is known, like a medication, its discontinuation may be enough to reverse the course of the disease [8–11, 18]. In cases of infectious or immunologic etiologies, treatment of the basic disease will abolish the inflammatory process in the kidneys too.

The main discussion is if and when to utilize corticosteroids. Studies in children are scarce [7, 10, 11, 22]. In adults, it was shown that early corticosteroid treatment, within 1–2 weeks after the disease started, may shorten the disease and result in better recovery, namely, higher rate of complete resolution [8, 9, 28]. Once it is decided to proceed with a corticosteroid course, 3 days of intravenous methylprednisolone followed by oral corticosteroids is recommended. While anecdotal cases reported success with the use of additional immunosuppressive medications, further studies are required to establish their efficacy in safety [29, 30].

Naturally, renal supportive therapy should be provided as indicated. Careful attention should be paid to fluid balance. Some patients may require renal replacement therapy until kidney function is restored.

17.7 Prognosis

In general, the prognosis of acute TIN is regarded as good. This is especially true when the etiology is diagnosed early and addressed promptly. It is also possible that early immunosuppressive therapy will enhance recovery and improve prognosis. Some patients nonetheless may progress to chronic kidney disease or end-stage kidney disease [8, 10, 11].

17.8 Summary

Acute TIN should be suspected in the patient with a rise in serum creatinine, normotension, and bland urine sediment. A thorough investigation of possible exposure to offending medications, systemic infectious or immunologic illness, and other possible etiologies should be conducted. Biochemical evaluation may detect segmental renal tubular dysfunction and at times eosinophilia and eosinophiluria. Urinary tract ultrasound will indicate renal parenchymal disease. Kidney biopsy is reserved to the more complicated cases. Treatment includes removal of the offending organism and treatment of coexisting underlying disease. In some cases the addition of corticosteroids may enhance recovery and improve prognosis. The latter is usually good with a few exceptions.

References

1. Eknoyan G. Tubulointerstitial nephropathies. In: Massry SG, Glassock RJ, editors. Textbook of nephrology. 3rd ed. Baltimore: Williams & Wilkins; 1995. p. 1036–46.
2. Rastegar A, Kashgarian M. The clinical spectrum of tubulointerstitial nephritis. Kidney Int. 1998;54:313–27.
3. Appel GB. Acute interstitial nephritis. In: Neilson EG, Couser WG, editors. Immunologic renal diseases. Philadelphia: Lippincott-Raven; 1997. p. 1221–34.
4. Neilson EG. Pathogenesis and therapy of interstitial nephritis. Kidney Int. 1989;35:1257–70.
5. Jones CL, Eddy AA. Tubulointerstitial nephritis. Pediatr Nephrol. 1992;6:572–86.
6. Hawkins EP, Berry PL, Silva FG. Acute tubulointerstitial nephritis in children: clinical, morphologic, and lectin studies. A report of the Southwest Pediatric Nephrology Study Group. Am J Kidney Dis. 1989;14:466–71.
7. Greising J, Trachtman H, Gauthier B. Acute interstitial nephritis in adolescents and young adults. Child Nephrol Urol. 1990;10:189–95.
8. Raghavan R, Eknoyan G. Acute interstitial nephritis – a reappraisal and update. Clin Nephrol. 2014;82:149–62.
9. Praga M, Gonzalez E. Acute interstitial nephritis. Kidney Int. 2010;77:956–61.
10. Joyce E, Glasner P, Ranganathan S, Swiatecka-Urban A. Tubulointerstitial nephritis: diagnosis, treatment and monitoring. Pediatr Nephrol. 2017;32:577–87.
11. Alon US. Pediatric tubulointerstitial nephritis. In: Avner ED, Harmon WE, Niaudet P, Yoshikawa N, Emma R, Goldstein SL, editors. Pediatric nephology. 7th ed. Berlin: Springer; 2016. p. 1407–28.
12. Baker RJ, Pusey CD. The changing profile of acute tubulointerstitial nephritis. Nephrol Dial Transplant. 2004;19:8–11.
13. Wolgast MA, Larson M, Nygren K. Functional characteristics of renal interstitium. Am J Phys. 1981;241(2):F105–11.
14. Lemley KV, Kriz W. Anatomy of the renal interstitium. Kidney Int. 1991;39:370–81.
15. Joss N, Morris S, Young B, Geddes C. Granulomatous interstitial nephritis. Clin J Am Soc Nephrol. 2007;2:222–30.
16. Cornell LD. IgG4-related tubulointerstitial nephritis. Kidney Int. 2010;78:951–3.
17. Praga M, Sevillano A, Aunon P, Gonzalez E. Changes in the aetiology, clinical presentation and management of acute interstitial nephritis, an increasingly common cause of acute kidney injury. Nephrol Dial Transplant. 2015;30:1472–9.
18. Perazella MA, Matkowitz GS. Drug-induced acute interstitial nephritis. Nat Rev Nephrol. 2010;6:461–70.
19. Vohra S, Eddy A, Levin AV, Taylor G, Laxer RM. Tubulointerstitial nephritis and uveitis in children and adolescents. Pediatr Nephrol. 1999;13:426–32.
20. Hettinga YM, Scheerlinck LM, Lilien MR, Rothova A, de Boer JH. The value of measuring urinary β2-microglobulin and serum creatinine for detecting tubulointerstitial nephritis and uveitis syndrome in young patients with uveitis. JAMA Ophthalmol. 2015;133:140–5.
21. Gallego N, Estepa R, Mampaso F. Tubulointerstitial nephritis and asymptomatic uveitis. J Nephrol. 2000;13:373–6.

22. Kobayashi Y, Honda M, Yoshikawa N, Ito H. Acute tubulointerstitial nephritis in 21 Japanese children. Clin Nephrol. 2000;54:191–7.
23. Levy M, Guesry P, Loirat C. Immunologically mediated tubulointerstitial nephritis in children. Contrib Nephrol. 1979;16:132–40.
24. Zhang H, Wang F, Xiao H, Yao Y. The ratio of urinary α1-microglobulin to microalbumin can be used as a diagnostic criterion for tubuloproteinuria. Intractable Rare Dis Res. 2018;7:46–50.
25. Nolan CR III, Anger MS, Kelleher SP. Eosinopliluria – a new method of detection and definition of clinical spectrum. N Engl J Med. 1986;315:1516–9.
26. Fletcher A. Eosinophiluria and acute interstitial nephritis. N Engl J Med. 2008;358:1760–1.
27. Faye M, Ganon RF. Acute allergic interstitial nephritis and eosinophiluria. Kidney Int. 2008;73:980–1.
28. Gonzalez E, Gutierrez E, Galeano C, de Sequera P, Bernis C, Parra EG, Delgado R. Early steroid treatment improves the recovery of renal function in patients with drug-induced acute interstitial nephritis. Kidney Int. 2008;73:940–6.
29. Zuliani E, Zwahlen H, Gilliet F, Marone C. Vancomycin-induced hypersensitivity reaction with acute renal failure: resolution following cyclosporine treatment. Clin Nephrol. 2005;64:155–9.
30. Preddie DC, Markowitz GS, Radhakrishnan J. Mycophenolate mofetil for the treatment of interstitial nephritis. Clin J Am Soc Nephrol. 2006;1:718–22.

Drug-Induced Nephrotoxicity 18

Deepa H. Chand and Meenal Patwardhan

18.1 Clinical Scenario

A 6-year-old female with a history of spina bifida is admitted for presumed acute pyelonephritis with fevers, vomiting, and abdominal pain. Her urine culture and sensitivity results are pending. She has a past medical history significant for a ventriculoperitoneal (VP) shunt, gastrostomy tube, and neurogenic bladder. She has been admitted several times in the past for pyelonephritis with bacteremia. Her baseline renal function equates to an estimated glomerular filtration rate (eGFR) of approximately 60 mL/min/1.73 m^2. You are consulted by the hospitalist to provide input regarding the choice of antibiotic and dosage to be prescribed.

18.2 Introduction

A critical consideration for the choice of antibiotic, or any drug for that matter, in this patient with chronic kidney disease should be guided by its potential for drug-induced nephropathy. Drug-induced nephrotoxicity has been reported to be responsible for approximately 20% of AKI events. Hundreds of medications have been implicated in drug-induced AKI in national and international databases, with antibiotics representing a preponderance of cases (40–50%) and aminoglycosides and amphotericin B as common offenders. Diuretics (18.5%) and agents affecting the renin-angiotensin system are also frequent causes of AKI (16.3%), with angiotensin receptor blockers more commonly associated with AKI than angiotensin converting

D. H. Chand (✉)
AbbVie, University of Illinois College of Medicine, Chicago, IL, USA

M. Patwardhan
Research and Development, Abbvie, Inc., North Chicago, IL, USA

S. K. Sethi et al. (eds.), *Critical Care Pediatric Nephrology and Dialysis: A Practical Handbook*, https://doi.org/10.1007/978-981-13-2276-1_18

enzyme inhibitors (ACEi) (8.4% vs. 7.9%, respectively). Antineoplastic agents (10.2%) and anti-inflammatory drugs (5.4%) have been reported frequently as well. Polypharmacy with multiple nephrotoxic agents significantly increases the risk of AKI. Notably, given the multitude of functions of the kidneys, namely, with reference to electrolyte and fluid balance, acute kidney injury (AKI) related to pharmacologic agents can play both causative and resultant roles. It is important to understand both of these roles when managing a patient with renal impairment.

In a hospitalized child, it is important to establish true renal function so as to determine the potential benefit vs. risk of prescribing any given medication. This can be best accomplished by estimating the glomerular filtration rate (GFR), with consideration of laboratory and clinical indicators. Traditionally, serum creatinine has been used to determine renal function; however, this measurement in absolute terms may not be accurate for a variety of reasons. However, the trend of increase or decrease prior to and during the hospital stay can be helpful. Similarly, the degree of oliguria can be an adjunct in determining the degree of renal impairment. The practitioner must also understand that oliguria may be absent or a late-stage finding in children with AKI. Specifically, if a molecule (i.e., pharmacologic agent) cannot be excreted due to lack of urine, it will accumulate and can potentially cause toxicity. Further, blood pressure should be monitored, with key attention to systemic hypotension, which can cause renal hypoperfusion, negatively impacting drug clearance.

18.3 Prevention of Drug-Induced AKI

Given that prevention of drug-induced renal toxicity is the optimal approach in this patient, a thorough review of the patient's past medical history should be conducted, with special attention to concomitant medications, which should be verified with the patient/family member on admission and on regular basis so as to avoid nephrotoxicity. Similarly, history of acute or chronic kidney disease should be noted, including if intervention was warranted as well as outcome. If available, recent vital signs and baseline renal function should be documented. Chronically used medications such as ACEi or nonsteroidal anti-inflammatory agents should be assessed for acute needs. For example, if the patient is hypotensive or if the serum creatinine is elevated, these medications should be discontinued until the patient is more stable. Similarly, the administration of radiographic contrast agents can contribute to renal injury, with gadolinium possibly causing irreversible injury. If contrast agent administration is required, nephrotoxicity should be anticipated to prevent associated injury.

Additionally, when prescribing medications in the presence of AKI, it is important to obtain known pharmacologic toxicity information from the US Package Insert (USPI), product monograph, product label, or country equivalent, which can summarize clinical trial adverse event findings as well as any previously known drug-drug interactions and potential organ toxicities. If necessary, relevant pharmacokinetic and metabolism information can be found in these documents as well.

A clinical pharmacist in the hospital setting can provide assistance as well regarding research of any prescribing nuances associated with the potential agent. While many pediatric institutions have PharmD professionals accompany intensive care unit rounds, they may not be involved in the care of non-critically ill children; however, they should still be consulted when necessary.

The estimated GFR should be used to determine if dose modification is necessary. This is particularly true in those with underlying chronic kidney disease (CKD) or other comorbidities. Similarly, if weight-based modifications, as in younger children, are necessary, these can be determined at the time of prescribing medications.

As mentioned previously, pharmacologic agents can play a causative role in AKI. However, the consequences of AKI on pharmacologic agents must be recognized and anticipated. During an acute episode of AKI, renal physiology is constantly evolving, and abnormalities can impair drug absorption, distribution, metabolism, and elimination based on circulating blood volume, intrinsic physiologic changes, and uremic changes impacting extrarenal organs in situations of abnormal renal function. For example, uremia can contribute to gastrointestinal malabsorption, thereby potentially decreasing medication absorption, resulting in a subtherapeutic effect. If significant systemic edema is present, the patient's volume of distribution may be compromised, as the altered increase in volume may result in lowered plasma drug concentrations. Drug metabolism may be compromised as well, especially due to the slowing of hydrolysis and various metabolic reactions. Similarly, if renal function is reduced, there may be significantly less clearance of a medication, potentially resulting in toxicity. With this in mind, many pharmacologic agents require dose adjustment based on renal impairment and the drug's biochemical properties.

18.4 Mechanisms of Drug-Induced AKI

Once AKI has been diagnosed and a drug is potentially implicated, injury minimization and reversal become the goals. It is imperative to understand the pathophysiology of injury mechanisms when approaching AKI due to drug nephrotoxicity. A summary of mechanisms and commonly associated agents is provided in Table 18.1. Of note, one class of medications may impact the kidney at various points, having multiple mechanisms of action. For example, aminoglycosides may cause both acute tubular necrosis and tubulointerstitial nephritis.

Prerenal AKI may be induced by medications that decrease renal perfusion. These can include diuretics which act systemically by decreasing intravascular volume. Other agents such as ACEi induce a hypoperfusion state by altering renal hemodynamics. This can be further evaluated by historical data including vital signs and temporal relationship to the medication. Again, medications administered prior to admission should be considered as potential etiologies, such as the use of NSAIDs as anti-pyrexia agents.

Table 18.1 Commonly used therapeutic agents and mechanism of action

Mechanism of injury	Therapeutic agent
Prerenal	
Hypoperfusion	Diuretics
	Nonsteroidal anti-inflammatory drugs
	Renin-angiotensin system inhibitors
Renal	
Acute tubular necrosis	Aminoglycosides
	Radiographic contrast dyes
Tubulointerstitial nephritis	Penicillins and cephalosporins
	Aminoglycosides
	Amphotericin B
	Macrolide antibiotics
	Quinolones
	Rifampin
	Sulfonamides
Drug-induced thrombotic microangiopathy	Calcineurin inhibitors
	Clopidogrel
	Indinavir
Vasculitis	Hydralazine
	Propylthiouracil
	Allopurinol
	Penicillamine
	Gemcitabine
	Mitomycin C
	Methamphetamines
	Calcineurin inhibitors
Post-renal	
Intraluminar (crystal) obstruction	Acyclovir
	Sulfonamides
	Indinavir
	Foscarnet
	Methotrexate
Nephrocalcinosis	Sulfonamides
	Triamterene
	Indinavir
	Thrombolytic agents
	Topiramate

Intrinsic renal AKI can be more complicated to evaluate. Possible mechanisms include acute tubular necrosis, tubulointerstitial nephritis, vasculitis, or acute glomerulonephritis. Rhabdomyolysis can cause indirect nephrotoxicity. The most common offenders of intrinsic AKI include ACEi and NSAIDs. Vascular injury can occur from thrombotic microangiopathy, commonly associated with calcineurin inhibitors (cyclosporine, tacrolimus), muromonab-CD3, and clopidogrel. Further, thrombolytics and anticoagulants can shower cholesterol emboli, which can damage blood vessels. Tubular damage can occur from aminoglycosides, ifosfamide, cisplatin, and radiographic contrast dyes. Immune-mediated drug reactions are common and include hypersensitivity reactions, tubule-interstitial nephritis, Stevens-Johnson syndrome, and "lupus-like syndrome" associated with hydralazine, procainamide, isoniazid, methyldopa, and chlorpromazine.

Post-renal AKI usually implies urinary tract obstruction. This can occur if the drug precipitates in the urinary system or urinary crystal excretion increases as a result. Examples of these include increased urinary calcium excretion with furosemide administration which can result in calcium oxalate renal calculi formation. Precipitation of medications such as acyclovir, methotrexate, and indinavir can cause direct crystal-induced kidney injury. Further, cyclophosphamide can cause hemorrhagic cystitis with resultant hematuria and blood clot excretion.

Drug-drug interactions are worth mentioning. For example, the combined use of vancomycin with piperacillin-tazobactam has been established to cause nephrotoxicity. Many medications are metabolized by the transporter P-glycoprotein (Pgp) and the enzymes cytochrome P450 (CYP) 3A4/5, thereby inhibiting or competing with each other, potentially resulting in alterations in drug levels as in the case of calcineurin inhibitors. Further, certain foods or herbal medications may alter drug metabolism as in the case of grapefruit and tacrolimus, and patient education is required. With known interactions, medical staff should be cautious when prescribing them and monitor renal function diligently.

18.5 Approach to Diagnosis and Management of Drug-Induced AKI

If a prerenal etiology is suspected, intravascular volume must be adequately restored. This may be challenging in a patient with total volume overload and intravascular volume depletion. Fluid must be shifted, if possible, to the intravascular compartment. Medications that could further deplete intravascular volume should be avoided and discontinued.

If drug administration is planned, such as in the case of radiographic contrast agents, appropriate pre-administration hydration should be provided. Some have reported the successful use of prophylactic n-acetylcysteine to prevent radiographic contrast nephropathy. Co-administration of mesna with cyclophosphamide can mitigate hemorrhagic cystitis. Administration of rasburicase with chemotherapy may prevent/treat hyperuricemia. Moreover, evaluating for possible drug-drug interactions prior to medication administration may prevent nephrotoxicity.

If a known nephrotoxic agent is suspected as the cause of AKI, a serum drug concentration may be obtained. However, if elevated, this may also be a consequence of decreased renal function from some other cause. Either way, the drug should be discontinued and levels monitored to determine if and when the agent should be readministered. The renal function should also be monitored as improvement is likely to result in increased drug metabolism/excretion, which may necessitate resumption of the drug and alterations in concomitant medication dosing. In neonates and infants, tubular and glomerular functions are significantly lower at baseline, and extreme caution must be utilized when prescribing medications. At birth, term neonates have approximately 20% of the renal function of an adult, and drug dosing must be personalized.

While changes in serum creatinine cannot differentiate between etiologies, further physical examination findings and laboratory evaluation can assist in determining the underlying etiology. The presence of associated rashes, fevers, and arthralgias may be suggestive of a vasculitis as seen in the "lupus-like syndrome." Laboratory evaluation should include a comprehensive metabolic profile, complete blood count, and urinalysis, at a minimum. Additional testing may be warranted, including, but not limited to, C-reactive peptide, antineutrophil antibody, etc., and should be based on clinical manifestations. Useful calculations include determination of an anion gap/non-anion gap metabolic acidosis as this may be indicative of volume depletion, diabetic ketoacidosis, lactic acidosis, etc. Calculation of a fractional excretion of sodium can help in sorting out prerenal vs. intrinsic renal etiologies. Evidence of fragmented red blood cells, or schistocytes, can point toward a hemolytic process. A urinalysis can further help evaluate fluid status (specific gravity), diabetic control (glucosuria), and proximal tubular function (aminoaciduria, glucosuria). Furthermore, the presence of certain casts (white blood cell casts, red blood cell casts, muddy brown casts (Fig. 18.1)) can be indicative of specific pathologies. The presence of "brown muddy casts" in the urine microscopy is representative of acute tubular necrosis. Eosinophiluria may be suggestive of interstitial nephritis if present. It is imperative to note that a manual microscopy is usually required to evaluate the urine. An automated laboratory urinalysis is unlikely to yield these significant results; therefore, it is recommended that the nephrologist inspect the urine microscopy personally. A renal ultrasound with Doppler should be obtained to exclude structural defects (including evaluation of renal sizes) as well as to assess for adequate renal blood flow and urinary obstruction. To definitely determine the histopathologic mechanism of injury, a renal biopsy may be required, especially if a rapidly progressive process is suspected or if multiple etiologies are implicated.

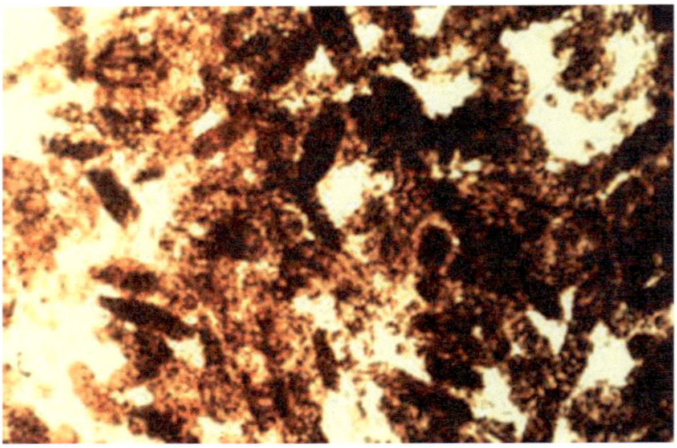

Fig. 18.1 Muddy Brown Cast suggestive of acute tubular necrosis

Once AKI has occurred, supportive therapy with discontinuation of the offending agent(s) remains the mainstay of management. For drug-induced interstitial nephritis, some have advocated the use of systemic corticosteroids; however, due to lack of clinical trials, supporting evidence for this is limited. Therefore, many practitioners recommend initiation of corticosteroid therapy if improvement is not seen within a few days after discontinuation of the offending agent.

If drug discontinuation does not result in improvement of renal function or if the potential benefit of the drug outweighs the risks, medical management should be optimized as per usual treatment of AKI. Eventually, renal replacement therapy should be considered if the patient meets clinical criteria.

Finally, it is noteworthy that if a new adverse drug reaction is suspected, this should be reported to the manufacturer. The case then be independently evaluated, and if a potential signal is identified, appropriate monitoring can occur, with ultimate changes to labelling, if warranted.

Clinical Scenario Discussion

In the case presentation mentioned above, it is imperative to recognize this child has baseline chronic kidney disease and is at increased risk of developing drug-induced AKI secondary to antimicrobial use. The situation is complicated by the fact that she has had multiple prior infections, making resistance very likely. She is also at risk for being infected with methicillin-resistant organisms. As such, she is likely to require empiric treatment with a combination of vancomycin and piperacillin-tazobactam. These should be "renally dosed" at a decreased dosing interval based on the USPI with vancomycin levels obtained regularly. Once the organism has been identified and sensitivities resulted, the treatment should be personalized so as to avoid unnecessary exposure to potentially nephrotoxic agents.

Suggested Readings

1. Pierson-Marchandise M, Gras V, Moragny J, Micallef J, Gaboriau L, Picard S, Choukroun G, Masmoudi K, Liabeuf S, French National Network of Pharmacovigilance Centres. The drugs that mostly frequently induce acute kidney injury: a case - noncase study of a pharmacovigilance database. Br J Clin Pharmacol. 2017;83(6):1341–9. https://doi.org/10.1111/bcp.13216.
2. Aronoff G, Berns J, Brier M, et al. Drug prescribing in renal failure. 4th ed. Philadelphia: American College of Physicians; 1999. p. 1–12.
3. Abouelkheir M, Alsubaie S. Acute kidney injury induced by concomitant use of vancomycin and piperacillin-tazobactam in pediatrics. Pediatr Int. 2018;60(2):136–41.
4. Wu H, Huang J. Drug-induced nephrotoxicity: pathogenic mechanisms, biomarkers and prevention strategies. Curr Drug Metab. 2018;19(7):559–67.
5. Nolin TD, Himmelfarb J. Mechanisms of drug-induced nephrotoxicity. In: Uetrecht J, editor. Adverse drug reactions. Handbook of experimental pharmacology, vol. 196. Berlin: Springer; 2010. p. 111–30.
6. Schetz M, Dasta J, Goldstein S, Golper T. Drug-induced acute kidney injury. Curr Opin Crit Care. 2005;11(6):555–65.
7. Pannu N, Nadim MK. An overview of drug-induced acute kidney injury. Crit Care Med. 2008;36(4 Suppl):S216–23. https://doi.org/10.1097/CCM.0b013e318168e375.

Acute Kidney Injury in Children Following Cardiopulmonary Bypass: A Call for Action

19

Rajit K. Basu

19.1 Introduction

Acute kidney injury (AKI) is a syndrome occurring frequently in critically ill patients. With remarkable consistency, AKI occurs in approximately one in four critically ill adults [1], children [2], and neonates [3]. In these recent large, multicenter population databases, the incidence of AKI and the association with poor outcomes were independent of severity of illness. In each cohort, compared to injury-free patients, patients with severe AKI suffered prolonged mechanical ventilation, longer duration of both intensive care unit (ICU) and hospital length of stay (LOS), and higher rates of mortality. A global meta-analysis of AKI data in all-age critically ill patients demonstrates a stepwise increase of poor outcome (notably mortality) in unison with increased AKI severity [4].

Nearly three decades' worth of data indicates AKI is a significant burden in children with complex congenital heart disease undergoing cardiopulmonary bypass (CPB) [5]. In this population, AKI occurs more frequently than in the general pediatric critically ill population but is similarly associated with worse patient outcome than the absence of AKI. An extensive number of ex vivo models of CPB have delineated numerous physiologic drivers putatively placing patients at risk for, or driving, AKI. More effort expended in the past decade to reduce the severity of AKI in these patients or lessen the disease prevalence has failed to slow the overall "progression" of this disease syndrome and its downstream sequelae for children.

In this chapter, the current paradigm of AKI in children following CPB will be challenged. In place of the existing strategy of reactive diagnostics and management,

R. K. Basu (✉)
Division of Critical Care Medicine, Children's Healthcare of Atlanta, Atlanta, GA, USA

Department of Pediatrics, Emory University School of Medicine, Atlanta, GA, USA
e-mail: Rajit.basu@choa.org; rkbasu@emory.edu

S. K. Sethi et al. (eds.), *Critical Care Pediatric Nephrology and Dialysis: A Practical Handbook*, https://doi.org/10.1007/978-981-13-2276-1_19

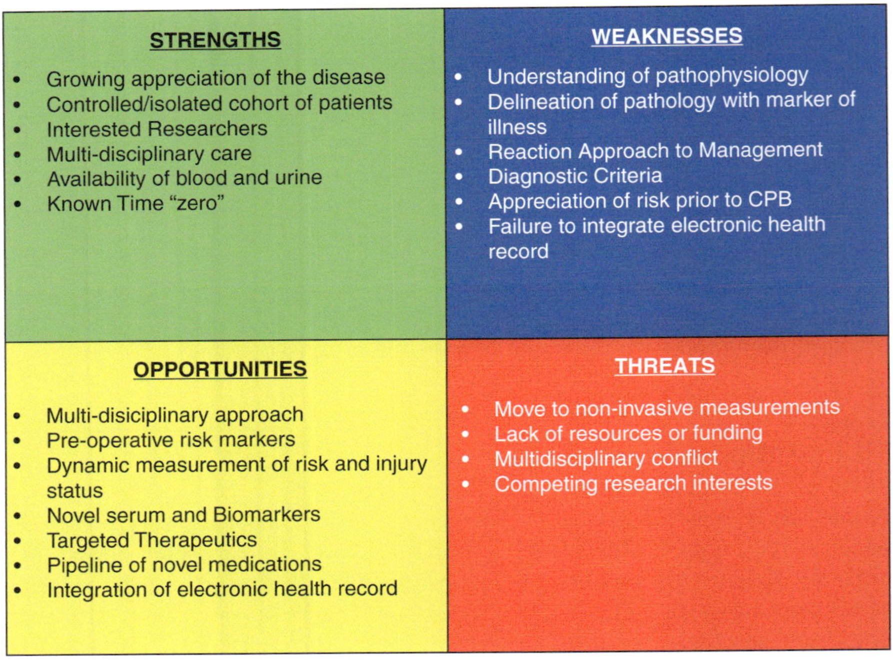

Fig. 19.1 The existing paradigm of acute kidney injury in children following cardiopulmonary bypass. The strengths, weaknesses, opportunities, and threats (SWOT) for the current, existing paradigm are described

a more predictive, proactive, and anticipatory diagnostic and recognition strategy will be described. Strengths, weaknesses, opportunities, and threats will be described (Fig. 19.1). The potential to move the needle and improve outcomes for children following cardiac surgery by reducing the burden of AKI is possible but requires multidisciplinary, collaborative, and sustained investment and effort.

19.2 Epidemiology: A Chance to Move the Needle

Acute kidney injury (AKI) is a syndrome with a significant disease burden in the critically ill patient. The recent AKI-EPI study performed in nearly 2000 adults demonstrated a high disease incidence and significant associations with increased ICU technology and death [1]. In pediatrics, the AWARE (Assessment of Worldwide Acute Kidney Injury, Renal Angina, and Biomarkers) uncovered a 26.9% AKI incidence rate in 4683 children, 11.6% severe AKI [2]. The patients with severe AKI suffered increased adjusted odds (1.77, 95% CI 1.17–2.68) for mortality and a higher death rate (11–2.5%) compared to patients without severe AKI. These findings remained consistent in the neonatal ICU as the AWAKEN (Assessment of Worldwide Acute Kidney Injury Epidemiology in Neonates) identified a 27% AKI rate in 2162 newborns [3]. In the United States, nearly a quarter of a million

(240,000) adults undergo cardiac surgery requiring CPB, and 25% patients in this population experience AKI (AKI-CPB). The most recent epidemiologic reports of AKI in children following CPB report an incidence of nearly 50%, slightly higher in neonates (65%) [5–7]. After adjustment for covariates, AKI-CPB is independently associated with both short-term and longer-term complications. The short-term sequelae associated with AKI-CPB include longer duration of mechanical ventilation, longer ICU and hospital length of stay (LOS), higher incidence of both low cardiac output syndrome and higher vasoactive medication requirements, and high rates of mortality. Longer-term sequelae include higher incidence of, and transition to, chronic kidney disease and longer-term mortality. It is notable that these findings are consistent regardless of patient age; similar findings are consistently demonstrated in adult AKI-CPB patients. When cost-estimate models are used to isolate the financial burden of AKI in this population, even patients with small changes in serum creatinine carry increased costs (1.6-fold) compared to disease-free patients [8] with a majority of costs increased by LOS and laboratory expenditures. By any measure, the epidemiology of AKI following CPB describes an epidemic with a wide range of associated negative consequences. Taken together, there is a significant need for innovation, discovery, and outcome improvement for these patients.

Identification of the at-risk patient for AKI-CPB has no objective methodology. The extensive data in adult and pediatric AKI-CPB has identified a long list of putative risk factors including, but not limited to, age, gender, surgical complexity, CPB time, cross-clamp time, preoperative ventilator support, diabetes mellitus, and hypertension [9]. When stratified by temporal relationship to CPB, the variables become more cleanly delineated into pre-, intra-, and post-CPB groups. The preoperative risks for AKI-CPB have expanded beyond simple demographic associations as genome-wide association studies (GWAS) and other genetic variant studies have uncovered a pattern of predisposing inherited mutations that confer added AKI risk [10]. Additionally, there is more appreciation in the preoperative period for comorbidities such as baseline chronic kidney disease, congestive heart failure, and diabetes (even in children) increasing the risk of postoperative AKI. Intraoperative variables associated with AKI-CPB have traditionally been focused exclusively on duration of bypass time and cross-clamp time. These variables have carried a direct relationship with increases in AKI rates and severity, that is, the longer the time of CPB or cross-clamp, the higher the incidence of severity of AKI. Additionally, other factors such as deep hypothermic arrest, intraoperative hypotension, and low hemoglobin have been associated with higher rates of AKI-CPB. Newer data, however, suggests an independence of AKI from CPB duration in patients controlled by age and surgical complexity. Newer, more sophisticated, and controlled data suggests the dogmatic belief in the direct relationship between AKI-CPB needs to be challenged as primary disease is more powerful in statistical modeling (controlling for confounders)—in adults following coronary artery bypass graft surgery [11], in children with a STAT (Society of Thoracic Surgeons-European Association for Cardiothoracic Surgery) score of at least three, and in homogenous neonates [12]. The postoperative variables associated with AKI-CPB have included the use of renal replacement therapy, the use of mechanical support, and volume status. Although the association of the former two with AKI is relatively intuitive, the latter is an important finding. The importance of volume status, as it relates to fluid accumulation, can be simultaneously a sign of, or a risk factor for, AKI. Early fluid accumulation is a harbinger of AKI in the pediatric CPB population [13, 14], and given the relationship with total body water, fluid accumulation may actually mask AKI recognition and diagnosis [12]. Several recent narrative documents describe phases of critical care and how each relates to net fluid balance [15]. Postoperative CPB data demonstrates a consistent association between avoidance of fluid accumulation (i.e., lower total net fluid balance) and improved patient outcomes.

Identifying the patient at risk for AKI prior to injury may ultimately improve outcome. Although no singular effective therapy has been identified to date, a prevailing sentiment in the critical care nephrology community is earlier diagnosis (or recognition) would expedite "management options" and lead to less deleterious associated effects of AKI. The parallel for this belief is the now routine assessment of cardiac angina or signs of impending and active stroke ("FAST") for recognition of unstable acute coronary syndrome (ACS) and cerebrovascular ischemia, respectively. Simply, the recognition of risk factors paired with tangible evidence of active injury leads a practitioner to institute immediate action. In the case of ACS, the action is confirmatory testing using troponin measurements and electrocardiogram with resultant notification and activation of the cardiac catheterization team. In the case of stroke, national guidelines are in place to regulate the ideal time for management of ischemic or hemorrhagic stroke from recognition of symptoms. These paradigms do not yet exist for AKI. Driven by the examples, however, the concept of renal angina has been described in the general pediatric ICU population [16, 17]. Similar to cardiac Prinzmetal's angina, renal angina (operationalized into the renal angina index) combines known risk factors for severe AKI with early signs of filtrative or tubular injury (small changes in creatinine or fluid accumulation) 12 h into an ICU admission for the purposes of identifying the patients at highest risk of severe AKI 3 days *after* admission [18]. Notably, biomarker incorporation into the model, meaning biomarkers tested in patients positive for renal angina, led to a significant improvement in the specificity of prediction [19]. Similar risk stratification tools are being tested in adult ICU patients [20].

Patients at risk of AKI after CPB can be identified earlier. Given the significant amount of data from both adults and children associating AKI-CPB with poor outcome, more attention should be given the recent literature describing the association of even early changes in creatinine and/or fluid accumulation with poor outcome. Risk factors for AKI after CPB are known. Prior to operative procedures, a patient's risk associated with genomic variants and past medical history and comorbidities can be incorporated into a subsequent management strategy (described later). A cardiac renal angina prodrome is currently being explored. Increasing appreciation of the epidemic postoperative burden from AKI (by cardiac intensivists and cardiologists) would raise the resting index of suspicion. Taken together, if moving the needle for the epidemiology of the disease, that is, if outcomes can actually be improved, it will rely on more vigilant and objective assessments of AKI risk.

19.3 Pathophysiology: Biology to Drive Diagnostics

The pathophysiology of AKI-CPB is multifactorial. Traditional thinking identifies, broadly, the categories of oxygen delivery, inflammation, and direct free radical or oxidative toxicity as drivers for reducing renal function for patients on and after CPB support. Renal blood flow can be impaired during CPB, particularly during aortic cross-clamp, leading to regional ischemia in the renal circulation. Concordant with ischemia is impairment in oxygen delivery to a system already under precise homeostatic control of regional oxygen tone. Study of animal models of AKI-CPB is limited to larger animals (as opposed to murine models) given technical complexity, but available data suggest homology in both perturbations in regional oxygen delivery and renal blood flow during CPB [21]. Clinical studies consistently demonstrate an association with noninvasive tissue oximetry and measurement of oxygen metabolism with the initiation, continuation, and discontinuation of CPB (changes occur in response to blood flow). Inflammation during and after CPB is secondary to liberation of humoral cytokines as blood interacts with an artificial surface such as a catheter or bypass surface. Numerous ex vivo and in vitro studies describe a pro-inflammatory cascade during this interaction (blood and surface), theoretically leading to an increase in systemic inflammation during and after CPB ultimately affecting the renal parenchyma and cellular integrity [22–24]. Central to the pro-inflammatory cascade is the transcription factor NF-kB [25], an intracellular mediator of upregulation of adhesins, selectins, and multiple immunoglobulins. Interestingly, evidence demonstrating a persistent regional upregulation of NF-kB-related gene products with downstream mediators of dysregulation in inflammation in the renal circulation or parenchyma is scant. The direct nephrotoxicity of CPB is felt to be associated with the liberation and transmigration of oxygen radicals and free oxygen moieties (again when red blood cells come in contact with and shear on the surface of artificial polymers) [26]. Renal tubular epithelial cell integrity can be compromised in the presence of high levels of superoxide and can undergo epithelial-mesenchymal transition to a more pro-fibrotic milieu in the presence of high circulating transforming growth factor-β, upregulated by oxidative conditions [24, 27]. The clinical parallel to these laboratory findings is difficult to isolate as existing diagnostic tools cannot differentiate between types of incipient or ongoing injury in the kidney.

Existing diagnostic criteria create an imprecise definition of AKI after CPB. The available markers of renal dysfunction are either increases in serum creatinine (SCr) or changes in urine output (UOP) as direct indices and changes in filtration, electrolyte imbalance, aberrant drug clearance, and loss of urinary concentrating ability or proteinuria. The markers are themselves flawed. Widespread data and innumerable reports discuss the limitations of SCr for the prediction or diagnosis of AKI, but the most problematic aspects in children are the dependency on muscle mass, the discrepancies between local laboratory standards and "steady state," and the effect of dilutional volume. The latter is a phenomenon initially described in a post hoc analysis of the Fluid and Catheter Treatment Trial for acute respiratory distress syndrome in adults [28]. Data from children suggests that correcting SCr for net fluid balance uncovers a refined creatinine-based diagnosis of AKI and associated sequelae [12]. Urine output is not reliably checked in the pediatric population without the presence of a Foley catheter. Initiatives to reduce the rate of catheter-associated urinary infections have made a priority of removing "unnecessary" Foley catheters; however, recent adult and pediatric data suggests following urine output closely in the initial days of ICU admission is vital to the accurate identification of AKI [2, 29, 30]. Outside of SCr and UOP, historic data lists serum and urine metrics for AKI diagnosis that have been relatively abandoned since the adoption of international AKI census criteria (RIFLE, AKIN, KDIGO) [31]. Unfortunately, the existing markers and the consensus diagnostic guidelines do little to advance the understanding of AKI or refine diagnosis. Creatinine and UOP still lead to imprecise nomenclature for AKI such as "prerenal" or "intrinsic renal/acute tubular necrosis." The former is flawed in the sense that patients diagnosed as prerenal may have injury occurring in the kidney, injury may be severe, injury may not be transient, and injury may not be responsive to volume (all of these are implied by the name). An apt example of an imprecise "prerenal" diagnosis is congestive heart failure. Concurrently, patients labeled as ATN often have no histologic evidence of tubular necrosis [32, 33], and more data suggests how inappropriate this terminology is from a pathophysiologic standpoint.

The precision of AKI diagnostics can be improved. A new analysis of creatinine suggests that static measures of creatinine are less indicative of glomerular filtration, instead supporting the case for a kinetic GFR based on change in creatinine over time [34]. In parallel fashion, urine output should be tracked and should likely be tracked in a dynamic state, flow rate change as a function of time. The critical care nephrology community has already issued statements to use more precise terminology such as "functional" or "damage-associated" AKI and to denote AKI phenotypes [35]. AKI biomarkers from the urine are able to delineate a more discrete location of AKI—glomerular, tubular, and mesenchymal—than the generic index reported by changes in creatinine or urine output. Although few novel biomarkers are broadly available for use at the current time, the development and introduction of these markers into clinical practice will facilitate a more precise understanding of the location and severity of AKI. Additionally, as has been well reported, many of these markers are more sensitive to injury, responding in a more temporally proximal nature to incipient or ongoing injury. The most widely reported data focuses on neutrophil gelatinase-associated lipocalin (NGAL), kidney injury molecule-1 (KIM-1), and tissue inhibitor of metalloproteinase-2/insulin-like growth factor-binding protein 7 (TIMP-2/IGFBP7). The pediatric CPB population has served as the ideal cohort of patients for discovery, isolation, derivation, and validation of these markers for prediction of AKI and diagnosis of AKI severity. Respectively, they confer information about tubular viability, mesenchymal or parenchymal damage, and molecular cell-cycle arrest at the level of the glomerulus. Taken together, these markers may render AKI phenotypes that are quite distinct, even though all may demonstrate similar "increases" of SCr from baseline. Literally what this means is testing of biomarkers in combination is likely the next step in biomarker adjudication [29]. Preliminary data indicates that a simple combination of a tubular injury marker and a glomerular filtration marker identifies distinct cohorts of patients—functional AKI or severe AKI [36]. Additionally, tracking biomarkers as they change over time may deliver information with regard to real-time fluid handling and also predict subsequent changes in creatinine, thereby filtration [37]. In addition to markers of kidney injury, testing the functional capacity of the kidney is possible. Applying standardized, objective criteria to urine production after a dose of furosemide, adult data identifies the value of the "furosemide stress test" (FST) for the prediction of severe AKI, AKI progression, and ultimately renal replacement therapy (RRT) utilization [38, 39]. By comparison, the FST is superior to biomarker prediction of AKI [40, 41]. Pediatric data supporting the predictive performance of the FST is beginning to emerge [42]. For the pediatric patient following CPB, the FST is particularly important. Precise control over fluid is emphasized in the perioperative period, and recent data suggests a benefit of early implementation of peritoneal dialysis over the use of furosemide (or continued use) [43]. The ability to use initial response to furosemide to predict AKI progression would potentially be a piece of actionable clinical decision support to the CICU provider making decisions with regard to fluid removal in the patient immediately postoperative from CPB.

Refined epidemiologic data may refine risk factors associated with AKI-CPB. Data controlled for age and surgical complexity now suggests AKI-CPB carries no association with CPB time or patient age [12, 14, 44]. Additionally, modeling suggests a lack of persistent inflammatory mediators in the nephron after 6 h following CPB (initial rise at 2 h with exponential decay)—suggesting a constant pro-inflammatory environment is potentially not contributing to progressive AKI.

Expedited diagnostics may lead to improved outcomes. A host of more contemporary diagnostics for AKI-CPB is available or soon will be (Fig. 19.2). Management bundles for AKI can be derived from the KDIGO AKI practice guideline. In adult

Past and Present

Time Frame	Marker
1960-1980s	Creatinine
1980s-1990s	Creatinine
2000s-2010s	Creatinine

Location	Marker
"Renal"	Creatinine

Population Age	Marker
Adults	Creatinine
Children	Creatinine
Neonates	Creatinine (or nothing)

Etiology	Marker
Ischemic	Creatinine
Septic	Creatinine
Nephrotoxic	Creatinine
Hypoxic	Creatinine
Obstructive	Creatinine

Severity/Progression	Marker
Low	Creatinine
High	Creatinine

Future

Time Frame	Marker
2020-2025	Creatinine, Urine Output & Biomarkers
2025-2030	Dynamic Biomarker Combinations
Beyond	Real-time functional tests & endotyping

Location	Marker
Glomerulus	Real-time GFR
Tubular Epithelium	Urine biomarker panel
Vasa recta	Renal oximetry
Collecting Duct	Kinetic Urine Output

Population Age	Marker
Variable	Age Specific Marker Panels

Etiology	Marker
Perfusion/Reperfusion	Real-time GFR
Apoptosis/Necrosis/Autophagy	Biomarker profile
Inflammation/Oxidative Stress	Bioenergetics panel
Chloride Transport	Furosemide stress Test

Severity/Progression	Marker
Low	Negative renal angina
Moderate	Renal angina+/Stable Biomarkers
Progressive/High	Renal angina+/Rising Biomarkers

Fig. 19.2 Diagnostic advances in AKI. The past, present, and future for the field of AKI diagnostics are depicted. The past and current paradigm is limited by essentially one diagnostic tool—expected to serve as a "do-all" and "be-all" marker. This is inappropriate. The future will offer the opportunity to refine the diagnosis of AKI, improving the precision of diagnosis and hopefully making a more tailored management approach to the disease possible

patients following CPB, stratification by TIMP-2/IGFBP7 levels post-op into receipt of AKI bundled care resulted in less AKI, less severe AKI, and improved patient outcomes (for those receiving the bundle) [45]. In total, diagnostic improvement for AKI following CPB is imminent. A combination of markers and functional tests, when used in the appropriate context of risk, should identify the patients at highest risk for AKI and certainly delineate levels of risk. The varying degrees of risk, or even incipient and ongoing injury, should naturally suggest more personalized and precise management plans.

19.4 Management: Defense to Offense

The paradigm of management for AKI has been centered on supportive care. Prior to the adoption of census criteria, a universally "accepted" approach lacking stratification included maintenance of mean perfusion pressure, adjustment of medications for renal clearance, avoidance of contrast or other iatrogenic sources of nephrotoxicity, and control of glycemia. The KDIGO guidelines created a tiered approach to management based on degree of AKI risk or severity. Although implementation of the guidelines has been slow, data has emerged demonstrating benefit to the incorporation of these steps in the management of patients with recognized AKI. In the patient with AKI-CPB, no published guidelines exist for management. Most clinicians would recognize the importance of the above stipulated tenets of care but would also incorporate fluid management and special care during the period of postoperative care when low cardiac output syndrome occurs at greatest frequency. The importance of control over fluid balance cannot be overemphasized. Repeated data from pediatric patients demonstrates the negative association of fluid accumulation in the post-CPB period with outcomes, even independent of AKI [46]. Notably, both small changes in SCr and small increases in fluid overload increase the odds for poor patient outcome [47]. Phases of fluid balance in the critically ill patient may be slightly different in the post-CPB patient, especially considering the widespread utilization of modified ultrafiltration during separation from bypass. As mentioned earlier, however, recognition of AKI by SCr can be masked by fluid accumulation, particularly in the small neonate following cardiac surgery. Correction of SCr for net fluid balance has been described in limited data sets and at the very least merits consideration for integration into routine practice (as infants are 75–80% total body water). Outside of these supportive care measures, however, there are few routine actions taken which prevent AKI or reduce AKI progression or severity. In total, the paradigm of AKI management, particularly in CPB, is reactive.

The electronic health record (EHR) can be incorporated into AKI management. Recent reports demonstrate the power of AKI sniffers and alert systems embedded within the EHR—expediting both recognitions for intensive care management teams but also triggering nephrology involvement [48]. The electronic record has several advantages—notably round-the-clock surveillance, objectified assessment, ability to instantaneously and simultaneously alert multiple providers, and the possibility of moving between institutions. As with other systems, EHR recognition systems are limited to some degree by the input variables requiring human. Interestingly, programming to algorithmically follow changes in urine output, or urine flow rate, can increase the rate of AKI prediction [49]. The use of these systems facilitates automatic incorporation or activation of AKI care bundles. Early reports of these systems are promising—demonstrating a reduction in AKI incidence, severity, and progression. As the ability to identify risk factors increases, the preoperative phase may be the time when the EHR serves the greatest utility. A mechanism to create an AKI-CPB risk score prior to CPB—and ultimately adjust intraoperative variables in proportion to the degree of risk or to specific aspects of risk—is how precision medicine will be oriented. Given the amount of pre-, intra-, and postoperative data available on pediatric CPB patients, the population seems ideal to derive and validate automated models of preventative AKI care.

Fluid control in the AKI-CPB patient can be proactive. Novel biomarkers may predict tubular dysfunction and the patients at risk for fluid retention. Early data suggests that the dynamic change of sequential tubular biomarkers can even predict who will be responsive to diuresis [37]. Additionally, retrospective data indicates early and persistent elevation in tubular markers—even in the absence of creatinine elevation, can predict fluid accumulation and the eventual initiation of renal replacement therapy [50]. Next-generation fluid removal machines can ultrafiltrate serum through peripheral catheters, eliminating the need for peritoneal dialysis drains or large central intravenous access in small patients [51]. The incorporation of these next steps will allow providers to be more “in control” of the fluid balance of their patients.

The care of children following cardiopulmonary bypass can move from reactive to proactive. The traditional mindset has followed a defensive, reactive paradigm—limitation of nephrotoxicity, supportive care of vital organs, fluid removal, and frequent assessment of filtration function by creatinine. A more offensive-minded approach is possible with current tools. Stratification of patients both preoperatively and immediately postoperatively into risk strata, linking risk to management bundles from the preoperative phase, early initiation of volume management to prevent fluid accumulation, and use of the electronic medical record to identify patients at risk or experiencing AKI is possible. AKI in the CPB patient is associated with long-term chronic kidney disease, parallel to the rise in chronic renal insufficiency in both adult survivors of AKI and survivors of critical illness in the general pediatric population. A more preventative approach is warranted.

19.5 Call to Action: Moving the Needle

The understanding and management of acute kidney injury following cardiopulmonary bypass in the pediatric patient is flawed. A combination of the poor understanding of the pathophysiology of disease and outdated and imprecise diagnostics leads to both a likely underestimate of disease incidence and underappreciation of associated sequelae. Problematically, all of these inadequacies synergistically handcuff management—creating a relatively ignorant and defensive approach. The needle can be moved and outcomes can be improved.

In this chapter, the path forward to improved patient outcomes in the pediatric AKI-CPB population has been outlined (Fig. 19.3). This cohort of patients should be risk stratified—and is an ideal population to understand from a genomic and pathophysiologic standpoint—how much risk exists at baseline. This means moving beyond a binary appreciation of risk—but moving to a quantified, objective calculation of risk. A cardiac renal angina score is a first step. Integration of urinary biomarkers for the purpose of assessment of baseline glomerular, tubular, and mesenchymal integrity would be valuable given the recent data describing the importance of sequential biomarker measurements. This should not come as a surprise as almost all of the meaningful metrics of critical illness are, in fact, more illustrative when tracked in dynamic fashion—over time (e.g., lactate, pH). The electronic health record must be integrated into the next generation of management strategies—leveraging the power of instantaneous alerts, data, and objective assessments. A patient-specific bundle of preventative measures can be instituted upon assessment of risk, and combinations of biomarkers can be used to not only help guide postoperative fluid management but also target cohorts of patients potentially responsive to "AKI therapies." Novel therapeutics were not discussed in this text but

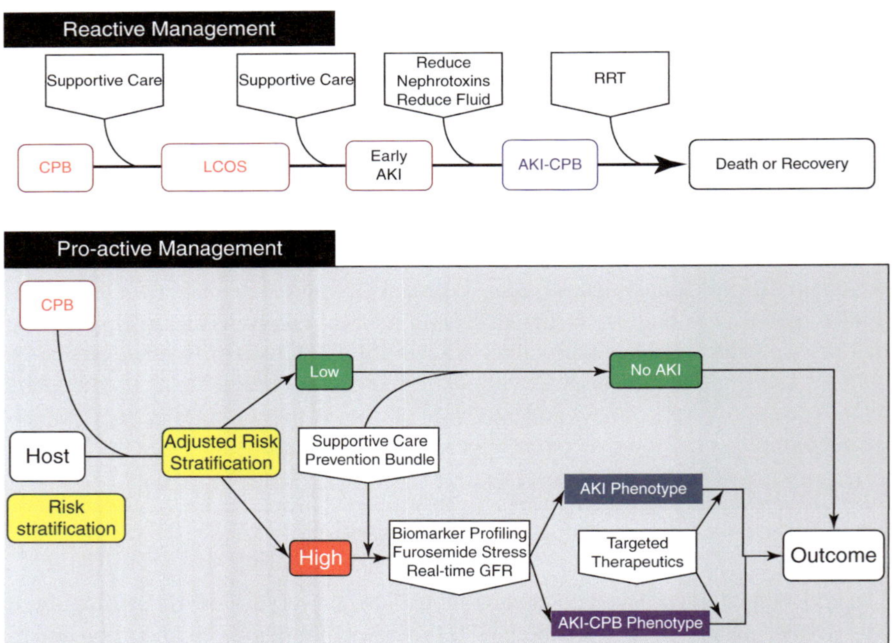

Fig. 19.3 Changing the paradigm. The needle for outcomes of children suffering AKI-CPB can be moved from an antiquated, defensive reactive paradigm to a more proactive and "offensive" approach. In this paradigm, patients are risk stratified prior to CPB and then recalibrated intra-and postoperatively. Patients are stratified by risk to receive proactive and preventative care, incorporating profiling and phenotyping of illness and ultimately targeted therapeutics

include a list of renal vasoactive medications, anti-inflammatory or apoptotic agents, stem cell therapy, and monoclonal therapeutics. Additionally, previous trials for AKI therapeutics including agents such as diuretics, steroids, sodium bicarbonate, and other commonly used medications may actually demonstrate a functional response in the appropriate, stratified groups of patients. Together, all of these approaches offer the potential to increase the recognition and awareness of the problem of AKI-CPB and associated patient outcome. To actually improve outcome, a multidisciplinary approach is required: intensivists, pediatricians, surgeons, cardiologists, nephrologists, pharmacists, and more are required to engage in collaborative prospective study—investing time, resources, and bandwidth to turn the tide against an epidemic.

References

1. Hoste EA, Bagshaw SM, Bellomo R, Cely CM, Colman R, Cruz DN, et al. Epidemiology of acute kidney injury in critically ill patients: the multinational AKI-EPI study. Intensive Care Med. 2015;41(8):1411–23.
2. Kaddourah A, Basu RK, Bagshaw SM, Goldstein SL, Investigators A. Epidemiology of acute kidney injury in critically ill children and young adults. N Engl J Med. 2017;376(1):11–20.
3. Jetton JG, Boohaker LJ, Sethi SK, Wazir S, Rohatgi S, Soranno DE, et al. Incidence and outcomes of neonatal acute kidney injury (AWAKEN): a multicentre, multinational, observational cohort study. Lancet Child Adolesc Health. 2017;1(3):184–94.
4. Susantitaphong P, Cruz DN, Cerda J, Abulfaraj M, Alqahtani F, Koulouridis I, et al. World incidence of AKI: a meta-analysis. Clin J Am Soc Nephrol. 2013;8(9):1482–93.
5. Li S, Krawczeski CD, Zappitelli M, Devarajan P, Thiessen-Philbrook H, Coca SG, et al. Incidence, risk factors, and outcomes of acute kidney injury after pediatric cardiac surgery: a prospective multicenter study. Crit Care Med. 2011;39(6):1493–9.
6. Sethi SK, Kumar M, Sharma R, Bazaz S, Kher V. Acute kidney injury in children after cardiopulmonary bypass: risk factors and outcome. Indian Pediatr. 2015;52(3):223–6.
7. Sethi SK, Goyal D, Yadav DK, Shukla U, Kajala PL, Gupta VK, et al. Predictors of acute kidney injury post-cardiopulmonary bypass in children. Clin Exp Nephrol. 2011;15(4):529–34.
8. Dasta JF, Kane-Gill SL, Durtschi AJ, Pathak DS, Kellum JA. Costs and outcomes of acute kidney injury (AKI) following cardiac surgery. Nephrol Dial Transplant. 2008;23(6):1970–4.
9. Jefferies JL, Devarajan P. Early detection of acute kidney injury after pediatric cardiac surgery. Prog Pediatr Cardiol. 2016;41:9–16.
10. Stafford-Smith M, Li YJ, Mathew JP, Li YW, Ji Y, Phillips-Bute BG, et al. Genome-wide association study of acute kidney injury after coronary bypass graft surgery identifies susceptibility loci. Kidney Int. 2015;88(4):823–32.
11. Schopka S, Diez C, Camboni D, Floerchinger B, Schmid C, Hilker M. Impact of cardiopulmonary bypass on acute kidney injury following coronary artery bypass grafting: a matched pair analysis. J Cardiothorac Surg. 2014;9:20.
12. Basu RK, Andrews A, Krawczeski C, Manning P, Wheeler DS, Goldstein SL. Acute kidney injury based on corrected serum creatinine is associated with increased morbidity in children following the arterial switch operation. Pediatr Crit Care Med. 2013;14(5):e218–24.
13. Hassinger AB, Wainwright MS, Lane JC, Haymond S, Backer CL, Wald E. Elevated preoperative serum asymmetrical dimethylarginine (ADMA) is associated with poor outcomes after pediatric cardiac surgery. Intensive Care Med. 2012;38(10):1697–704.
14. Hassinger AB, Backer CL, Lane JC, Haymond S, Wang D, Wald EL. Predictive power of serum cystatin C to detect acute kidney injury and pediatric-modified RIFLE class in children undergoing cardiac surgery. Pediatr Crit Care Med. 2012;13(4):435–40.

15. Hoste EA, Maitland K, Brudney CS, Mehta R, Vincent JL, Yates D, et al. Four phases of intravenous fluid therapy: a conceptual model. Br J Anaesth. 2014;113(5):740–7.
16. Basu RK, Zappitelli M, Brunner L, Wang Y, Wong HR, Chawla LS, et al. Derivation and validation of the renal angina index to improve the prediction of acute kidney injury in critically ill children. Kidney Int. 2014;85(3):659–67.
17. Basu RK, Chawla LS, Wheeler DS, Goldstein SL. Renal angina: an emerging paradigm to identify children at risk for acute kidney injury. Pediatr Nephrol. 2012;27(7):1067–78.
18. Basu RK, Wang Y, Wong HR, Chawla LS, Wheeler DS, Goldstein SL. Incorporation of biomarkers with the renal angina index for prediction of severe AKI in critically ill children. Clin J Am Soc Nephrol. 2014;9(4):654–62.
19. Menon S, Goldstein SL, Mottes T, Fei L, Kaddourah A, Terrell T, et al. Urinary biomarker incorporation into the renal angina index early in intensive care unit admission optimizes acute kidney injury prediction in critically ill children: a prospective cohort study. Nephrol Dial Transplant. 2016;31(4):586–94.
20. Cruz DN, Ferrer-Nadal A, Piccinni P, Goldstein SL, Chawla LS, Alessandri E, et al. Utilization of small changes in serum creatinine with clinical risk factors to assess the risk of AKI in critically ill adults. Clin J Am Soc Nephrol. 2014;9(4):663–72.
21. Murphy GJ, Lin H, Coward RJ, Toth T, Holmes R, Hall D, et al. An initial evaluation of post-cardiopulmonary bypass acute kidney injury in swine. Eur J Cardiothorac Surg. 2009;36(5):849–55.
22. Sellke FW, DiMaio JM, Caplan LR, Ferguson TB, Gardner TJ, Hiratzka LF, et al. Comparing on-pump and off-pump coronary artery bypass grafting: numerous studies but few conclusions: a scientific statement from the American Heart Association council on cardiovascular surgery and anesthesia in collaboration with the interdisciplinary working group on quality of care and outcomes research. Circulation. 2005;111(21):2858–64.
23. Okusa MD. The inflammatory cascade in acute ischemic renal failure. Nephron. 2002;90(2):133–8.
24. Haase M, Bellomo R, Haase-Fielitz A. Novel biomarkers, oxidative stress, and the role of labile iron toxicity in cardiopulmonary bypass-associated acute kidney injury. J Am Coll Cardiol. 2010;55(19):2024–33.
25. Paparella D, Yau TM, Young E. Cardiopulmonary bypass induced inflammation: pathophysiology and treatment. An update. Eur J Cardiothorac Surg. 2002;21(2):232–44.
26. Westhuyzen J, McGiffin DC, McCarthy J, Fleming SJ. Tubular nephrotoxicity after cardiac surgery utilising cardiopulmonary bypass. Clin Chim Acta. 1994;228(2):123–32.
27. Yap SC, Lee HT. Acute kidney injury and extrarenal organ dysfunction: new concepts and experimental evidence. Anesthesiology. 2012;116(5):1139–48.
28. Macedo E, Bouchard J, Soroko SH, Chertow GM, Himmelfarb J, Ikizler TA, et al. Fluid accumulation, recognition and staging of acute kidney injury in critically-ill patients. Crit Care. 2010;14(3):R82.
29. McCullough PA, Shaw AD, Haase M, Bouchard J, Waikar SS, Siew ED, et al. Diagnosis of acute kidney injury using functional and injury biomarkers: workgroup statements from the tenth acute dialysis quality initiative consensus conference. Contrib Nephrol. 2013;182:13–29.
30. Kellum JA, Sileanu FE, Murugan R, Lucko N, Shaw AD, Clermont G. Classifying AKI by urine output versus serum creatinine level. J Am Soc Nephrol. 2015;26(9):2231–8.
31. Sampaio MC, Maximo CA, Montenegro CM, Mota DM, Fernandes TR, Bianco AC, et al. Comparison of diagnostic criteria for acute kidney injury in cardiac surgery. Arq Bras Cardiol. 2013;101(1):18–25.
32. Langenberg C, Gobe G, Hood S, May CN, Bellomo R. Renal histopathology during experimental septic acute kidney injury and recovery. Crit Care Med. 2014;42(1):e58–67.
33. Langenberg C, Bagshaw SM, May CN, Bellomo R. The histopathology of septic acute kidney injury: a systematic review. Crit Care. 2008;12(2):R38.
34. Chen S. Retooling the creatinine clearance equation to estimate kinetic GFR when the plasma creatinine is changing acutely. J Am Soc Nephrol. 2013;24(6):877–88.

35. Murray PT, Mehta RL, Shaw A, Ronco C, Endre Z, Kellum JA, et al. Potential use of biomarkers in acute kidney injury: report and summary of recommendations from the 10th acute dialysis quality initiative consensus conference. Kidney Int. 2014;85(3):513–21.
36. Basu RK, Wong HR, Krawczeski CD, Wheeler DS, Manning PB, Chawla LS, et al. Combining functional and tubular damage biomarkers improves diagnostic precision for acute kidney injury after cardiac surgery. J Am Coll Cardiol. 2014;64(25):2753–62.
37. Varnell CD Jr, Goldstein SL, Devarajan P, Basu RK. Impact of near real-time urine neutrophil gelatinase-associated lipocalin assessment on clinical practice. Kidney Int Rep. 2017;2(6):1243–9.
38. Chawla LS, Davison DL, Brasha-Mitchell E, Koyner JL, Arthur JM, Shaw AD, et al. Development and standardization of a furosemide stress test to predict the severity of acute kidney injury. Crit Care. 2013;17(5):R207.
39. Chawla LS. The furosemide stress test to predict renal function after continuous renal replacement therapy. Authors' response. Crit Care. 2014;18(3):429.
40. Koyner JL, Davison DL, Brasha-Mitchell E, Chalikonda DM, Arthur JM, Shaw AD, et al. Furosemide stress test and biomarkers for the prediction of AKI severity. J Am Soc Nephrol. 2015;26(8):2023–31.
41. Koyner JL, Chawla LS. Use of stress tests in evaluating kidney disease. Curr Opin Nephrol Hypertens. 2017;26(1):31–5.
42. Borasino S, Wall KM, Crawford JH, Hock KM, Cleveland DC, Rahman F, et al. Furosemide response predicts acute kidney injury after cardiac surgery in infants and neonates. Pediatr Crit Care Med. 2018;19(4):310–7.
43. Kwiatkowski DM, Goldstein SL, Cooper DS, Nelson DP, Morales DL, Krawczeski CD. Peritoneal dialysis vs furosemide for prevention of fluid overload in infants after cardiac surgery: a randomized clinical trial. JAMA Pediatr. 2017;171(4):357–64.
44. Gist KM, Goldstein SL, Wrona J, Alten JA, Basu RK, Cooper DS, et al. Kinetics of the cell cycle arrest biomarkers (TIMP-2*IGFBP-7) for prediction of acute kidney injury in infants after cardiac surgery. Pediatr Nephrol. 2017;32(9):1611–9.
45. Meersch M, Schmidt C, Hoffmeier A, Van Aken H, Wempe C, Gerss J, et al. Prevention of cardiac surgery-associated AKI by implementing the KDIGO guidelines in high risk patients identified by biomarkers: the PrevAKI randomized controlled trial. Intensive Care Med. 2017;43(11):1551–61.
46. Alobaidi R, Morgan C, Basu RK, Stenson E, Featherstone R, Majumdar SR, et al. Association between fluid balance and outcomes in critically ill children: a systematic review and meta-analysis. JAMA Pediatr. 2018;172(3):257–68.
47. Hassinger AB, Wald EL, Goodman DM. Early postoperative fluid overload precedes acute kidney injury and is associated with higher morbidity in pediatric cardiac surgery patients. Pediatr Crit Care Med. 2014;15(2):131–8.
48. James MT, Hobson CE, Darmon M, Mohan S, Hudson D, Goldstein SL, et al. Applications for detection of acute kidney injury using electronic medical records and clinical information systems: workgroup statements from the 15(th) ADQI consensus conference. Can J Kidney Health Dis. 2016;3:9.
49. Song Y, Kim DW, Kwak YL, Kim BS, Joo HM, Ju JW, et al. Urine output during cardiopulmonary bypass predicts acute kidney injury after cardiac surgery: a single-center retrospective analysis. Medicine (Baltimore). 2016;95(22):e3757.
50. Klein SJ, Brandtner AK, Lehner GF, Ulmer H, Bagshaw SM, Wiedermann CJ, et al. Biomarkers for prediction of renal replacement therapy in acute kidney injury: a systematic review and meta-analysis. Intensive Care Med. 2018;44(3):323–36.
51. Askenazi D, Ingram D, White S, Cramer M, Borasino S, Coghill C, et al. Smaller circuits for smaller patients: improving renal support therapy with Aquadex. Pediatr Nephrol. 2016;31(5):853–60.

Sepsis-Associated Acute Kidney Injury 20

Rashid Alobaidi and Sean M. Bagshaw

20.1 Introduction

Acute kidney injury (AKI) is commonly encountered and contributes to high burden of morbidity and mortality during critical illness. On the other hand, sepsis remains highly prevalent and the leading cause of non-trauma-related mortality in children. Sepsis carries a strong association with the development of AKI and accounts for approximately quarter of the cases of pediatrics AKI. Sepsis-associated acute kidney injury (SA-AKI) is a serious complication that exacerbates an already less than favorable outcome in patients with sepsis. Several pathophysiological mechanisms have been described to suggest that SA-AKI represents a distinct subclass of AKI precipitated by alterations in renal microvascular mechanisms and immune-mediated injury. There is no single modality of treatment that can alter the natural course of SA-AKI, making it a challenging clinical problem. The general principals of SA-AKI management focus on early risk identification, fluid resuscitation, and appropriate antimicrobial administration, followed by a strategy of limiting injury, avoiding life-threatening complications, eliminating any potential contributors to worsening kidney function and facilitating recovery.

R. Alobaidi
Department of Pediatrics, Division of Pediatric Critical Care Medicine, Faculty of Medicine and Dentistry, University of Alberta, Edmonton, AB, Canada

S. M. Bagshaw (✉)
Department of Critical Care Medicine, Faculty of Medicine and Dentistry, University of Alberta, Edmonton, AB, Canada
e-mail: bagshaw@ualberta.ca

S. K. Sethi et al. (eds.), *Critical Care Pediatric Nephrology and Dialysis: A Practical Handbook*, https://doi.org/10.1007/978-981-13-2276-1_20

20.2 Case History

A previously well 3-year-old girl presented to her local hospital having been unwell with fever for 2 days. On examination, the child was febrile and tachycardic with poor perfusion. Petechial rash involving the lower limbs and trunk was noted on examination of her skin. Intravenous ceftriaxone and vancomycin were administered, in addition to 10 mL/kg aliquots of crystalloid boluses. The child became more lethargic with worsening hemodynamics. Further crystalloid boluses were given for a total of 60 mL/kg, and epinephrine infusion was commenced. Initial blood tests were significant for white blood cell count of 16.3×10^9/L, platelet 95×10^9/L, and hemoglobin 109 g/L. Venous blood gas showed metabolic acidosis with pH 7.21, PCO_2 34 mm HG, and HCO_3 13.4 mmol/L. Lactate was 4.4 mmol/L. Electrolyte panel was within normal range. Creatinine was 52 μmol/L, while urea was 11.1 mmol/L. Blood culture grew gram negative bacteria (later identified as Neisseria Meningitidis).

The child was admitted to the pediatric intensive care where she received respiratory and hemodynamic support. She had minimal urine output in the first 24 h (0.3 mL/kg/h). She had worsening metabolic acidosis and electrolytes imbalance. By the end of the second day, her creatinine had doubled, and urine output continued to be minimal. She appeared overly edematous with signs of pulmonary edema and pleural effusion on chest X-ray. Cumulative fluid balance was more than 10% of admission weight. The decision was made to start continuous renal replacement therapy (CRRT). Over the following 4 days, her clinical status improved, and she was weaned off inotropic support and extubated. She continued to receive CRRT until day 7 of her stay, and then transitioned to intermittent hemodialysis every 2–3 days. Her kidney function recovered by the third week of her hospital stay and she was subsequently liberated from dialysis.

20.3 SA-AKI Epidemiology

Several pediatric studies have described sepsis to be a common trigger of AKI. Sepsis was the primary risk factor for the development of AKI in approximately a quarter of pediatric patients with AKI (Table 20.1). In a study of over 2000 critically ill children, AKI developed in 18% of the patients. In those, infection was identified as an independent risk factor (adjusted odds ratio [OR] 1.92, 95% CI 1.23–2.99) [1]. In a large cohort of children with severe sepsis, AKI (defined as doubling creatinine) was present in 16% [2].

20.4 SA-AKI Outcomes

Accumulating data suggest that SA-AKI portends a worse prognosis. ICU and in-hospital mortality rates have consistently been described as higher for SA-AKI compared with non-septic AKI (ICU mortality, 19.8% vs. 13.4%; in-hospital

Table 20.1 Summary of selected pediatric studies describing AKI and sepsis

Study	Year	Design	Population (n)	AKI definition	AKI incidence	SA-AKI proportion
Volpon et al. [35]	2016	Prospective, two centers	General PICU (160)	KDIGO criteria	46%	49%
Mehta et al. [36]	2012	Prospective, single center	General PICU (108)	AKIN criteria	36%	25%
Alkandari et al. [1]	2011	Retrospective, two centers	General PICU (2106)	AKIN criteria	18%	11%
Duzova et al. [37]	2010	Prospective, single center	Hospitalized patients with AKI (472)	pRIFLE criteria	N/A	18%
Plotz et al. [38]	2008	Retrospective, single center	Intubated PICU (103)	pRIFLE criteria	58%	21%
Akcan-Arikan et al. [39]	2007	Prospective, single center	Intubated PICU (123)	pRIFLE criteria	82%	27%
Bailey et al. [40]	2007	Prospective, single center	General PICU (1047)	Cr doubling	4.5%	22%

mortality, 29.7% vs. 21.6%). When patients were stratified as per the severity of AKI, it was noted that there is stepwise increase in ICU, in hospital, and long-term morality.

Data suggest that patients with SA-AKI stay longer in the ICU compared to those with AKI without sepsis or sepsis alone. The duration of hospital stay in septic patients with AKI may be up to twice as long as those without AKI [3]. The length of hospital stay increases in a stepwise fashion depending on severity of AKI. When patients with SA-AKI progressed from RIFLE–Injury to RIFLE–Failure stage, the median length of ICU stay increased from 3.1 to 4.8 days [4]. The recovery of renal function was similar for patients with AKI irrespective of the presence of sepsis. It was noted that renal function recovered completely in a mean time of 10.1 ± 8 days in 97% of 315 sepsis AKI patients [5].

20.5 SA-AKI Pathophysiology

Evolving evidence suggest that SA-AKI is precipitated by unique and complex mechanisms. Sepsis-mediated kidney hypoperfusion causing ischemic injury and "acute tubular necrosis" has been often described as the mechanism of renal injury in sepsis. However, recent clinical investigations have challenged this explanation. Autopsy studies have shown that in patients with clinically defined SA-AKI, only 22% of 184 patients showed features of tubular necrosis on histopathological examination [6]. Recent experimental and clinical evidence have identified several alternative triggers of kidney damage and dysfunction in sepsis (Fig. 20.1).

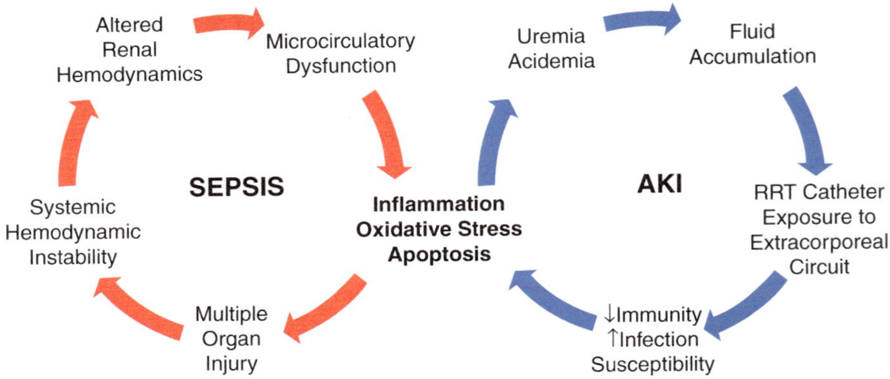

Fig. 20.1 The pathophysiologic interaction between sepsis and AKI (from: Pathophysiology and management of septic acute kidney injury. Romanovsky et al. Pediatr Nephrol (2014) 29:1–12 with permission)

20.5.1 Alternation in Renal Hemodynamics

Experimental animal models have shown that sepsis is associated with abnormal hyperdynamic renal blood flow. In humans, renal vein thermodilution measurement of renal blood flow (RBF) in septic critically ill patients showed preservation of renal plasma flow [7]. There was no correlation between decrease in GFR and changes in renal blood flow, or vice versa. So on the whole, renal blood flow appears to have less contribution to renal perfusion during sepsis. The changes taking place in glomerular perfusion pressure and relative intrarenal shunting instead appear to be the primary aberration occurring early during sepsis.

20.5.2 Renal Microcirculatory Dysfunction

Numerous factors can disrupt renal microcirculation in sepsis. Loss of the endothelial glycocalyx contributes to altered vascular permeability, excess fluid extravasation, and renal tissue edema. Cellular debris, including leukocytes, platelets, and coagulation activation, further contributes to endothelial disruption and occlusion. These factors contribute to impaired microcirculatory perfusion and may be further exacerbated by elevated intrarenal pressure and elevated renal venous pressure and/or excessive intra-abdominal pressure.

20.5.3 Immune-Mediated Injury

The systemic host immune response to sepsis has the potential to lead to end organ injury. Elevated circulating levels of selected inflammatory mediators in sepsis are known to be associated with development of SA-AKI. An experiment comparing

SA-AKI versus ischemia–perfusion models in mice showed that SA-AKI models had histology consistent more with renal cell apoptosis associated with rise in IL-10 expression and proliferation of regulatory T-cells [8]. When specimens from kidney biopsies performed postmortem from adults with septic shock were compared with those without sepsis and those with trauma, it was seen that septic patients had increased renal tubular cell apoptosis and leucocyte infiltration which was not observed in non-septic group [9].

20.6 SA-AKI Diagnosis

The delay in recognizing renal injury leads to increased risk of poor outcomes associated with SA-AKI. The mainstay of therapy is early initiation of supportive care that targets the drivers of injury. To institute this prompt support, there is a need of risk identification and timely diagnosis of injury (Table 20.2).

20.6.1 Serum Creatinine and Urine Output

Azotemia and oliguria are the key diagnostic criteria of SA-AKI. The recent diagnostic and staging criteria by the Kidney Disease: Improving Global Outcomes (KDIGO) use changes (both absolute and relative) in serum creatinine and urine output to define and assess the severity of kidney injury. Although this definition is important and has provided an advance in the field of AKI, it come with well-recognized limitations. Serum creatinine is insensitive and can vary widely between different clinical settings. Septic patients typically receive aggressive fluid resuscitation, which can have a dilutional effect on serum creatinine. Similarly, sepsis has been shown to reduce the muscular production and/or release

Table 20.2 Utility and limitations of tests used in AKI diagnosis

Criteria/test	Utility	Limitations
Serum creatinine	Cheap, easily measured, well-known relationship to disease	Slow to change in response to injury, insensitive—no change until >50% loss of function
Serum cystatin C	Experience from chronic kidney disease	Similar to creatinine
Urine sediment	Can help identify specific cause of AKI	Not standardized and usually nonspecific
Kidney damage markers (uKIM1, uNGAL)	Measure cellular injury rather than organ function	Not standardized nor completely validated in humans
AKI risk markers (uTIMP2, pNGAL)	Measure of kidney stress or systemic inflammation states rather than injury per se	Not standardized nor completely validated in humans

Modified from Bellomo et al. Acute kidney injury in sepsis. Intensive Care Med. 2017;43:816–828 [41]

of creatinine, even in the absence of any changes in weight, hematocrit, or extracellular fluid volume [10]. These pitfalls impair the sensitivity of serum creatinine and limit its efficacy in the early detection of SA-AKI.

20.6.2 Urine Biochemistry

The role of classic urine biochemistry and derived indices in the diagnosis and discrimination of AKI remains controversial. Various criteria, particularly urine sodium (Una), and fractional excretion of sodium and urea (Fe Na, Fe U) still have poor operational value in providing information of the diagnosis and to support clinical decision-making [11]. Valuable information may be obtained from urine sediment examination, where the presence of casts and renal epithelial cells provides information about the risk of worsening AKI. A prospective evaluation of a urine microscopy score derived from renal tubular cells and casts correlated with urinary neutrophil gelatinase-associated lipocalin (NGAL) levels and with severity of AKI [12].

20.6.3 Novel Kidney Damage Biomarkers

The precise role of novel kidney damage biomarkers, such as: cystatin C; neutrophil gelatinase-associated lipocalin (NGAL); insulin-like growth factor-binding protein 7 (IGFBP7) and tissue inhibitor of metalloproteinases-2 (TIMP-2); kidney injury molecule-1; interleukin-18; L-type fatty acid binding protein, detectable in the blood and urine for the diagnosis of AKI and for clinical decision support, while very promising, is still undergoing investigation. These newer biomarkers have demonstrated an ability to identify AKI before the changes in creatinine levels set in. It has been seen in a study involving 83 patients that plasma and urine NGAL levels were significantly higher at 0, 12, and 24 h in patients with SA-AKI as compared to those without sepsis [13]. While other studies showed inconsistent findings, a systematic review that included 15 studies evaluating plasma and urine NGAL in septic patients suggested that they have good precision in diagnosing SA-AKI and predicting outcome including receipt of RRT and mortality [14].

20.6.4 Risk Prediction Tools

Various risk prediction tools help identify patients at greater risk of developing overt or worsening AKI. For example, the concept of renal angina index (RAI), a composite based on risk factors and early signs of kidney injury, has shown good predictive performance (Table 20.3) [15].

Table 20.3 The Renal Angina Index (RAI) to predict risk of AKI among critically ill children

Risk criteria		×	*Injury criteria*		
Admission to ICU	1		Serum creatinine	Fluid overload %	Score
Transplantation	3		No change	<5	1
Ventilation, vasoactive support, or both	5		Increase >1–1.49 times	5–10	2
			Increase >1.5–1.99 times	11–15	4
			Increase ≥2 times	>15	8

The RAI calculation is assessed 12 h after a patient is admitted to an intensive care unit and used for prediction of severe acute kidney injury 72 h (3 days) later. The RAI is calculated by multiplying the patient risk score by the injury score (scores 1–40). The higher score for either of the injury criteria (creatinine or fluid overload) is used. A RAI product of ≥8 fulfills the renal angina classification. Transplantation refers to solid organ or stem cell transplantation

20.7 SA-AKI Management

The general principles in the evaluation and management of SA-AKI are aimed at early resuscitation targets to physiological endpoints, source control, and antimicrobial administration, followed by strategy of limiting injury, avoiding life-threatening complications (Table 20.4), and eliminating any potential contributors to worsening kidney function.

20.7.1 Fluid Resuscitation

Soon after shock is identified, it is important to optimize intravascular volume by administering fluid and vasoactive therapy and titrate them to physiological endpoints. Optimizing systemic and kidney hemodynamics should always be a priority, as reestablishment of adequate intravascular volume and perfusion pressure using early aggressive fluid administration and vasoactive support can be lifesaving. Recent trials evaluating early goal-directed therapy (EGDT) compared to usual care suggest that EGDT is not associated with improved mortality or benefits to renal function [16]. Following the acute resuscitation phase, patients who do not respond to fluids should be carefully evaluated for signs of fluid overload. Fluid overload is associated with less favorable outcomes including higher mortality, higher incidence of AKI, and prolonged mechanical ventilation and PICU length of stay [17].

When considering the type of fluid to be used for acute resuscitation of patients with sepsis, there is an additional insight provided from recent data. In randomized trials of fluid resuscitation in septic patients, the use of synthetic colloid hydroxyethyl starch (HES) compared with crystalloids was associated with increased risk of AKI, greater RRT utilization, and increased mortality [18]. Based on these data, the use of HES fluids for resuscitation in sepsis are discouraged. The use of albumin in acute resuscitation remains controversial. A secondary analysis of the SAFE study

Table 20.4 Summary approach to SA-AKI

Early identification of risk
• Early recognition of sepsis • Clinical risk prediction scores (example: Renal Angina index) • Automated electronic alerts system • Novel kidney injury biomarkers
Early and effective resuscitation
• Early and appropriate antibiotic administration coupled with source control • Fluid and vasoactive support to restore hemodynamics and perfusion • Early goal-directed therapy protocol carries no added renal benefit compared to standard of care • Excessive fluid resuscitation leading to fluid overload is not beneficial to kidney function and may lead to harm • Crystalloid solutions are generally preferred over colloid solutions • Artificial colloid solutions should be avoided • Balanced crystalloid solutions maybe safer than 0.9% saline • Epinephrine or Norepinephrine are the first-line vasoactive drugs depending on the presentation of pediatric septic shock • Vasopressin has some potential renal benefits in adults; however, the routine use in pediatric patients is not advisable
Renal replacement therapy
• In the absence of absolute indications, the optional timing of RRT initiation remains unknown • Higher fluid accumulation at the time of CRRT initiation is associated with worse outcomes • CRRT is the preferred first-line renal support in septic shock • RRT intensity of 20–25 mL/kg/h of solute clearance is suggested
Supportive care
• Routine and close monitoring of renal function and fluid status • Unnecessary fluid loading and transfusions should be avoided • Minimize exposure to nephrotoxins • Adjust medications for renal clearance

and a systematic review have shown that use of albumin solutions is associated with reduced mortality, however no significant difference in the incidence of AKI [19, 20]. Although the ALBIOS trial showed that albumin replacement in sepsis was not associated with survival benefit, a post hoc analysis suggested that albumin-containing solutions may improve the hemodynamic profile, reduce fluid volumes, organ dysfunction, and survival in patients with septic shock [21]. However, there remain a number of uncertainties regarding the routine use of albumin for resuscitation in septic shock.

The composition of crystalloid solutions and the risk of adverse kidney sequelae have also been examined. It has been seen that risk of iatrogenic metabolic acidosis decreases when balanced crystalloid solutions (e.g., Plasmalyte and ringers lactate) are preferred for use. A recent large randomized cross-over trial showed the use of balanced crystalloids to be associated with lower occurrence of composite outcome (mortality, RRT, and persistent renal dysfunction) [22]. The issue of the ideal crystalloid solution for acute resuscitation to optimize kidney and patient survival remains to be definitively proven.

20.7.2 Antimicrobial Therapy

Early antibiotic administration has been shown to improve outcome in sepsis. An independent predictor of development of SA-AKI is a delay in administration of appropriate antimicrobial therapy [23]. There is a direct increase in SA-AKI incidence as well as severity when there is an additional delay in instituting appropriate antimicrobial therapy after the onset of hypotension. For every 1-h delay in administering antibiotics, the odds of AKI increased by >40% (OR 1.41; 95% CI, 1.10–1.20, $P < 0.001$). In another study, early administration of antimicrobials was associated with greater likelihood of recovery of SA-AKI within 24 h from admission [24].

20.7.3 Vasoactive Support

There is limited pediatric data to suggest the optimal vasoactive therapy approach in septic shock. Recent pediatric guidelines recommend the use of epinephrine or dopamine for children with cold shock, and norepinephrine in vasodilatory shock that remains refractory to fluid therapy. Specific to AKI, the use of "renal-dose" dopamine has not proven effective for preventing the development of AKI [25]. Fenoldopam (selective Dopamine receptor-1 agonist) was found to have protective effect against the development of SA-AKI in a small RCT; however, that did not show survival benefit, suggesting the need for further verification in high-quality trials [26].

Some adult data suggest potential renal benefits from using vasopressin in septic shock including minimizing the progression of AKI and less utilization of RRT. However, these findings were not associated with significant decrease in mortality. The use of vasopressin in pediatric vasodilatory shock was evaluated in a multicenter RCT [27]. The study showed a nonsignificant trend of increased mortality in the vasopressin group. There was no difference in creatinine level between the two groups. Based on the lack of observed clinical benefits and potential of harm, the routine use of vasopressin in pediatric septic shock is currently not advisable. Use of recombinant angiotensin II (ANGII) infusion as a novel vasopressor has shown kidney-specific benefits in experimental sepsis models. A recent phase 3 RCT evaluating the use of ANGII showed significant improvements in mean arterial pressure in patients with catecholamine-resistant vasodilatory shock compared to placebo [28]. Further trials are anticipated to evaluate whether these findings can further translate to survival and kidney benefits.

20.7.4 Renal Replacement Therapy (RRT)

Despite supportive therapy, kidney function might be lost and RRT might be indicated. The decision to start RRT is often complex and shows considerable variability. RRT should be initiated when confronted with life-threatening complications attributed to AKI (Table 20.5). It currently remains uncertain whether the earlier initiation of RRT in critical illness before the onset of overt complications of AKI can improve outcomes. Accumulating evidence from observational pediatric studies demonstrate

Table 20.5 Summary of classic or absolute indications for initiation of RRT

Conventional ("rescue") indications
• Oliguria or anuria
• Azotemia (serum urea >36 mmol/L or uremic organ complications)
• Metabolic acidosis/acidemia (pH <7.15)
• Hyperkalemia (K+ >6.5 mEq/L and/or rapidly rising and/or cardiac toxicity)
• Volume overload (clinically significant, diuretic unresponsive organ edema)
• Sodium disorders (progressive and/or uncontrolled dysnatremia)
• Overdose with dialyzable toxin
• Thermoregulation (uncontrolled hyper- or hypothermia)
Relative (expanded) indications
• Rapidly worsening AKI or illness severity in the setting of reduced renal reserve
• Allow delivery of adequate nutritional support
• Fluid removal or prevention of excessive fluid accumulation
• Chemotherapy-induced organ injury and/or transfusion support
• Refractory acidosis in acute respiratory distress syndrome
• Hypercatabolism
• Immunomodulation and restoration of immune responsiveness in sepsis

strong and consistent association between fluid accumulation at the time of RRT initiation and worse outcomes [17]. Based on these findings, percent fluid overload (%FO) of higher than 10% should be considered when evaluating the timing for CRRT initiation. The formula used to calculate %FO is: [(Total fluid in – Total fluid out)/Admission weight * 100]. In adults, selected data from observational studies suggested that early or preemptive RRT initiation may be associated with improved survival. However, two recent RCTs in adult critically ill patients showed conflicting results [29, 30]. These inconsistent findings will hopefully be further clarified with the completion of two ongoing large multicenter RCTs.

The RRT modality most commonly used early in the course of hemodynamically unstable patients is continuous renal replacement therapy (CRRT). CRRT offers the advantages of adaptability to the patient condition, achievement of more consistent hemodynamic tolerance, and metabolic and fluid homeostasis. Recent data have suggested a beneficial effect of using CRRT to facilitate recovery of renal function to RRT independence and reduce the long-term risk of chronic kidney disease, when used as initial supportive modality. However, the evidence does not support a survival advantage of using one modality over another [31].

It was seen from earlier data that using higher intensity RRT may be potentially beneficial. However, the same could not be seen on evidence generated subsequently. Rather, it was noted that lower intensity RRT may be associated with fewer metabolic complications [32]. The evidence remains inconclusive in regard to the role of plasma exchange in sepsis. While results from small trials showed some promise in improving sepsis outcomes, further evidence from more rigorous RCT is needed [33]. A number of additional extracorporeal blood purification techniques are being actively investigated as potential adjuvant therapies in sepsis, including novel membranes and hemofilters, sorbent technologies (i.e., polymyxin B hemoperfusion).

Table 20.6 Selected potential novel therapeutic agents in the prevention and treatment of SA-AKI

Agent	Proposed mechanism of action
Fenoldopam	Dopamine-1 receptor agonist Increase renal blood flow
Low-dose vasopressin	Glomerular efferent arteriolar vasoconstriction Catecholamine sparing
Alkaline phosphatase	Anti-inflammatory activity Dephosphorylation of endotoxins Conversion of adenosine triphosphate to adenosine
Caspase 3 inhibitors	Suppressing apoptotic pathways
Ghrelin	Anti-inflammatory activity Reduce cytokine levels Decrease serum nitric oxide levels
Soluble thrombomodulin	Anti-inflammatory and anticoagulant effects Reduce microvascular endothelial injury Improve microvascular perfusion
Resveratrol	Anti-inflammatory activity Reduce cytokine levels Minimize endothelial injury Suppress macrophage activity Decrease reactive nitrogen species
Adenosine-receptor agonists	Anti-inflammatory activity
Erythropoietin	Anti-apoptotic and antioxidant activity
Temsirolimus	Promote autophagy and kidney recovery

While these agents have shown potential role in the prevention and treatment of SA-AKI, further evidence assessing their clinical use is needed

20.7.5 Targeted Molecular and Cellular Therapies

Multiple factors are now known to be involved in pathogenesis of SA-AKI, including apoptotic, immune, and inflammatory pathways. There may be value of therapeutic potential of various newer therapies directed at these factors and pathways. Some of these are summarized in (Table 20.6); however, further evidence in assessing their beneficial effect in SA-AKI patients is needed.

20.8 Supportive Care and Prevention

Septic patients are at high risk of developing AKI. They require heightened monitoring of kidney function including frequent assessments of serum creatinine, continuous urine output monitoring, and accurate assessment of fluid status. Considering the harmful impact of fluid overload, unnecessary and non-beneficial fluid loading and transfusions should be avoided.

It is of utmost importance to realize that avoidance of nephrotoxins takes a priority in preventing worsening of AKI. When there are no options but to use nephrotoxic medications, one should utilize therapeutic drug monitoring and careful dose adjustment be done, after consulting with the pharmacy. In cases where the patient requires administration of contrast agents for imaging purposes, the benefits and risk of the same should be weighed and wherever applicable one may delay the procedure or resort to an alternative imaging modality.

Certain modern clinical information systems may be designed to generate a trigger and alert the clinicians regarding those who are exposed to unnecessary nephrotoxins or are developing early AKI.

A quality improvement project based on electronic health record screening of nephrotoxin exposure in hospitalized children was effective in reducing nephrotoxin exposure rate by 38% with associated decrease of AKI rate by 64% [34].

20.9 Conclusion

The development of AKI in sepsis is not a trivial complication. Current evidence suggest that SA-AKI is associated with worse prognosis.

Although the diagnosis of AKI is still based on clinical assessment and use of KDIGO criteria which involves use of urine output and serum creatinine measurement, the use of clinical risk scores, electronic alerting systems, more robust monitoring, and newer damage-specific markers would help early identification of those at risk, early diagnosis, and institution of a bundle of interventions which would aim at reversing the course of SA-AKI.

Early aggressive resuscitation, vasoactive support to restore adequate perfusion, coupled with appropriate antimicrobial administration remains the mainstay of SA-AKI management. As our understanding of the pathobiology of SA-AKI expands, additional rigorous investigation is needed to develop novel and effective preventative and therapeutic interventions.

References

1. Alkandari O, Eddington KA, Hyder A, Gauvin F, Ducruet T, Gottesman R, et al. Acute kidney injury is an independent risk factor for pediatric intensive care unit mortality, longer length of stay and prolonged mechanical ventilation in critically ill children: a two-center retrospective cohort study. Crit Care. 2011;15(3):R146.
2. Weiss SL, Fitzgerald JC, Pappachan J, Wheeler D, Jaramillo-Bustamante JC, Salloo A, et al. Global epidemiology of pediatric severe sepsis: the sepsis prevalence, outcomes, and therapies study. Am J Respir Crit Care Med. 2015;191(10):1147–57.
3. Hoste EA, Lameire NH, Vanholder RC, Benoit DD, Decruyenaere JM, Colardyn FA. Acute renal failure in patients with sepsis in a surgical ICU: predictive factors, incidence, comorbidity, and outcome. J Am Soc Nephrol. 2003;14(4):1022–30.
4. Bagshaw SM, George C, Bellomo R, Committee ADM. Early acute kidney injury and sepsis: a multicentre evaluation. Crit Care. 2008;12(2):R47.
5. Lopes JA, Jorge S, Resina C, Santos C, Pereira A, Neves J, et al. Acute kidney injury in patients with sepsis: a contemporary analysis. Int J Infect Dis. 2009;13(2):176–81.
6. Langenberg C, Bagshaw SM, May CN, Bellomo R. The histopathology of septic acute kidney injury: a systematic review. Crit Care. 2008;12(2):R38.

7. Brenner M, Schaer GL, Mallory DL, Suffredini AF, Parrillo JE. Detection of renal blood flow abnormalities in septic and critically ill patients using a newly designed indwelling thermodilution renal vein catheter. Chest. 1990;98(1):170–9.
8. Lee SY, Lee YS, Choi HM, Ko YS, Lee HY, Jo SK, et al. Distinct pathophysiologic mechanisms of septic acute kidney injury: role of immune suppression and renal tubular cell apoptosis in murine model of septic acute kidney injury. Crit Care Med. 2012;40(11):2997–3006.
9. Lerolle N, Nochy D, Guerot E, Bruneval P, Fagon JY, Diehl JL, et al. Histopathology of septic shock induced acute kidney injury: apoptosis and leukocytic infiltration. Intensive Care Med. 2010;36(3):471–8.
10. Doi K, Yuen PS, Eisner C, Hu X, Leelahavanichkul A, Schnermann J, et al. Reduced production of creatinine limits its use as marker of kidney injury in sepsis. J Am Soc Nephrol. 2009;20(6):1217–21.
11. Bagshaw SM, Bennett M, Devarajan P, Bellomo R. Urine biochemistry in septic and non-septic acute kidney injury: a prospective observational study. J Crit Care. 2013;28(4):371–8.
12. Bagshaw SM, Haase M, Haase-Fielitz A, Bennett M, Devarajan P, Bellomo R. A prospective evaluation of urine microscopy in septic and non-septic acute kidney injury. Nephrol Dial Transplant. 2012;27(2):582–8.
13. Bagshaw SM, Bennett M, Haase M, Haase-Fielitz A, Egi M, Morimatsu H, et al. Plasma and urine neutrophil gelatinase-associated lipocalin in septic versus non-septic acute kidney injury in critical illness. Intensive Care Med. 2010;36(3):452–61.
14. Zhang A, Cai Y, Wang PF, Qu JN, Luo ZC, Chen XD, et al. Diagnosis and prognosis of neutrophil gelatinase-associated lipocalin for acute kidney injury with sepsis: a systematic review and meta-analysis. Crit Care. 2016;20(1):41.
15. Basu RK, Zappitelli M, Brunner L, Wang Y, Wong HR, Chawla LS, et al. Derivation and validation of the renal angina index to improve the prediction of acute kidney injury in critically ill children. Kidney Int. 2014;85(3):659–67.
16. Investigators P, Rowan KM, Angus DC, Bailey M, Barnato AE, Bellomo R, et al. Early, goal-directed therapy for septic shock - a patient-level meta-analysis. N Engl J Med. 2017;376(23):2223–34.
17. Alobaidi R, Morgan C, Basu RK, Stenson E, Featherstone R, Majumdar SR, et al. Association between fluid balance and outcomes in critically ill children: a systematic review and meta-analysis. JAMA Pediatr. 2018;172(3):257–68.
18. Zarychanski R, Abou-Setta AM, Turgeon AF, Houston BL, McIntyre L, Marshall JC, et al. Association of hydroxyethyl starch administration with mortality and acute kidney injury in critically ill patients requiring volume resuscitation: a systematic review and meta-analysis. JAMA. 2013;309(7):678–88.
19. Investigators SS, Finfer S, McEvoy S, Bellomo R, McArthur C, Myburgh J, et al. Impact of albumin compared to saline on organ function and mortality of patients with severe sepsis. Intensive Care Med. 2011;37(1):86–96.
20. Delaney AP, Dan A, McCaffrey J, Finfer S. The role of albumin as a resuscitation fluid for patients with sepsis: a systematic review and meta-analysis. Crit Care Med. 2011;39(2):386–91.
21. Caironi P, Tognoni G, Masson S, Fumagalli R, Pesenti A, Romero M, et al. Albumin replacement in patients with severe sepsis or septic shock. N Engl J Med. 2014;370(15):1412–21.
22. Semler MW, Self WH, Wanderer JP, Ehrenfeld JM, Wang L, Byrne DW, et al. Balanced crystalloids versus saline in critically ill adults. N Engl J Med. 2018;378(9):829–39.
23. Bagshaw SM, Lapinsky S, Dial S, Arabi Y, Dodek P, Wood G, et al. Acute kidney injury in septic shock: clinical outcomes and impact of duration of hypotension prior to initiation of antimicrobial therapy. Intensive Care Med. 2009;35(5):871–81.
24. Sood MM, Shafer LA, Ho J, Reslerova M, Martinka G, Keenan S, et al. Early reversible acute kidney injury is associated with improved survival in septic shock. J Crit Care. 2014;29(5):711–7.
25. Bellomo R, Chapman M, Finfer S, Hickling K, Myburgh J. Low-dose dopamine in patients with early renal dysfunction: a placebo-controlled randomised trial. Australian and New Zealand Intensive Care Society (ANZICS) Clinical Trials Group. Lancet. 2000;356(9248):2139–43.

26. Morelli A, Ricci Z, Bellomo R, Ronco C, Rocco M, Conti G, et al. Prophylactic fenoldopam for renal protection in sepsis: a randomized, double-blind, placebo-controlled pilot trial. Crit Care Med. 2005;33(11):2451–6.
27. Choong K, Bohn D, Fraser DD, Gaboury I, Hutchison JS, Joffe AR, et al. Vasopressin in pediatric vasodilatory shock: a multicenter randomized controlled trial. Am J Respir Crit Care Med. 2009;180(7):632–9.
28. Khanna A, English SW, Wang XS, Ham K, Tumlin J, Szerlip H, et al. Angiotensin II for the treatment of vasodilatory shock. N Engl J Med. 2017;377(5):419–30.
29. Zarbock A, Kellum JA, Schmidt C, Van Aken H, Wempe C, Pavenstadt H, et al. Effect of early vs delayed initiation of renal replacement therapy on mortality in critically ill patients with acute kidney injury: the ELAIN randomized clinical trial. JAMA. 2016;315(20):2190–9.
30. Gaudry S, Hajage D, Schortgen F, Martin-Lefevre L, Pons B, Boulet E, et al. Initiation strategies for renal-replacement therapy in the intensive care unit. N Engl J Med. 2016;375(2):122–33.
31. Bonnassieux M, Duclos A, Schneider AG, Schmidt A, Benard S, Cancalon C, et al. Renal replacement therapy modality in the ICU and renal recovery at hospital discharge. Crit Care Med. 2018;46(2):e102–10.
32. Joannes-Boyau O, Honore PM, Perez P, Bagshaw SM, Grand H, Canivet JL, et al. High-volume versus standard-volume haemofiltration for septic shock patients with acute kidney injury (IVOIRE study): a multicentre randomized controlled trial. Intensive Care Med. 2013;39(9):1535–46.
33. Rimmer E, Houston BL, Kumar A, Abou-Setta AM, Friesen C, Marshall JC, et al. The efficacy and safety of plasma exchange in patients with sepsis and septic shock: a systematic review and meta-analysis. Crit Care. 2014;18(6):699.
34. Goldstein SL, Mottes T, Simpson K, Barclay C, Muething S, Haslam DB, et al. A sustained quality improvement program reduces nephrotoxic medication-associated acute kidney injury. Kidney Int. 2016;90(1):212–21.
35. Volpon LC, Sugo EK, Consulin JC, Tavares TL, Aragon DC, Carlotti AP. Epidemiology and outcome of acute kidney injury according to pediatric risk, injury, failure, loss, end-stage renal disease and kidney disease: improving global outcomes criteria in critically ill children-a prospective study. Pediatr Crit Care Med. 2016;17(5):e229–38.
36. Mehta P, Sinha A, Sami A, Hari P, Kalaivani M, Gulati A, et al. Incidence of acute kidney injury in hospitalized children. Indian Pediatr. 2012;49(7):537–42.
37. Duzova A, Bakkaloglu A, Kalyoncu M, Poyrazoglu H, Delibas A, Ozkaya O, et al. Etiology and outcome of acute kidney injury in children. Pediatr Nephrol. 2010;25(8):1453–61.
38. Plotz FB, Bouma AB, van Wijk JA, Kneyber MC, Bokenkamp A. Pediatric acute kidney injury in the ICU: an independent evaluation of pRIFLE criteria. Intensive Care Med. 2008;34(9):1713–7.
39. Akcan-Arikan A, Zappitelli M, Loftis LL, Washburn KK, Jefferson LS, Goldstein SL. Modified RIFLE criteria in critically ill children with acute kidney injury. Kidney Int. 2007;71(10):1028–35.
40. Bailey D, Phan V, Litalien C, Ducruet T, Merouani A, Lacroix J, et al. Risk factors of acute renal failure in critically ill children: a prospective descriptive epidemiological study. Pediatr Crit Care Med. 2007;8(1):29–35.
41. Bellomo R, Kellum JA, Ronco C, Wald R, Martensson J, Maiden M, et al. Acute kidney injury in sepsis. Intensive Care Med. 2017;43(6):816–28.

Management of Intoxications in Pediatrics

21

Rupesh Raina, Stephanie Lam, Hershita Raheja, Michelle Bestic, and Martha Blackford

21.1 Introduction

Poisonings in pediatrics remains a consistent cause for presentation to emergency departments. According to the 2016 34th annual report of the American Association of Poison Control Centers', children <3 years of age accounted for 34.7% of all exposures and children ≤5 years of age accounted for 50% of all exposures. The top three most common poisonings were analgesics, household cleaning substances, and cosmetics/personal care products. Overall, compared to the 2015 data, there was an overall decline in number of reported fatalities in children <20 years old. In children <6 years of age, there were 24 reported deaths. Most common causes were fumes/gases/vapors. Among children between 6 and 12 years old, there were seven reported deaths with the most common cause listed as analgesic exposure. In adolescents aged 13–19 years old, there were 42 reported fatalities with the most common cause listed as analgesics [1] (see Table 21.2).

Currently, there is little literature regarding renal replacement therapy in pediatric poisonings. Our objective was to review the literature and create a resource for pharmacokinetics, toxicity, and treatment of common pediatric poisonings.

R. Raina (✉)
Department of Nephrology, Cleveland Clinic Akron General and Akron Children's Hospital, Akron, OH, USA

Akron Nephrology Associates/Cleveland Clinic Akron General, Akron, OH, USA
e-mail: RRaina@akronchildrens.org

S. Lam · M. Bestic · M. Blackford
Department of Pediatrics, Akron Children's Hospital, Akron, OH, USA

H. Raheja
Akron Nephrology Associates/Cleveland Clinic Akron General, Akron, OH, USA

S. K. Sethi et al. (eds.), *Critical Care Pediatric Nephrology and Dialysis: A Practical Handbook*, https://doi.org/10.1007/978-981-13-2276-1_21

21.2 Modes of Drug Removal

21.2.1 Single Pass Albumin Dialysis

Single pass albumin dialysis (SPAD) removes protein-bound substances through a high-influx membrane using an albumin-containing dialysate. The dialysate solution is mixed with 20% human albumin and run as a countercurrent to the patient's flow across a dialysate membrane [2]. Albumin dialysate solution removes protein-bound substances by diffusion. This system binds free toxins that cross the dialyzer membrane by the concentration gradient [2]. Once the toxin binds to the dialysate-side albumin, the concentration gradient is restored, more blood-side toxin will dis-associate, cross the membrane into the dialysate, and then bind to dialysate-side albumin [3]. These contents are then removed from the system after a single pass, resulting in an overall loss of toxins [4]. Hemodialysis and SPAD are combined to remove water-soluble products simultaneously. Typically, SPAD runs for 6-h long cycles, totaling 5 cycles over a 5-day time period.

Acute liver failure, hepatic encephalopathy, hepatitis, and Wilson's disease can all cause liver failure resulting in decreased clearance of protein-bound substances. SPAD improves clearance of protein-bound substances like bile salts, copper, and conjugated bilirubin. It also removes water-soluble substances such as ammonia, urea, and uric acid. Medications removed by SPAD include: carbamazepine, methotrexate, phenobarbital, phenytoin, and valproic acid [4, 5].

21.2.2 SPAD Protocol with Hemodialysis

1. Obtain a standard continuous renal replacement therapy machine and a pediatric line set.
2. Obtain central vascular access:
   (a) Newborns:
   - IJ/Femoral 7F or 8F dual lumen catheter in IJ or femoral vein
   - 5.0–8.5F UVC for blood return, but arterial access cannot be accessed by either UACs or UVCs
   - 7F or 8F dual lumen catheter in the subclavian vein

   (b) Older children/adolescents: Choose catheter appropriate for their body size.
3. Prepare a dialysate solution containing standard bicarbonate-buffered dialysate enhanced with 20% human albumin:
   (a) Remove 1100 mL of standard dialysis solution (Hemosol B0) from the 5 L bag and replace 1100 mL of 20% human albumin.
   (b) The prepared dialysate has a final albumin concentration of 4–5% (40–50 g/L).
4. Prime the circuit with dilute blood in all patients <15 kg or if hemodynamically unstable:
   (a) Obtain a unit of diluted packed red blood cells (hematocrit 35%).
   (b) Use heparinized normal saline to prime the circuit then reprime with non-heparinized normal saline.

   (c) Use the diluted packed red blood cells to prime the dialysis circuit.
   (d) The blood is warmed by recirculation for 5–10 min.
5. While machine is recirculating, obtain blood samples and blood gas.
6. Blood flow rate (Qb) set at 3–5 mL/min/kg body weight.
7. Albumin dialysate flow rate (Qd) set at 20–60 mL/kg/h.
8. Combined SPAD and HD dialysate flow rate set higher at 500–800 mL/min.
9. Prepare heparin anticoagulation infusion:
   (a) Infants: Prepare infusion with 50 units/mL heparin concentration.
   (b) Check activated clotting time (ACT) promptly after beginning dialysis.
   (c) If ACT<200, administer a heparin bolus 25–50 units/kg IV.
   (d) Continuous heparin infusion at a rate of 10–25 units/kg/h.
   (e) Check ACT every 15–30 min and adjust heparin infusion if needed.
   (f) Maintain ACTs 180–220 s.
   (g) ACT guidelines:

ACT (s)	Action
<160	Heparin bolus 10 units/kg via circuit Increase heparin drip by 20%
160–180	Heparin bolus 5 units/kg via circuit Increase heparin drip by 10%
180–220	No action
220–260	Decrease heparin drip by 10%
>260	Decrease heparin drip by 20%

10. Check serum osmolality, electrolytes, calcium, and phosphorus every 2 h.
11. Each session runs for 3–5 h.
12. When withdrawing HD, if the circuit was primed with blood then clamp the lines and discard the entire apparatus containing the blood.
13. Once the treatment is complete, repeat all blood tests.

Calculations
The fraction of drug, toxin, or protein-bound substance that crosses the hemodialyzer during continuous hemodialysis is expressed as the extraction coefficient (EC). To determine EC and transmembrane clearance (Cl) of each solute, the following equations are used [4]:

Extraction coefficient (EC) = D/A
Continuous hemodialysis transmembrane clearance = EC × Qd
A = solute plasma concentration obtained from the pre-hemodialyzer port
D = solute spent dialysate concentration obtained from the spent dialysate port
Qd = dialysate flow rate

21.2.3 SPAD Protocol with CRRT

1. Obtain a standard CRRT machine and a pediatric line set.
2. Obtain central vascular access:

   (a) Newborns:
      - IJ/Femoral 7F or 8F dual lumen catheter in IJ or femoral vein
      - 5.0–8.5F UVC for blood return, but arterial access cannot be accessed by either UACs or UVCs
      - 7F or 8F dual lumen catheter in the subclavian vein
   (b) Older children/adolescents: Choose catheter appropriate for their body size.
3. Prepare a dialysate solution containing standard bicarbonate-buffered dialysate enhanced with 20% human albumin:
   (a) Remove 500 mL of standard dialysis solution (Gambro) from the 5 L bag and replace 250 mL of 20% human albumin.
   (b) The prepared dialysate has a final albumin concentration of 2%.
4. Prime the circuit with dilute blood in all patients <15 kg or if hemodynamically unstable:
   (a) Obtain a unit of diluted packed red blood cells (hematocrit 35%).
   (b) Use heparinized normal saline to prime the circuit then reprime with non-heparinized normal saline.
   (c) Use the diluted packed red blood cells to prime the dialysis circuit.
   (d) The blood is warmed by recirculation for 5–10 min.
5. Obtain blood samples and blood gas while machine is recirculating.
6. Blood flow rate (Qb) set at 6 mL/min/kg body weight.
7. Albumin dialysate flow rate (Qd) set at 500 mL/h (2000 $cm^3/1.73\ m^2$).
8. Preparing heparin anticoagulation infusion (10 U/kg/h):
   (a) Infants: Prepare infusion with 50 units/mL heparin concentration.
   (b) Check ACT promptly after beginning dialysis.
   (c) If ACT <200, administer a heparin bolus 25–50 units/kg IV.
   (d) Continuous heparin infusion at a rate of 10–25 units/kg/h.
   (e) Check ACT every 15–30 min and adjust heparin infusion if needed.
   (f) Maintain ACTs 180–220 s.
   (g) ACT guidelines:

ACT (s)	Action
<160	Heparin bolus 10 units/kg via circuit Increase heparin drip by 20%
160–180	Heparin bolus 5 units/kg via circuit Increase heparin drip by 10%
180–220	No action
220–260	Decrease heparin drip by 10%
>260	Decrease heparin drip by 20%

9. Check serum osmolality, electrolytes, calcium, and phosphorus every 2 h.
10. Each session runs approximately 8 h.
11. When withdrawing CVVHD, if the circuit was primed with blood then clamp the lines and discard the entire apparatus containing the blood.
12. Once the treatment is complete, repeat all blood tests.

21.2.4 Molecular Adsorbent Recirculating System (MARS)

The Molecular Absorbent Recirculating System (MARS) uses an albumin-containing dialysate to clear protein-bound substances including hydrophobic bile acids, bilirubin, and plasmatic nitric oxide [2, 6]. MARS is composed of three circuits: (1) blood circuit, (2) albumin circuit, and (3) an open-loop single pass dialysate circuit. In addition to a standard dialysis or CVVH machine for the blood and dialysate circuits, this technique requires a MARS monitor for the albumin circuit. The indications for MARS are similar to the indications for SPAD including: MARS improves clearance of protein-bound toxins and decomposition of liver diseases. Uses for MARS include: increased intracranial pressure, hepatic encephalopathy, liver synthesis dysfunction, a bridge while awaiting liver transplantation, and renal and cerebral blood perfusion enhancement [6].

SPAD is preferred over MARS because SPAD requires less training, less specialized personnel, and less specialized equipment. SPAD is more versatile and can be operated in various hospital locations [6].

21.2.5 Hemoperfusion

Hemoperfusion is an extracorporeal technique designed to detoxify contaminated blood. Blood passes through a cartridge that contains an absorbent covered with a thin and semipermeable membrane. A commonly used absorbent is activated charcoal; it efficiently competes with plasma proteins, like albumin, for the bound drug [7]. When exposed to charcoal, the bound substance dissociates from the plasma protein, allowing it to be absorbed and discarded from circulation [8]. Unlike other detoxification techniques, such as hemodialysis and hemofiltration, hemoperfusion does not require a dialysate or other replacement fluid circuits. Hemoperfusion is used less frequently than hemodialysis. According to the American Association of Poison Control Centers National Poison Data System 2016 annual report, hemoperfusion was used 3 times in children aged 3–19 whereas hemodialysis was used 145 times [1].

Hemoperfusion targets heavier, water-insoluble, lipid-soluble, and protein-bound drugs when compared to hemodialysis. Hemoperfusion is indicated in severe intoxications with substances that cannot be easily eliminated or in cases of liver and kidney impairment preventing drug excretion. Theophylline, carbamazepine, organophosphates, and methotrexate are well-established substances cleared by hemoperfusion [9, 10]. Hemoperfusion is specifically indicated for severe versus mild overdose in both carbamazepine and organophosphate.

Hemodialysis remains the primary treatment of choice because it is widely available and of its ability to improve acid/base abnormalities, to clear small water-soluble substances, and to cause fewer complications [9].

The primary disadvantage of hemoperfusion is that it is not readily available due to its narrow indications, limited shelf life, and expensive cost related to numerous cartridge use [9]. Heparin is absorbed alongside the toxins so cartridges tend to easily clot and require frequent replacement. With that said, hemoperfusion requires additional heparin use compared to hemodialysis [11]. Adverse events encountered during hemoperfusion use include: mild thrombocytopenia, mild leucopenia, low fibrinogen, hypothermia, hypocalcaemia, and hypoglycemia [9].

Calculations

The method used to measure the clearance of a drug/toxin is

CL = Qb (1-Hematocrit) × [(Ca − Cv)/Ca)]

Qb = blood flow rate through the column

Ca = pre-column plasma concentration

Cv = post-column plasma concentration

Therefore, [(Ca − Cv)/Ca)] = the extraction ratio (ER)

The higher the calculated extraction ratio indicates a larger proportion of drug has been discarded.

21.2.6 Hemoperfusion (HP) Protocol

1. Obtain required material: Dialysis equipment and blood lines, a blood pump, pressure gauges, cartridge, and a column containing 100–300 gr of activated charcoal:
   (a) Choose small cartridge size for pediatric patients (check expiration date).
   (b) Pressure gauges detect rises in pressure within the machine, this can arise as clots form within the cartridges.
2. Choose dialyzer according to patient weight:
   (a) Neonates <3 kg use F4.
   (b) Neonates >3 kg use F6.
   (c) Older children use the largest possible dialyzer.
3. Coat the charcoal column with a thin porous membrane (this will decrease risk of thrombocytopenia and improve efficacy of the charcoal columns):
   (a) Membrane thickness typically 0.05–0.5 μm.
4. Obtain central vascular access via a large bore dual lumen catheter.
5. Connect the catheter and dialyzer to dialysis machine.
6. Prime the circuit with dilute blood in all patients <15 kg or if hemodynamically unstable:
   (a) Obtain a unit of diluted packed red blood cells (hematocrit 35%).
   (b) Use heparinized (2000 U/h) normal saline to prime the circuit then reprime with non-heparinized normal saline.
   (c) Use the diluted packed red blood cells to prime the dialysis circuit.
   (d) The blood is warmed by recirculation for 5 min.
7. Blood flow rates (Qb) maintain at 300–350 mL/min:
   (a) The blood will pass through a disposable column, filtered, and the purified blood flows back to the patient via a dialyzer.

8. Activated clotting time (ACT) is similar to the HD protocol.
   (a) Infants: Prepare infusion with 50 units/mL heparin concentration.
   (b) Check ACT promptly after beginning dialysis.
   (c) If ACT <200, administer a heparin bolus 25–50 units/kg IV.
   (d) Continuous heparin infusion at a rate of 10–25 units/kg/h.
   (e) Check ACT every 15–30 min and adjust heparin infusion if needed.
   (f) Maintain ACTs 180–220 s.
   (g) ACT guidelines:

ACT (s)	Action
<160	Heparin bolus 10 units/kg via circuit Increase heparin drip by 20%
160–180	Heparin bolus 5 units/kg via circuit Increase heparin drip by 10%
180–220	No action
220–260	Decrease heparin drip by 10%
>260	Decrease heparin drip by 20%

9. Duration of each HP session is about 3–4 h; cartridges should be changed every 4 h.
10. Monitor vitals and electrolyte levels given potential adverse effects (hypothermia, hypocalcaemia, and hypoglycemia).
11. Obtain repeat drug/toxin serum concentration.
12. When withdrawing HP, if the circuit was primed with blood then clamp the lines and discard the entire apparatus containing the blood.

21.2.6.1 Plasmapheresis

Plasmapheresis, also known as therapeutic plasma exchange (TPE), is an extracorporeal technique used to purify plasma. There are two types of techniques: membrane and centrifugal plasmapheresis. Membrane plasmapheresis is therapeutic, performed in dialysis centers. Centrifugal plasmapheresis is performed at transfusion departments to separate components from donor blood [12].

TPE is indicated in severe toxicity of drugs that have high plasma protein binding and low volume of distribution. Plasmapheresis may be used in drug removal that conventional extracorporeal techniques, like hemodialysis or hemoperfusion, cannot remove efficiently. This technique reduces circulating antibodies, immune complexes, and accumulation of drugs/toxins [13].

21.2.6.2 Plasmapheresis Prescription

Each session lasts approximately 1.5–3 h. Frequency of sessions depends on the level of toxicity. Plasmapheresis removes 40–60 mL/kg of plasma during each procedure and replenished with replacement fluid. Normal saline, 4.5–5% isotonic human albumin solution or fresh frozen plasma can all be used as replacement fluids. One plasma volume exchange removes 63% of intravascular components. Two plasma volume exchanges remove 78% of intravascular components. Anticoagulation is commonly combined with citrate given typical calcium accumulation.

Calculations

The following equation is used to calculate plasma volume exchanged:

Estimated plasma volume (in liters) = 0.07 × Body Weight (kg) × (1-hematocrit)

21.3 Drugs

21.3.1 Ethylene Glycol

21.3.1.1 Pharmacokinetics

Ethylene glycol (EG), a toxic alcohol found in antifreeze and pesticides, is a water-soluble substance with a molecular weight of approximately 62 Da and a volume of distribution of 0.5–0.8 L/kg. It is quickly absorbed in the GI tract reaching peak levels within 1–4 h following ingestion [14–17] (see Table 21.1). Alcohol dehydrogenase, aldehyde dehydrogenase, and lactate dehydrogenase (glycolic acid oxidase) metabolize ethylene glycol into glycolaldehyde, glycolic acid, and glyoxylic acid, respectively. Glyoxylic acid is metabolized to oxalic acid [18].

21.3.1.2 Toxicity

Symptoms of toxicity may be categorized by time of onset: (1) 0–12 h: CNS abnormalities such as nausea/vomiting, ataxia, areflexia, dizziness, lethargy, coma, and seizures, (2) 12–24 h: cardiopulmonary dysfunction including: hypertension, tachycardia, pulmonary edema, and dyspnea, and (3) 24–72 h: renal dysfunction with flank pain, hypocalcemia, and acute kidney injury. Calcium oxalate crystals are formed when oxalic acid complexes with calcium. This accumulates in the renal tubules causing acute kidney injury. The hypocalcemia may cause QT prolongation and thus, ventricular arrhythmias [16–19].

Patients with ethylene glycol toxicity can present with an anion gap or a non-anion gap metabolic acidosis. The glycolic acid metabolite contributes to the metabolic acidosis [18, 20].

21.3.2 Treatment

Nonrenal replacement therapies include gastric decontamination, pyridoxine, thiamine, ethanol, and fomepizole. Gastric decontamination via nasogastric lavage should be performed within 1–2 h of ingestion and activated charcoal may be used in doses of 1 g/kg in cases of co-ingestion. Pyridoxine and thiamine provide an alternative pathway for glyoxylic acid metabolism [16]. Antidotes, ethanol and fomepizole, competitively inhibit alcohol dehydrogenase (ADH) and prevent accumulation of toxic metabolites. Both have a stronger affinity for ADH than EG, but fomepizole has an 8000 times higher affinity than ethanol [16]. Ethanol is administered first with a loading dose of 0.6–1.2 g/kg followed by maintenance of 0.1–0.12 g/kg/h, with goal level 100 mg/dL [16, 21, 22]. Loading dose of fomepizole is

Table 21.1 Toxicokinetics of drugs

Drug	Molecular weight	Volume of distribution	Therapeutic range	Toxic/lethal range	Peak serum levels	% Protein binding	Toxic metabolite	Δsosm (mOsm/L) per 10 mg/dL Δ serum [alcohol]	Water soluble
Ethylene glycol	62 Da	0.5–0.8 L/kg	–	>0.1 mL/kg	Within 1–4 h	0%	Glycolic acid, and calcium oxalate	1.6	Yes
Methanol	32 Da	0.6–0.7 L/kg	–	>0.2 g/L (20 mg/dL)	Within 20–60 min	0%	Formic acid, lactic acid, and ketones	3.09	Yes
Ethanol	46 Da	0.7 L/kg	–	3 g/kg (lethal)	Within 30–90 min	0%	Beta-hydroxybutyric acid and acetoacetic acid	2.12	Yes
Isopropanol	60 Da	0.7 L/kg	–	>4 g/L (severe)	Within 30 min	0%	Isopropanol	1.66	Yes
Lithium	7 Da	0.7–0.9 L/kg	0.8–1.2 mEq/L	>1.2–1.4 mEq/L	Within 1–3 h	0%	Lithium	–	Yes
Vancomycin	1449 Da	0.4–1 L/kg	5–10 mg/L	>15 mg/L	–	55%	Vancomycin	–	Yes
Theophylline	180 Da	0.5 L/kg	5–15 mg/L	>20 mg/L	Within 1–2 h	50–60%	Theophylline	–	Yes
Short-acting barbiturate (pentobarbital)	226 Da	0.5–1 L/kg	15–30 μg/mL	>30 μg/mL	–	35–70%	Pentobarbital, and 3-hydroxypentobarbital	–	No
Long-acting barbiturate (phenobarbital)	232 Da	0.25–1.2 L/kg	10–25 μg/mL	>25 μg/mL	–	20–60%	Alpha-ethyl-benzeneacetamide	–	No
Acetaminophen	151 Da	0.75–1 L/kg	10–25 μg/mL	Varies depending on Rumack–Matthew nomogram	Within 30 min-4 h	20–50%	*N*-acetyl-*p*-benzoquinone imine	–	Yes

(continued)

Table 21.1 (continued)

Drug	Molecular weight	Volume of distribution	Therapeutic range	Toxic/lethal range	Peak serum levels	% Protein binding	Toxic metabolite	Δsosm (mOsm/L) per 10 mg/dL Δ serum [alcohol]	Water soluble
Metformin	129 Da	1.1 L/kg	0.5–2.5 μg/mL	–	Within 1.8–4.1 h (immediate release); within 6–8 h (extended release)	Minimal	Metformin	–	Yes
Carbamazepine	236 Da	0.8–1.4 L/kg	4–12 mg/L	>12 mg/L	Within 6–24 h	75–80%	Carbamazepine-10,11-epoxide	–	No
Salicylates	138 Da	0.1–0.2 L/kg	10–30 mg/dL	>40 mg/dL	Within 1 h	80–90%	Salicylate	–	Yes
Methotrexate	454 Da	0.4–0.8 L/kg	Varies depending on route	Varies depending on route	Within 0.7–4 h (oral)	50%	Methotrexate	–	
Valproic acid	144 Da	0.1–0.5 L/kg	50–100 μg/mL	>200 mg/kg (toxic) >1000 mg/L (lethal)	–	94% (in therapeutic range) and 15% in concentrations >1000 mg/L	Valproic acid	–	Yes
Aminoglycoside (i.e., gentamicin)	477 Da	0.5–0.7 L/kg	5–12 μg/mL	> 12 μg/mL	Within 30–90 min	<30%	Unchanged form	–	
Phenytoin	252 Da	0.6–0.8 L/kg	10–20 μg/mL	>20 μg/mL	1.5–3 h (immediate release); 4–12 h (extended-release)	87–93%	Phenytoin	–	

15 mg/kg, followed by repeated infusions of 10 mg/kg every 12 h or every 4 h during dialysis [16, 22, 23]. If acid–base abnormality is corrected and EG levels have decreased with antidotal therapy, then RRT is not indicated.

Indications for hemodialysis include EG levels >25–50 mg/dL, severe acidosis (pH <7.25–7.3), presence of renal dysfunction, hemodynamic instability, and persistent toxicity despite non-RRT [16, 22]. Hemodialysis should continue until EG levels are <20 mg/dL, electrolytes are corrected, and renal function is recovered [16].

Hirsch et al. developed an equation to determine the time required for dialysis treatment [24]:

$$\text{Time Estimate} = \frac{-V \ln\left(5/A\right)}{\left(0.06k\right)}$$

where V is in liters, Time is in hours, A is in mmol/L, and k is in mL/min.

21.3.2.1 Case Series

Schwerk et al. discussed a comatose 7-year-old boy presenting with anion gap metabolic acidosis and calcium oxalate crystals on urine microscopy. Suspecting ethylene glycol intoxication, ethanol therapy was started (0.6 g/kg in 1 h, then 0.1 g/kg/h) with symptomatic improvement within an hour and complete resolution of EG on toxicological labs within 6 h. Hemodialysis was not required [20]. In more severe cases, as in a suicide attempt of a 12-year-old with initial serum EG of 88 mg/dL, a combination of antidotal and RRT therapy was efficient in toxin removal and treatment of metabolic abnormalities [22].

Stapenhorst et al. discussed the use of ethanol in combination with 3.5 h of hemodialysis. This decreased the concentrations to 40 mg/dL. After hemodialysis was withdrawn, ethanol treatment continued to decrease EG levels. Likewise, Cox et al. discussed 16-year-old who required intubation following antifreeze ingestion. He was treated with a combination of fomepizole, thiamine, pyridoxine, and hemodialysis for 6.5 h with drastic improvement [14]. Brent et al. compared 10 patients, 5 months old to 16 years old, who presented with ethylene glycol concentrations ranging 130–3840 mg/L. Of the 10 patients, 8/10 patients were treated with fomepizole therapy, while 2/10 patients were hemodialyzed. All 10 patients' metabolic acidosis improved, symptomatically recovered with no fatalities, and eventually was discharged despite treatment option [25]. Although the morbidity of intoxication is high, the mortality in pediatrics remains low given early intervention with antidotes such as ethanol and fomepizole in conjunction with hemodialysis, if necessary.

21.3.3 Methanol

21.3.3.1 Pharmacokinetics

Methanol is a small, water-soluble alcohol with relatively low volume of distribution, see Table 21.1 [17, 26]. It is a colorless solvent present in industrial, car, and home products. Methanol is hepatically metabolized by alcohol dehydrogenase and forms formaldehyde. Formaldehyde dehydrogenase converts formaldehyde to the toxic metabolite formic acid. Formic acid is further metabolized to a hydrogen ion and formate, which is converted into carbon dioxide and water. This process is driven by dietary folic acid and tetrahydrofolate. Similar to ethanol, methanol undergoes nonlinear elimination [27].

21.3.3.2 Toxicity

Methanol toxicity can cause visual, GI, and CNS disturbances. Initially, patients will have an osmolar gap that transitions to an anion gap as methanol is metabolized. Visual changes, which can be transient or permanent, range from cloudy or blurred vision to complete blindness [28]. GI effects include nausea, vomiting, and abdominal pain. CNS symptoms can range between headache, vertigo, lethargy, and confusion in mild–moderate toxicity to coma and seizure in severe toxicity [27]. With severe poisoning, patients can also develop multiorgan dysfunction including acute renal failure, metabolic acidosis, hypotension, electrolyte abnormalities, arrhythmias, and pancreatitis [29]. If patients co-ingest ethanol, the symptoms from methanol toxicity can be delayed due to alcohol dehydrogenase having a higher affinity for ethanol [27].

21.3.3.3 Treatment

Nonrenal replacement therapies include: folate, bicarbonate, ethanol, and fomepizole. Both ethanol and fomepizole inhibit methanol metabolism due to being competitive agonists for alcohol dehydrogenase. Fomepizole has been shown to be safe and effective in children without the side effects produced by ethanol (i.e., hypoglycemia, and intoxication). Folate facilitates the breakdown of formate into carbon dioxide and water [25, 27].

ECTR is indicated in severe poisoning, impaired renal function, and in cases of toxic methanol concentration >50 mg/dL. If fomepizole is being administered in conjunction with dialysis, the dosing interval will need to be adjusted because fomepizole is also removed by dialysis. After review of the literature, intermittent hemodialysis is most recommended in severe methanol toxicity. CRRT may be used if intermittent hemodialysis is not available [29].

21.3.3.4 Case Series

Brown et al. described a 5-year-old male who presented with worsening confusion, tachypnea, and abdominal pain 60 min after an unknown quantity of methanol (40% methanol solution stored in a sports drink bottle). Initial methanol concentration was 35 mg/dL. At 8 h post-ingestion, fomepizole was started. A repeat level at this time was 29 mg/dL. At 14 h post-ingestion, repeat level was 28 mg/dL. Hemodialysis was started and the patient underwent a total of 4 h of hemodialysis. Post-dialysis concentration was 0 mg/dL and the patient was later discharged [30].

Loza et al. described a 6-year-old girl initially treated for severe dehydration from food poisoning who was found to have methanol poisoning in the context of respiratory failure requiring ventilator support, depressed mental status, and severe mixed acidosis. After fluid resuscitation and IV sodium bicarbonate, her methanol concentration was 1.47 mg/dL. While not specifically indicated by the author, she likely received two 1-h hemodialysis sessions for persistent encephalopathy. She was later discharged with no long-term sequelae [26].

21.3.4 Ethanol

21.3.4.1 Pharmacokinetics

Ethanol, also known as ethyl alcohol or more commonly as alcohol, is one of the most commonly used xenobiotics in the world. Other than its well-known use in alcoholic beverages, the drug can also be found in a variety of products including household products like mouthwash, perfumes, and hand sanitizers as well as medicinal products such as liquid cough and cold preparations. It has a molecular weight of 62 Da and a volume of distribution of 0.7 L/kg. Ethanol is water-soluble and reaches peak blood concentration levels within 30–90 min after consumption [21] (see Table 21.1). While multiple mechanisms exist, ethanol is largely metabolized in the liver by the alcohol dehydrogenase pathway. Alcohol dehydrogenase metabolizes ethanol to acetaldehyde, which is further metabolized to acetate by aldehyde dehydrogenase. Normally, acetate is converted into acetylcoenzyme A, which enters the Krebs cycle where it is broken down into carbon dioxide and water. When alcohol dehydrogenase becomes saturated, ethanol elimination changes from first-order to zero-order kinetics [18].

Given their smaller relative size and limited ability to metabolize alcohol, children will have a higher blood alcohol concentration relative to quantity of ethanol ingested when compared to adults. Children, especially those <5 years old, have a low concentration of alcohol dehydrogenase [21, 31].

21.3.4.2 Toxicity

Symptoms of acute ethanol intoxication range from nausea/vomiting, slurred speech, and hypothermia to more severe presentations such as lactic acidosis, ketoacidosis, electrolyte disturbances, hypoglycemia, and CNS or respiratory depression [32]. Patients with equivalent serum ethanol levels may present with vastly different symptoms, owing to functional tolerance. In general however, at lower doses, ethanol is a CNS depressant, but with increasing concentrations, it causes an overall depression. It also inhibits gluconeogenesis. Children are more likely to develop ethanol-induced hypoglycemia due to fewer overall hepatic glycogen stores [18].

21.3.4.3 Treatment

Supportive care with temperature regulation, glucose monitoring, and airway protection should be started at initial presentation. Nonrenal replacement therapies include: gastric decontamination, IV dextrose or fructose, flumazenil, and naloxone. Gastric decontamination may be considered in select patients, such as those with co-ingestions. Administering IV fructose can decrease blood ethanol concentrations by 25% [31]. Renal replacement therapy is indicated in patients with blood alcohol level >300 mg/dL, hemodynamic instability, or worsening CNS or respiratory depression. Although hemodialysis effectively and rapidly clears ethanol from the serum, it is invasive and not routinely recommended in children [32].

21.3.4.4 Case Series

Gibson et al. reported a 12.5-kg 3-year-old who ingested 600 mL of rum (180 g of ethanol). On arrival to the ED, he had shallow respirations, no gag reflex, and was unarousable. He was quickly intubated and started on non-RRT. Within 6 h, the patient was more alert. Within 13 h, he was extubated and breathing independently. Despite his high level on arrival, ethanol's rate of elimination is rapid in children and in 19 h, his blood alcohol concentration was <0.1 g/L [31].

In severe toxicity, hemodialysis can rapidly correct acidosis and eliminate toxic metabolites. Gormley et al. reported a 17-year-old immunosuppressed and depressed patient, who ingested ethanol-based hand sanitizer through his gastrostomy tube. His serum ethanol level was 720 mg/dL 6 h after onset of symptoms. Given his levels, increasing serum osmolality, and his declining neurological state, he underwent hemodialysis. The patient became increasingly alert within hours and was extubated the following day [32].

21.3.5 Isopropanol

21.3.5.1 Pharmacokinetics

Isopropanol, a toxic alcohol found in rubbing alcohol, hair sprays, hand sanitizers, and cleaning agents, has a molecular weight of 60 Da and a volume of distribution of 0.7 L/kg. It is water-soluble and reaches peak blood concentration levels within 30 min post-consumption. Isopropanol poisoning may occur through mechanisms including: ingestion, inhalation, and dermal or rectal exposure. Metabolism mainly occurs in the liver where isopropanol is converted to acetone via alcohol dehydrogenase [33] (see Table 21.1).

21.3.5.2 Toxicity

The exact mechanism of isopropanol has not been fully elucidated, but like other alcohols, it is a CNS depressant. Other toxicity includes GI irritation, respiratory depression, and cardiovascular collapse. Patients may present with lethargy, stupor, ataxia, hyporeflexia, tremor, emesis, abdominal pain, rhabdomyolysis, or gastritis. Ketosis without metabolic acidosis is a pathognomonic finding of isopropanol toxicity [18]. Severe symptoms of intoxication include respiratory compromise, hypothermia, and hypotension [33, 34].

21.3.5.3 Treatment

Supportive care with airway protection, fluid resuscitation, temperature regulation, antiepileptics, cardiorespiratory monitoring is recommended as initial therapy [33]. While isopropanol's properties of low molecular weight, low volume of distribution, and low protein binding make it a dialyzable drug, renal replacement therapy is rarely used as patients generally improve with supportive care [35].

Hemodialysis may be considered when levels reach >200–400 mg/dL as patients are at risk for severe cardiovascular collapse and coma or in patients who do not respond to supportive therapies or continue to deteriorate. Unlike treatment of methanol and ethylene glycol toxicity, ethanol and fomepizole are contraindicated. These antidotes will inhibit isopropanol metabolism into acetone and prolong severe neurologic, respiratory, and cardiovascular depression [33].

21.3.5.4 Case Series

Stremski et al. conducted a retrospective review of 91 cases of isopropanol ingestion in children <6 years old. The majority of patients (62/91) were classified as asymptomatic, while 26 patients exhibited symptoms of toxicity (altered mental status, apnea, ataxia, seizure, or spontaneous emesis). Only three patients presented with both symptoms of toxicity and toxic isopropanol levels (>25 mg/dL). One patient required mechanical ventilation. No patients required hemodialysis. All were discharged to home without long-term sequelae [36].

21.3.6 Lithium

21.3.6.1 Pharmacokinetics

Lithium is a small cation with a moderate volume of distribution used in the treatment of bipolar disorder. See Table 21.1 for detailed pharmacokinetic information. While the exact mechanism of action is unknown, it is clear that lithium alters signal transduction pathways in the CNS, where it exerts its main toxic effects. Additionally, it decreases norepinephrine and dopamine release and may increase serotonin release. It is available either as lithium citrate (as a solution) or lithium carbonate in immediate- or controlled-release formulations. Lithium undergoes multiple compartment pharmacokinetics, which explains, in part, why toxicity does not always correlate well with levels. The rate of distribution of lithium into and out of the intracellular compartment is slow when compared to its rate of elimination. Distribution into the CNS is slow. Lithium is freely filtered in the glomerulus and completely excreted in the urine [37, 38].

21.3.6.2 Toxicity

Lithium has a narrow therapeutic range. Toxicity is categorized into acute, chronic, or acute-on-chronic poisoning. In acute poisoning, lithium-naïve individuals present with EKG changes, GI disturbances such as nausea, vomiting, and diarrhea, and minimal neurological effects. It takes several weeks of regular lithium use before chronic poisoning occurs. Manifestations of chronic and acute-on-chronic toxicity include neurologic effects such as lethargy, ataxia, confusion, agitation, neuromuscular excitability, and seizures including nonconvulsive status epilepticus [37].

Lithium-induced nephrogenic diabetes insipidus presents as polyuria and polydipsia. Patients with continued polyuria can develop hypovolemic acute kidney injury. Hypovolemia increases serum lithium through increased proximal reabsorption [39].

21.3.6.3 Treatment

Supportive care includes IV fluids, airway management, and GI decontamination. Whole bowel irrigation with polyethylene glycol can help prevent absorption of sustained release lithium. Although lithium levels are not accurate in predicting the severity of toxicity, serial lithium levels should be obtained as absorption may be delayed and to ensure the patient's ability to clear the agent. Steady-state lithium levels at least 12 h post-ingestion can be obtained. Sodium polystyrene sulfonate has been proposed as an adjunct in cases of chronic lithium poisoning where ECTR is not available. However, its role is not well defined [37].

Lithium is a highly dialyzable drug. ECTR is indicated when kidney failure is present and in patients with seizures, life-threatening arrhythmias, or depressed level of consciousness. High-efficiency hemodialysis is recommended as it can clear lithium up to 180 mL/min. Intermittent hemodiafiltration and sustained low-efficiency hemodialysis and continuous venovenous hemodialysis (CVVHD) may also be used [38]. Peritoneal dialysis has been reported, but not recommended as its lithium clearance rate is only 9–15 mL/min [40].

Lithium redistribution into the extracellular compartment or ongoing gastrointestinal absorption, especially seen with extended-release formulations, can cause rebound phenomenon following initial ECTR removal. Further intermittent HD or CVVHD as a hybrid therapy may be used to remove lithium in the rebound period [37, 38, 40–42].

Typically, each HD session runs for 2–4 h. A CT 190 dialyzer with cellulose triacetate (1.92 m^2) membrane should be used in clearance of small molecules like lithium. Settings include: blood flow rate (Qb) at 200–325 mL/min (4–5 mL/min/kg) and dialysate rate (Qd) of 30–40 L/h. Lithium clearance is proportional to blood flow; therefore, clearance of the drug increases as blood flow rates increase. Lithium concentration should be monitored every 2–4 h to evaluate for rebound. Monitoring frequency can be spaced to every 6–12 h if downward trend is noted. Hemodialysis should be repeated until levels are <1.0 mmol/L for at least 6–8 h to account for rebound [41, 43].

Following hemodialysis, CRRT can be initiated in hybrid therapy to control post-dialysis rebound. CRRT settings include: blood flow rate (Qb) at 200–250 mL/min (~2.5 mL/min/kg) and dialysate flow rate (Qd) at 2.0 L/h/1.73 m^2. After initiating CRRT, drug concentration should be monitored every 2–4 h until a downward trend is established at which frequency can be spaced to every 6–12 h. CRRT should be continued up to >24 h or until lithium concentrations have returned below therapeutic range [41, 44].

21.3.6.4 Case Series

Meyer et al. described chronic toxicity in a 14-year-old female with bipolar disorder, attention deficit hyperactivity disorder, and oppositional defiant disorder. She presented with lethargy, ataxia, and slurred speech after taking naproxen for joint pain. Lithium level on presentation was 5.4 mEq/L, unclear if this was steady-state or random level. Fluid resuscitation was initiated with decrease in level to 4.86 mEq/L. At this time, she developed neurologic symptoms and high-flux hemodialysis was performed for 2.5 h. Mental status improved and hemodialysis was stopped. Levels were 2.3 mEq/L. In anticipation of rebound following hemodialysis, 32 h of countercurrent CVVHD was used and final lithium level was 0.91 mEq/L. Meyer et al. also described a 16-year-old with paranoid schizophrenia, obsessive compulsive disorder, and depression presenting with somnolence and slurred speech after intentional toxic ingestion of prescribed medications chlorpromazine hydrochloride and lithium. Lithium level on admission was 4.81 mEq/L. Following supportive care, he received 4 h of hemodialysis and 22 h of countercurrent CVVHD. His lithium concentration decreased to 1.34 mEq/L after hemodialysis and to 0.81 mEq/L after CVVHD [41].

21.3.7 Acetaminophen

21.3.7.1 Pharmacokinetics

Acetaminophen (APAP) is an analgesic/antipyretic agent that functions by inhibiting prostaglandins in the CNS and by blocking peripheral pain nerve impulses. APAP is metabolized via the liver to nontoxic metabolites by glucuronidation (~50%), sulfation (~40%), and to the toxic metabolite n-acetyl-p-benzoquinoneimine (NAPQI) by CYP1A2 and 2E1 (<10%) which is rapidly detoxified by glutathione. However, in an acute overdose more APAP is metabolized to the toxic metabolite and glutathione stores can become depleted, potentially resulting in hepatotoxicity. Peak APAP serum concentrations occur within 1–2 h after therapeutic doses but are delayed in overdose [45].

21.3.7.2 Toxicity

While the most significant and well-known adverse event of APAP is hepatic failure, other significant effects including acute renal tubular necrosis can occur as well. Typically, APAP toxicity undergoes four phases:

Phase 1: (within 0.5–24 h) anorexia, nausea/vomiting, lethargy, and diaphoresis.

Phase 2: (within 24–72 h) right upper quadrant pain, liver enlargement, oliguria, bilirubin and liver enzyme elevation, prothrombin time prolongation phase 1 symptoms become less pronounced.

Phase 3: (within 72–96 h) phase 1 symptoms reappear plus signs of hepatic failure like jaundice, hypoglycemia, encephalopathy, and renal and cardiac failure may develop.

Phase 4: (within 4–14 days) patient will either recover and progress to liver failure or even die.

Furthermore, high levels of toxicity metabolic acidosis, hypothermia, shock, and CNS depression can manifest [46].

21.3.7.3 Treatment

Following acute APAP ingestion, it is essential to obtain serum concentrations 4 h after ingestion. The Rumack–Mathew nomogram plots this serum concentration and assesses the risk of hepatotoxicity [47]. The Rumack–Matthew's nomogram fails to take into account if extended-release APAP products are ingested or combination products with drugs that slow GI motility (e.g., anticholinergics, and opioids) and high-risk individuals (e.g., patients on CYP2E1-inducing drugs). In these cases, serial APAP serum concentrations should be monitored to assess the potential for hepatotoxicity.

Nonrenal replacement therapies aim to either quickly absorb acetaminophen or reduce NAPQI accumulation. GI decontamination, via activated charcoal, can be considered in acute ingestions or co-ingestion with other drugs to enhance absorption of the toxin [45]. N-acetylcysteine (NAC) reduces hepatotoxicity, replenishes glutathione, and thus producing more nontoxic metabolites while reducing NAPQI production [45]. Ideally, NAC is given within 8–10 h of an acute ingestion. However, even delayed treatment (within 16–24 h) with NAC is beneficial in decreasing hepatotoxicity as well as the need for vasopressors when begun after onset of fulminant hepatic failure. NAC has also enhanced oxygen delivery to extrahepatic organs and decreased the incidence of cerebral edema and even death [48]. Generally, IV and oral NAC efficacy is similar; thus, IV NAC should be utilized in cases of contraindications to oral therapy like risk of aspiration or persistent vomiting.

The prescription for oral NAC administration includes 140 mg/kg loading dose of NAC then a maintenance dose of 70 mg/kg every 4 h. The prescription for IV NAC administration in patients weighing >30 kg is a loading dose of 150 mg/kg, then a second dose 50 mg/kg over 4 h, and a third dose 100 mg/kg over 16 h. The prescription for IV NAC administration in patients weighing <30 kg requires a dilution of 20% NAC in 5% dextrose solution resulting in a final concentration of 40 mg/mL by mixing 50 mL of 20% NAC with 200 mL of 5% dextrose. The loading dose is 150 mg/kg (3.75 mL/kg), then 50 mg/kg (1.25 mL/kg) over 4 h, and finally a third dose of 100 mg/kg (2.5 mL/kg) over 16 h. Continue to closely monitor blood concentration levels, liver enzymes, and acid–base abnormalities. Withdraw treatment when there is no detection of acetaminophen or at least <10 μg/mL [46].

RRT management is indicated in severe cases that involve: coma, acidosis, concentrations >1000 μg/mL, hemodynamic instability, or persistent elevated concentrations despite non-RRT [47].

21.3.7.4 Case Series

Data from an observational study based on pediatric acute liver failure, the recovery rate approximated 94% in children of acetaminophen overdose when properly treated [45, 49]. Ogilvie et al. described the case of a 22-day-old male who received 200 mg/kg acetaminophen in error. Four-hour acetaminophen level was 1243 μmol/L which was in the probable toxicity range on the Rumack–Matthew nomogram. NAC was started within 8 h of ingestion. At the end of third bag of NAC, no acetaminophen was detectable and NAC was discontinued. He was discharged to home with no adverse effects [45].

Ghannoum et al. described an 18-year-old female who presented to the ED following intentional ingestion of 100 g acetaminophen, handful of ibuprofen tablets, and unknown amount of ethanol. Venous blood gas on arrival showed lactic acidosis and stable hepatic enzymes. She was intubated for airway protection and given 50 g activated charcoal after intubation. Initial acetaminophen level was 6496 μmol/L measured 90 min post-ingestion. Ethanol level was 3.9 mmol/L and ibuprofen was not measured. Hemodialysis was started along with NAC therapy. During hemodialysis, NAC infusion rate was maintained at 12.5 mg/kg/h to compensate for losses in the dialysate. She completed 6.5 h of hemodialysis (acetaminophen level decreased from 3315.7 μmol/L at start to 384 mcmol/L at end). NAC was continued at 6.25 mg/kg/h until concentration was undetectable [50].

21.3.8 Salicylates

21.3.8.1 Pharmacokinetics

Salicylates, similar to the NSAIDs, have analgesic, anti-inflammatory, and antipyretic properties. Salicylates mediate fever and inflammation through inhibition of cyclooxygenase thereby decreasing prostaglandins and thromboxane A2. The most common salicylates include aspirin (acetylsalicylic acid), a phenolic ester, and methyl salicylate (oil of wintergreen), a carboxylic acid ester. Most of the understanding of the pharmacokinetic properties of salicylates comes from aspirin. It is assumed that the remaining salicylates have similar kinetics after being converted to the common metabolite, salicylic acid. Aspirin undergoes most of its absorption in the stomach, where it is mainly nonionized via passive diffusion. Slowed, but continued, absorption continues in the small bowel. It is metabolized in the liver and eliminated by the kidneys [18]. At higher doses, oxidative phosphorylation uncoupling occurs, inducing pyruvic and lactic acid accumulation and heat release as well as stimulating the medullary respiratory center [18, 51].

21.3.8.2 Toxicity

Symptoms of mild or early salicylate toxicity include nausea, vomiting, and tinnitus. Tachypnea occurs fairly early on in the presentation following direct stimulation of the respiratory center. A primary respiratory alkalosis predominates in early toxicity. Later, labs show respiratory alkalosis with anion gap metabolic acidosis. Clinical symptoms, in some more severe cases, include worsening tachypnea, hyperpyrexia, sweating, dehydration loss of coordination, and restlessness. In severe poisoning, hallucinations, stupor, convulsions, cerebral edema, renal failure, cardiovascular failure, and coma can be seen [52]. As ingestions of enteric-coated or delayed-release formulations may initially present asymptomatically; serial salicylate measurements should be made [53, 54]. Further, care should be taken to assess the affect that co-ingestions may have on the presentation of the salicylate-poisoned patient (i.e., alcohol or benzodiazepines blunting the central respiratory drive).

21.3.8.3 Treatment

Multidose activated charcoal (MDAC) can reduce GI absorption of salicylates. However, MDAC may not be practical in large ingestions; a 10:1 ratio of activated charcoal to ingested salicylate is needed to be efficacious. Serum and urine alkalinization with IV sodium bicarbonate removes the weak acid, salicylic acid, from the CNS and prevents passive reabsorption in the kidney. Urine alkalinization goal pH is 7.5–8.0 [18].

ECTR is recommended in severe poisoning: salicylate level >100 mg/dL, altered mental status, pulmonary or cerebral edema, renal failure, severe fluid and electrolyte disturbances, deterioration in vital signs, and poisoning refractory to other treatment [54]. After extensive review of the literature, intermittent hemodialysis is the preferred mode of ECTR [55]. Intermittent HD is preferred as it can rapidly correct fluid, electrolyte, and acid–base abnormalities [54]. Intermittent hemoperfusion, continuous renal replacement therapy, and exchange transfusion in neonates may be used [55].

21.3.8.4 Case Series

Muniandy et al. reported a 16-month-old boy who ingested massage oil (methyl salicylate). On presentation, he was lethargic. He had an elevated anion gap metabolic acidosis and salicylate level of 112.15 mg/dL. Despite activated charcoal and bicarbonate infusion, repeat salicylate level 4 h later was 98.7 mg/dL. Hemodialysis was started and salicylate level at time of discharge was zero [56]. Papacostas et al. reported a 16-year-old male presenting with altered mental status and subsequent tonic-clonic seizure following ingestion of 135 g (1901 mg/kg) of enteric-coated aspirin. Four hours after ingestion, salicylate level was 90.6 mg/dL. Despite bicarbonate infusion, 8.5 h after ingestion, the salicylate level was 92.2 mg/dL. He received 5.5 h of hemodialysis. Levels were 87.7 mg/dL and 37.4 mg/dL before and after hemodialysis, respectively. CVVHDF was initiated, and then stopped after 12.5 h after symptoms resolved and QTC normalized. Salicylate level peaked 3 h after CVVHDF was stopped to 32.8 mg/dL, but then decreased to undetectable levels [57].

21.3.9 Theophylline

21.3.9.1 Pharmacokinetics

The methylxanthines, theophylline, aminophylline, and caffeine are structural analogs of adenosine, resulting in antagonism of adenosine receptors. It is thought that as adenosine modulates histamine release and causes bronchoconstriction, blockade of these receptors is responsible for the drugs' effectiveness in treating bronchospasm. Additionally, they provide adrenergic stimulation through direct catecholamine release and phosphodiesterase inhibition, which increases intracellular cyclic adenosine monophosphate [58, 59]. Theophylline and aminophylline were once the mainstay of asthma therapy and related conditions, but have since fallen out of first-line therapy with the introduction of agents with fewer side effects and more selectivity such as the beta-2 agonists. Caffeine continues to be the treatment of neonatal apnea. The levels of oral immediate-release theophylline typically peak ~2 h after ingestion, whereas sustained release preparations can be delayed until 8–10 h post-ingestion. Approximately, 60% is bound to serum proteins with a volume of distribution of ~0.5 L/kg. In neonates, 50% of theophylline is excreted unchanged in the urine because of immature hepatic function whereas only ~10% of the drug is excreted unchanged in patients >3 months old. Variability in theophylline clearance may be secondary to inherent single nucleotide polymorphisms of CYP1A2 and co-ingestion of phenytoin, phenobarbital, erythromycin, and fluoroquinolones [60]. The elimination half-life is 13–26 h in newborns and 3–4 h in pediatric patients [61], but can be highly variable based on age, hepatic function, cardiac function, smoking history, disease state, and concurrent medications. Clearance increases by 10% per year from ages 1 to 15 [60]. At high concentrations, theophylline, like ethanol and salicylates, exhibits Michaelis–Menten kinetics, resulting in a significantly longer half-life.

21.3.9.2 Toxicity

Theophylline has a narrow therapeutic range (5–15 mg/L) with adverse effects seen in high serum concentrations (>20 mg/L). Although it can be difficult to correlate toxicity with serum concentrations, in general, life-threatening toxicity occurs following an acute single overdose at levels of 90–100 mg/L, whereas it occurs at levels 40–60 mg/L in chronic intoxication. Mild toxicity includes headache, nausea, vomiting, abdominal pain, restlessness, and gastroesophageal reflux. With severe toxicity, metabolic acidosis, hypokalemia, hypotension, ventricular arrhythmias, and seizures may occur [60, 61].

21.3.9.3 Treatment

Management includes supportive care measures—airway, breathing, circulation, and maintaining hemodynamic stability. Multidose activated charcoal (MDAC) employs the principle of gut dialysis. However, its use is limited by intractable vomiting often associated with theophylline toxicity. Extracorporeal therapy is recommended in the following situations: theophylline levels >90–100 mg/L, significant dysrhythmias, seizures, mental status changes, and rising theophylline levels despite optimal therapy or clinical deterioration despite optimal therapy. Both hemoperfusion and hemodialysis have been recommended [59].

Hemodialysis, hemoperfusion, continuous venovenous hemodiafiltration (CVVHDF), peritoneal dialysis, and plasma exchange can all be used as extracorporeal treatment. The combination of hemodialysis and hemoperfusion in series is preferred for most effective clearance. In one prospective study, hemoperfusion and hemodialysis methods were compared in patients with severe theophylline toxicity. There was no statistical difference in outcome. However, there were significant procedure-related complications in the hemoperfusion group. Cessation of extracorporeal therapy is recommended when theophylline <15 mg/L [61].

21.3.9.4 Case Series

Yaman et al. report the case of an unintentional theophylline ingestion by a previously healthy 3-year-old girl. Prior to admission, she took an unknown quantity of her grandmother's sustained release theophylline and indapamide tablets. Six hours following ingestion, she began vomiting and was in status epilepticus for 4 h. She was given midazolam and phenytoin (phenytoin later stopped as it is contraindicated in theophylline toxicity) and intubated. First serum theophylline level was 54 μg/mL on admission. CVVHD was started 3 h after arrival to the hospital (27 h after ingestion). CVVHD was administered using a hemofilter HF 20 circuit and circuit was primed with 5% albumin to avoid hypotension. Blood-pump flow rate was 6 mL/kg/min. Dialysate fluid rate was run at 20 mL/kg/h. Replacement fluid rate was 2000 mL/m^2/1.73/h. CVVHD was run over 9 h and discontinued when theophylline level was 10 μg/mL. Seizures continued to be difficult to control with brain edema seen on CT scan. Patient was discharged with severe neurological disability [61].

21.3.10 Barbiturates

21.3.10.1 Pharmacokinetics

Barbiturates act on the gamma-aminobutyric acid (GABA) mediated chlorine receptors, similar to benzodiazepines. However, they bind to a different site on the channel and increase the duration the channel is open. Barbiturates can be used for seizures, sedation, and hypnosis. Barbiturates are classified as short-acting (i.e., pentobarbital, and secobarbital) or long-acting (i.e., phenobarbital, and barbital). Their biological half-life does not always correlate with their classification of short, intermediate, or long-acting due to redistribution and active metabolites. Barbiturates are hepatically cleared and several are CYP450 enzyme inducers (see Table 21.1) [62].

21.3.10.2 Toxicity

Barbiturates exert their effects on the CNS, respiratory, and cardiovascular system. At low doses, barbiturates cause sedation and hypnosis. At moderate doses, patients exhibit sluggishness, lack of coordination, slow speech, faulty judgment, and drowsiness. Shallow breathing and coma occur in severe poisoning because barbiturates can affect the GABA receptor independently. Barbiturates induce respiratory depression through suppression of the medullary respiratory center. Cardiac vascular tone and contractility are affected at higher doses, which can be seen clinically as hypotension and reduced cardiac output [62].

21.3.10.3 Treatment

Nonrenal replacement therapy with multiple-dose activated charcoal (MDAC) may enhance elimination, but is limited in improvements in clinical outcome. MDAC (15–20 g orally every 6 h) may be administered if airway is protected and patient is hemodynamically stable [62].

Extracorporeal therapy is recommended in patients with clinical signs and symptoms of severe barbiturate toxicity: prolonged coma is present/expected, fluid refractory shock, toxicity/elevated barbiturate levels despite MDAC therapy, and respiratory failure requiring mechanical ventilation. Indications for ECTR include patients with signs and symptoms of severe poisoning that carry a poor prognosis and failure to improve with medical management. Long-acting barbiturates are better cleared by hemodialysis compared to short-acting barbiturates. Short-acting barbiturates have a larger volume of distribution and greater lipid solubility. Intermittent hemodialysis is the preferred mode of renal replacement therapy. Hemodialysis removes electrolytes and water and replaces bicarbonate if the patient has coexisting kidney failure. Hemoperfusion and CRRT are acceptable alternatives if hemodialysis is not available [62].

21.3.10.4 Case Series

Soylemezoglu et al. used extracorporeal therapy in a 9-month-old boy who ingested 450 mg of phenobarbital. On admission, plasma phenobarbital level was 120 μg/mL. A gambro AK 10 and hollow-fiber type dialyzer with a surface area of 0.6 m^2 was used. Repeat phenobarbital level was 64.2 μg/mL after 6 h of hemodialysis. Dialysis was discontinued at this time [63]. Kihitir et al. described a 7-month-old with seizure disorder who was prescribed 100 mg phenobarbital in error. His peak drug levels measured >140 μg/mL. Given the drug's high percentage of protein-binding capacity (60%), SPAD was initiated. After 6 h, repeat phenobarbital level was 62 μg/mL. Dialysis was discontinued and the patient was discharged without complication [64].

21.3.11 Carbamazepine

21.3.11.1 Pharmacokinetics

Carbamazepine is a lipophilic antiepileptic drug that primary inhibits voltage-gated sodium channels, but it also has weak anticholinergic activity. Due to its anticholinergic effects, carbamazepine can have delayed absorption. It is a major substrate for CYP3A4 and forms the 10,11 epoxide active metabolite while it is a minor substrate for CYP2C8. Epoxide hydrolase catalyzes the active metabolite into the inactive metabolite carbamazepine-diol. Carbamazepine does induce its own metabolism due to inducing CYP3A4 in addition to CYP2B6, CYP1A2, and UGT1A1. Therapeutic concentrations range from 4 to 12 mg/L. It is available in immediate-release and controlled-release formulations [18] (see Table 21.1).

21.3.11.2 Toxicity

Carbamazepine toxicity can manifest as CNS depressant effects and/or anticholinergic symptoms, which can occur with serum concentrations >12 mg/L. Acute carbamazepine toxicity can cause nystagmus, ataxia, dysarthria, seizures, mental status changes, prolonged QRS, prolonged QT, hyponatremia, and respiratory depression. Compared to adults, children have fewer EKG changes; instead, children have higher rates of dystonic reactions, choreoathetosis, and seizures. Chronic carbamazepine toxicity can cause headaches, diplopia, and ataxia [18]. Carbamazepine can form a bezoar following an overdose, which can prolong absorption. Carbamazepine is structurally similar to tricyclic antidepressants (TCA) and may cause a false-positive TCA screen.

21.3.11.3 Treatment

Supportive therapy following an overdose includes monitoring for EKG changes, airway management, and benzodiazepines for seizures [18]. Single-dose or multiple-dose activated charcoal should be carefully considered because, although it may decrease carbamazepine absorption and minimize enterohepatic recirculation, it is controversial since carbamazepine can cause CNS depression and decreased GI motility.

Renal replacement therapy may be used in severe cases (serum concentrations >40 mg/L) resulting in refractory seizures, life-threatening dysrhythmias, prolonged coma, or respiratory depression or if carbamazepine levels are persistently high despite MDAC and other supportive care measures. Carbamazepine is a small, highly protein-bound molecule with relatively low volume of distribution. Hemodialysis is the preferred mode of renal replacement therapy. Given its protein-bound nature, carbamazepine is more efficiently removed with continuous venovenous hemodialysis when compared to conventional hemodialysis [3, 65]. Intermittent hemoperfusion and continuous renal replacement therapy can also be used. Both resin and charcoal hemoperfusion can remove carbamazepine. Hemodialysis is preferred due to its cost and its familiarity with more nurses and physicians. Renal replacement therapy should be continued until clinical improvement or serum levels <10 mg/L [66].

21.3.11.4 Case Series

Yildiz et al. used continuous venovenous hemodiafiltration (CVVHDF) in a 2-year-old boy who presented after generalized tonic-clonic seizure to the emergency department 20 h after ingesting 2 g (166 mg/kg) of his grandmother's controlled-release carbamazepine. On arrival, he was noted to be unconscious with reactive pupils with carbamazepine levels >20 μg/mL. He underwent bowel irrigation, gastric lavage, and activated charcoal. Two hours later, he developed mydriasis, nonreactive pupils, and seizure. He was intubated. Due to his labile state, a double-lumen catheter was placed into the left femoral vein and CVVHDF was started at the 46th hour at blood flow rate of 80 mL/min using dialysate rate of 1000 mL/h. After 10 h of hemodiafiltration, his circuit clotted. A second 8-h session of hemodiafiltration was performed using a new circuit. Serum carbamazepine levels prior to CVVHDF were unavailable due to laboratory error. Serum carbamazepine levels following CVVHDF were 0.25 μg/mL. He made a full recovery and was discharged on hospital day 5 [67]. Askenazi et al. reported the use of continuous venovenous hemodialysis (CVVHD) with 4.5% albumin dialysate to treat carbamazepine intoxication in a 10-year-old girl with peak drug levels of 44.8 μg/mL. For children using carbamazepine chronically, the half-life of drug elimination is typically 12–20 h; however, with the albumin-enhanced CVVHD serum carbamazepine levels declined significantly with a new half-life of drug elimination of 7–8 h [3]. Plasmapheresis can also be used to remove carbamazepine. Duzova et al. reported a 15-year-old ingesting a lethal dose of carbamazepine. After no neurological improvement after 20 h of admission, plasmapheresis was performed. Both his toxic levels and symptoms improved and he was discharged.

21.3.12 Phenytoin

21.3.12.1 Pharmacokinetics

Phenytoin is a hydantoin antiepileptic that inhibits sodium channels by reducing their capacity for recovery after inactivation through increased activation of gamma-aminobutyric acid (GABA) [68]. Phenytoin is a small, highly protein-bound (~90%) molecule with small volume of distribution between 0.6 and 0.8 L/kg, see Table 21.1. Phenytoin is metabolized by CYP2C9, CYP2C19, and CYP3A4 and one of its major metabolites, HPPA, undergoes enterohepatic recirculation. Phenytoin follows Michaelis–Menten kinetics, similar to aspirin, theophylline, and ethanol which is dose-dependent and can dramatically affect the apparent half-life. This can occur even with therapeutic dosing. Phenytoin has a narrow therapeutic index, 10–20 μg/mL, and toxicity can occur when concentrations are slightly elevated or if more free drug is available than anticipated, as in the case of hypoalbuminemia [8, 68].

The prodrug IV formulation is fosphenytoin, which is converted to phenytoin by plasma esterases. Using the prodrug for IV dosing allows for faster infusion rates because IV phenytoin is formulated with propylene glycol and has been associated with cardiotoxicity with faster infusion rates (hypotension, bradycardia, and cardiac arrest) [18, 69].

21.3.12.2 Toxicity

Phenytoin toxicity can result from acute overdoses or chronic supratherapeutic dosing. With mild toxicity, patients may experience nausea, vomiting, diplopia, agitation, nystagmus, and ataxia [18]. Severe toxicity manifests as stupor, coma, and respiratory arrest however fatalities are rare. In the 2016 AAPCC Poison Data, there were five reported deaths. See Table 21.2 for 2016 AAPCC Poison Data. Seizures have infrequently been reported with phenytoin toxicity. Therefore, other etiologies or co-ingestions should be considered if seizures do occur.

21.3.12.3 Treatment

Management includes supportive care with airway protection and fluid resuscitation. In cases of IV phenytoin toxicity, cardiac stabilization is necessary. Activated charcoal may be given soon after ingestion. In severe toxicity, extracorporeal therapies may be used. After review literature, we recommend using intermittent hemodialysis with high-efficiency filters for phenytoin removal. Because phenytoin is highly protein bound, intermittent hemoperfusion may also be considered. While plasmapheresis can remove phenytoin from the vascular compartment, it does so slowly and is less preferred than intermittent hemodialysis and hemoperfusion [68].

21.3.12.4 Case Series

Singh et al. presented a 4-year-old female who presented with altered mental status after ingestion of an unknown amount of her mother's phenytoin tablets. After 7 days of supportive care with no improvement and elevated phenytoin levels (74 μg/mL), tandem sessions of plasmapheresis and hemodialysis were started. She completed three sessions of plasmapheresis followed by 3 h of hemodialysis with

Table 21.2 2016 AAPCC annual report data

	≤5 years old	6–12 years old	13–19 years old	Unknown child age	Total
Ethylene glycol	541	187	515	13	1256
Methanol (single agent)	309	57	121	3	490
Ethanol (single agent, excluding rubbing alcohol)	3329	293	1141	15	4778
Isopropanol (single agent, excluding rubbing alcohol)	5606	399	472	15	6492
Lithium (medication)	132	63	431	1	627
Lithium (batteries)	72	14	9	0	95
Theophylline	13	0	5	0	18
Short-acting barbiturate (pentobarbital)	2	0	4	0	6
Long-acting barbiturate (phenobarbital)	201	36	40	0	277
Acetaminophen (single agent)	26,185	2627	7079	37	35,928
Salicylates	104	8	11	0	123
Phenytoin	92	13	33	0	138
Biguanides (includes metformin)	830	125	305	2	1262
Tetrahydrocannabinol (THC) homologs	15	11	479	1	506
Amitriptyline	308	93	475	0	876
Carbamazepine	213	57	132	1	403
Valproic acid	316	176	381	1	874
Methotrexate	–	–	–	–	–
Aminoglycoside	–	–	–	–	–
Fatalities	24	7	42	0	73
Therapies					
– Hemodialysis	8	4	133	0	
– Hemoperfusion	0	0	3	0	
– Charcoal, multiple doses	53	11	297	0	

Acetaminophen = alone, pediatric dosage; Methanol = excluding automotive products and cleaning products

high-flux hemodialyzer. At the end of the third session, mental status was regained and serum phenytoin level was 25 μg/mL. Plasmapheresis removed the highly protein-bound drug, while hemodialysis removed excess phenytoin. She made a full recovery [70]. Kumar et al. reported on the case of a 4-year-old female with altered mental status and involuntary head nodding who was found to have an elevated phenytoin concentration (88 μg/mL) 42 h after the onset of symptoms. Supportive care was provided, however, after a week, her concentration remained elevated (94 μg/mL) and dialysis options were discussed. Charcoal hemoperfusion was performed four times until her serum concentration was 12 μg/mL 24 h after her last session. The patient developed mild thrombocytopenia during the first session, but tolerated the remaining sessions. She recovered without any sequelae from the phenytoin toxicity and was eventually discharged home [8].

21.3.13 Amitriptyline

21.3.13.1 Pharmacokinetics

Amitriptyline is a tricyclic antidepressant (TCA) that, at therapeutic doses, inhibits presynaptic reuptake of norepinephrine and serotonin. Amitriptyline competitively antagonizes muscarinic acetylcholine receptors, peripheral and central histamine receptors, GABAa receptors, and peripheral alpha-1 receptors. However, it is the drug's blockade of cardiac calcium channels that is responsible for most of the morbidity and mortality associated with amitriptyline overdoses [18].

With a normal therapeutic dose, amitriptyline has rapid and near complete absorption with peak concentrations reached between 2 and 4 h. However, at supratherapeutic concentrations, the drug's anticholinergic effects can slow GI absorption. The drug undergoes extensive first pass metabolism (FPE) resulting in overall low bioavailability. It is important to consider that, in overdose, the enzymes responsible for FPE may become saturated, which can further increase absorption. It is highly lipophilic weak base and varies in volume of distribution. In the acidotic state, amitriptyline becomes ionized and binds the sodium channel [18, 71]. See Table 21.1 for detailed pharmacokinetics.

21.3.13.2 Toxicity

Amitriptyline has a narrow therapeutic index. Overdose is associated with doses >15–30 mg/kg/dose. Toxicity includes lethargy, seizures, coma, and ventricular or supraventricular tachyarrhythmias. Cardiotoxicity includes PR and QT prolongation, widened WRS, sinus tachycardia, sinus arrest, idioventricular rhythm, premature ventricular contractions, ventricular tachycardia, and ventricular fibrillation.

21.3.13.3 Treatment

Initial management involves airway protection, cardiac stabilization, and hemodynamic support. Activated charcoal may be used early in treatment because peak concentrations occur 6–8 h after ingestion. Serum alkalinization with hypertonic sodium bicarbonate therapy is cardioprotective. Lidocaine is recommended in treatment of arrhythmias that do not respond to bicarbonate. Extracorporeal therapies include hemoperfusion and plasmapheresis. Although hemoperfusion is not routinely recommended due to amitriptyline's large volume of distribution and high protein-binding capacity, it may be considered early on in severe intoxication. Plasmapheresis can eliminate amitriptyline in severe intoxication. Lipid emulsion therapy has been described in amitriptyline removal. The lipid emulsion reduces toxicity; infusion into the bloodstream effectively sequesters lipophilic compounds, making them less available to tissues [72].

21.3.13.4 Case Series

Donmez et al. discussed hemoperfusion in the context of a 17-month-old girl presenting with multifocal clonic seizures and lethargy 2 h after ingesting 75 mg/kg amitriptyline. On arrival, she had a Glasgow coma score 3 with mydriasis and hypotension. EKG showed ventricular tachycardia and wide QRS complexes. She was fluid resuscitated, started on multidose activated charcoal therapy, and treated with lidocaine and sodium bicarbonate for cardiac arrhythmias and for alkalinization. She continued to have cardiac arrhythmias and seizures despite alkalinization with sodium bicarbonate infusion. Arrhythmias and seizures stopped on the day 2 of hospital stay. She was discharged to home on the ninth hospital day [71]. Prior to hemoperfusion, serum amitriptyline level was 1299 μg/L. Following 2 h of hemoperfusion (10 h after admission), level decreased to 843 μg/L. She was cardioverted six times while undergoing hemoperfusion. Mutlu et al. used charcoal hemoperfusion to treat an 18-month-old male who ingested 57 mg/kg amitriptyline 2 h prior to presentation. He was intubated and treated with adenosine and amiodarone for narrow complex tachycardia. He subsequently developed seizures which were treated with midazolam and phenytoin. At fourth hour of hospital admission, he completed 4 h of hemoperfusion with resolution of arrhythmia and seizures [73]. In a large case study of 20 children between 1.5 and 15 years old, charcoal hemoperfusion successfully resolved severe cardiotoxicity and respiratory depression with reduction of morbidity and mortality [74].

Kolsal et al. used plasmapheresis in a 2-year-old who presented with seizures and lethargy 6 h after ingestion of 70 mg/kg of amitriptyline. She was intubated, started on sodium bicarbonate infusion and activated charcoal, and given midazolam. Ventricular tachycardia and seizures persisted so plasmapheresis was initiated. She completed two 3-h sessions for a total of 6 h. Plasma amitriptyline levels before the first plasmapheresis session was 4.87 μg/mL. After second plasmapheresis, level was 0.02 μg/mL. She was discharged home on hospital day 4 [75]. Plasmapheresis was used to treat toxicity in a 15-year-old girl who ingested 22 mg/kg amitriptyline 4 h prior to emergency department. On arrival, she was intubated for poor respiratory effort and GCS 5. Plasma amitriptyline level was 112.78 ng/mL. After activated charcoal and gastric irrigation, sodium bicarbonate was started. Plasmapheresis was performed for 4 h. Following completion, she was extubated and repeat plasma amitriptyline levels were 9.23 ng/mL. She was discharged home without complication [76]. Lipid emulsion therapy was used in a 13-year-old girl who was intubated on arrival to emergency department for acute encephalopathy following ingestion of unknown amount of amitriptyline. Following cardiopulmonary resuscitation and seizure management with sodium bicarbonate, epinephrine, lidocaine, magnesium sulfate, and midazolam, lipid emulsion therapy was initiated. She was given two boluses of 1.5 mL/kg intralipid 20% and started on continuous infusion of intralipid at 0.25 mL/kg/min for 30 min. Although she developed hypertriglyceridemia and pancreatitis, arrhythmias resolved and she was eventually discharged to home with no residual deficits [72].

21.3.14 Valproic Acid

21.3.14.1 Pharmacokinetics

Valproic acid (VPA) is a simple branched chain carboxylic acid that is used as an antiepileptic agent and is also used in the management of different psychiatric disorders. It has small molecular mass, low volume of distribution, and is highly protein bound, see Table 21.1. It undergoes hepatic metabolism via glucuronic acid conjugation (~30–50%), mitochondrial beta-oxidation (~40%), cytosolic omega-oxidation (~10%), and also a minor substrate of several CYP450 enzymes. At therapeutic doses (50–100 μg/mL), VPA undergoes first-order elimination. However, with significantly elevated VPA concentrations (>300 μg/mL), protein-binding sites become saturated and free valproic acid can accumulate [77, 78].

21.3.14.2 Toxicity

VPA can cause toxicity both at therapeutic concentrations and supratherapeutic concentrations following an acute overdose. Hyperammonemia can develop with or without elevated VPA concentrations. Signs and symptoms of mild to moderate toxicity include vomiting, CNS depression, ataxia, lethargy, and hypotension with tachycardia. More severe ingestions can result in respiratory depression, coma, and electrolyte abnormalities such as hypernatremia, hypocalcemia, and anion gap metabolic acidosis [78].

21.3.14.3 Treatment

Supportive management includes GI decontamination with activated charcoal and airway protection for patients who present within the first 2 h. Serum concentrations should be obtained upon presentation and redrawn every 4–6 h until levels trend downward [18]. In children with severe toxicity, carnitine is recommended. L-carnitine theoretically augments mitochondrial beta-oxidation and limits cytosolic omega oxidation to reduce the accumulation of toxic metabolites. Both chronic therapeutic valproic acid use and overdose are thought to deplete carnitine stores. Toxic metabolites include 2-propl-2-pentenoic acid, 2-propyl-4-pentenoic acid, and propionic acid, which are thought to cause cerebral edema, hepatotoxicity, and hyperammonemia, respectively. Carnitine can be given either enterally or IV, depending on if patients are asymptomatic or symptomatic, respectively, from hyperammonemia and/or hepatotoxicity. The IV carnitine loading dose is 100 mg/kg (max 6 g) over 30 min followed by 15 mg/kg over 10–30 min every 4 h, while enteral carnitine can be dosed at 100 mg/kg/day in divided doses [18, 79].

Despite VPA being highly protein bound, extracorporeal removal can be considered when serum VPA concentrations are >850 μg/mL since the free fraction increases due to saturation. After review of the literature, we recommend using intermittent hemodialysis or hemodiafiltration in severe poisoning. Hemodialysis also removes ammonia efficiently [77].

21.3.14.4 Case Series

Tsai et al. reported a 14-year-old female with seizure disorder who presented with dizziness and generalized malaise after restarting 25 mg/kg/day (1000 mg/day) 3 weeks prior. Ammonia level was 184 μmmol/L and valproate level was 182 μg/mL. Due to worsening encephalopathy, she received 3 h of hemodialysis. Mental status improved and ammonia level decreased to 1 μmmol/L 1 day after dialysis. Valproate level was 24 μg/mL 2 days after dialysis [80]. Dharnidharka et al. reported two patients with valproic acid toxicity. The first patient was an 18-year-old female with seizure disorder found unresponsive after intentional ingestion of unknown amount of valproic acid. She was given activated charcoal, intubated, and found to have a valproic acid level of 633 μg/mL on arrival. She received 4 h of high-flux hemodialysis. The second patient was a comatose 18-month-old girl who ingested an unknown amount of valproic acid. After activated charcoal and intubation, initial valproic acid level drawn was 922 μg/mL. She received 5 h of conventional hemodialysis. In both cases, levels dropped quickly with no rebound noted after hemodialysis was discontinued [81].

References

1. Gummin DD, et al. 2016 annual report of the American Association of Poison Control Centers' National Poison Data System (NPDS): 34th annual report. Clin Toxicol (Phila). 2017;55(10):1072–252.
2. Rademacher S, Oppert M, Jorres A. Artificial extracorporeal liver support therapy in patients with severe liver failure. Expert Rev Gastroenterol Hepatol. 2011;5(5):591–9.
3. Askenazi DJ, Goldstein SL, Chang IF, Elenberg E, Feig DI. Management of a Severe Carbamazepine Overdose Using Albumin-Enhanced Continuous Venovenous Hemodialysis. Pediatrics. 2004;133(2):406–9.
4. Churchwell MD, Pasko DA, Smoyer WE, Mueller BA. Enhanced clearance of highly protein bound drugs by albumin supplemented dialysate during modeled continuous hemodialysis. Nephrol Dial Transplant. 2009;24:231–8.
5. Collins KL, Roberts EA, Adeli K, Bohn D, Harvey EA. Single pass albumin dialysis (SPAD) in fulminant Wilsonian liver failure: a case report. Pediatr Nephrol. 2008;23:1013–6.
6. Mitzner SR, Stange J. Albumin dialysis with molecular adsorbent recirculating system in the treatment of liver failure. In: Critical care nephrology. Philadelphia: Saunders; 2008. p. 1539–43.
7. Harbord N, Feinfeld DA, Winchester JF. Hemodialysis, hemofiltration, and hemoperfusion in acute intoxication and poisoning. In: Critical care nephrology. Philadelphia: Saunders; 2008. p. 919–25.
8. Kumar PP, et al. Charcoal hemoperfusion for phenytoin intoxication. Indian Pediatr. 2012;49(2):152–3.
9. Shalkham AS, et al. The availability and use of charcoal hemoperfusion in the treatment of poisoned patients. Am J Kidney Dis. 2006;48(2):239–41.
10. Nemoto T, et al. Effect of charcoal hemoperfusion for removal of plasma methotrexate in a patient with acute renal failure. Pediatr Hematol Oncol. 2009;26(7):520–5.
11. Borkan SC. Extracorporeal therapies for acute intoxications. Crit Care Clin. 2002;18:393–420.
12. Misanovic V, et al. Plasmapheresis in pediatric intensive care unit. Med Arch. 2016;70(5):332–5.
13. Nenov VD, Marinov P, Sabeva J, Nenov DS. Current applications of plasmapheresis in clinical toxicology. Nephrol Dial Transplant. 2003;18(Suppl 5):v56–8.
14. Cox RD, Phillips WJ. Ethylene glycol toxicity. Mil Med. 2004;169(8):660–3.

15. Kuang D, Ronco C, NA H. Poisoning: kinetics to therapeutics. In: Critical care nephrology. Philadelphia: Saunders; 2008. p. 931–54.
16. Wiley JF. Novel therapies for ethylene glycol intoxication. Curr Opin Pediatr. 1999;11(3):269–73.
17. Jacobsen D, Hovda KE. Methanol, ethylene glycol, and other toxic alcohols. In: Haddad and Winchester's clinical management of poisoning and drug overdose. Philadelphia: Saunders; 2007. p. 605–21.
18. Goldfrank LR, et al. Goldfrank's toxicologic emergencies. 8th ed. New York: McGraw Hill; 2006.
19. Tadokoro M, et al. A case of acute renal failure due to ethylene glycol intoxication. Nihon Jinzo Gakkai Shi. 1995;37(6):353–6.
20. Schwerk N, et al. Successful therapy of paediatric ethylene glycol poisoning: a case report and annual survey by a regional poison centre. Acta Paediatr. 2007;96(3):461–3.
21. Litovitz T. The alcohols: ethanol, methanol, isopropanol, ethylene glycol. Pediatr Clin N Am. 1986;33(2):311–23.
22. Stapenhorst L, Hesse A, Hoppe B. Hyperoxaluria after ethylene glycol poisoning. Pediatr Nephrol. 2008;23(12):2277–9.
23. Brent J. Current management of ethylene glycol poisoning. Drugs. 2001;61(7):979–88.
24. Hirsch DJ, et al. A simple method to estimate the required dialysis time for cases of alcohol poisoning. Kidney Int. 2001;60(5):2021–4.
25. Brent J. Fomepizole for the treatment of pediatric ethylene and diethylene glycol, butoxyethanol, and methanol poisonings. Clin Toxicol (Phila). 2010;48(5):401–6.
26. Loza R, Rodriguez D. A case of methanol poisoning in a child. Case Rep Nephrol. 2014;2014:652129.
27. Barceloux DG, et al. American Academy of Clinical Toxicology practice guidelines on the treatment of methanol poisoning. J Toxicol Clin Toxicol. 2002;40(4):415–46.
28. Sutton TL, Foster RL, Liner SR. Acute methanol ingestion. Pediatr Emerg Care. 2002;18(5):360–3.
29. Roberts DM, et al. Recommendations for the role of extracorporeal treatments in the management of acute methanol poisoning: a systematic review and consensus statement. Crit Care Med. 2015;43(2):461–72.
30. Brown MJ, et al. Childhood methanol ingestion treated with fomepizole and hemodialysis. Pediatrics. 2001;108(4):E77.
31. Gibson PJ, Cant AJ, Mant TG. Ethanol poisoning. Acta Paediatr Scand. 1985;74(6):977–8.
32. Gormley NJ, et al. The rising incidence of intentional ingestion of ethanol-containing hand sanitizers. Crit Care Med. 2012;40(1):290–4.
33. Slaughter RJ, et al. Isopropanol poisoning. Clin Toxicol (Phila). 2014;52(5):470–8.
34. Church AS, Witting MD. Laboratory testing in ethanol, methanol, ethylene glycol, and isopropanol toxicities. J Emerg Med. 1997;15(5):687–92.
35. Wiener SW. Toxic alcohol. In: Goldfrank's Toxicologic emergencies. New York: McGraw-Hill; 2014. p. 1346–53.
36. Stremski E, Hennes H. Accidental isopropanol ingestion in children. Pediatr Emerg Care. 2000;16(4):238–40.
37. Baird-Gunning J, et al. Lithium poisoning. J Intensive Care Med. 2017;32(4):249–63.
38. Decker BS, et al. Extracorporeal treatment for lithium poisoning: systematic review and recommendations from the EXTRIP workgroup. Clin J Am Soc Nephrol. 2015;10(5):875–87.
39. Bruns AS, Sebestyen J. Twelve-year-old female with nausea, vomiting, edema, tremor, and slurred speech. Clin Pediatr (Phila). 2015;54(2):194–6.
40. McLean MM, et al. A 17-year-old female patient with a Lithium overdose. Air Med J. 2015;34(4):162–5.
41. Meyer RJ, et al. Hemodialysis followed by continuous hemofiltration for treatment of lithium intoxication in children. Am J Kidney Dis. 2001;37(5):1044–7.
42. Groleau G. Lithium toxicity. Emerg Med Clin North Am. 1994;12(2):511–31.
43. Fischbach M, et al. Hemodialysis in children: general practical guidelines. Pediatr Nephrol. 2005;20(8):1054–66.

44. Tolwani A. Continuous renal-replacement therapy for acute kidney injury. N Engl J Med. 2012;367(26):2505–14.
45. Ogilvie JD, Rieder MJ, Lim R. Acetaminophen overdose in children. CMAJ. 2012;184(13):1492–6.
46. Marzullo L. An update of N-acetylcysteine treatment for acute acetaminophen toxicity in children. Curr Opin Pediatr. 2005;17(2):239–45.
47. Shannon M, Borron S, Burns M. Haddad and Winchester's clinical management of poisoning and drug overdose. Philadelphia: Saunders; 2007. p. 825–31.
48. Keays R, et al. Intravenous acetylcysteine in paracetamol induced fulminant hepatic failure: a prospective controlled trial. BMJ. 1991;303(6809):1026–9.
49. Squires RH, et al. Acute liver failure in children: the first 348 patients in the pediatric acute liver failure study group. J Pediatr. 2006;148(5):652–8.
50. Ghannoum M, et al. Massive acetaminophen overdose: effect of hemodialysis on acetaminophen and acetylcysteine kinetics. Clin Toxicol (Phila). 2016;54(6):519–22.
51. Mirrakhimov AE, et al. The role of renal replacement therapy in the management of pharmacologic poisonings. Int J Nephrol. 2016;2016:3047329.
52. Dargan PI, Wallace CI, Jones AL. An evidence based flowchart to guide the management of acute salicylate (aspirin) overdose. Emerg Med J. 2002;19(3):206–9.
53. Rivera W, et al. Delayed salicylate toxicity at 35 hours without early manifestations following a single salicylate ingestion. Ann Pharmacother. 2004;38(7–8):1186–8.
54. Lugassy D. Salicylates. In: Hoffman R, Howland M, Lewin N, Nelson L, Goldfrank L, editors. Goldfrank's toxicologic emergencies. New York: McGraw-Hill; 2015.
55. Juurlink DN, et al. Extracorporeal treatment for salicylate poisoning: systematic review and recommendations from the EXTRIP workgroup. Ann Emerg Med. 2015;66(2):165–81.
56. Muniandy RK, Sinnathamby V. Salicylate toxicity from ingestion of traditional massage oil. BMJ Case Rep. 2012;2012. https://doi.org/10.1136/bcr-2012-006562.
57. Papacostas MF, et al. Use of continuous renal replacement therapy in salicylate toxicity: a case report and review of the literature. Heart Lung. 2016;45(5):460–3.
58. Fisher J, Graudins A. Intermittent haemodialysis and sustained low-efficiency dialysis (SLED) for acute theophylline toxicity. J Med Toxicol. 2015;11(3):359–63.
59. Ghannoum M, et al. Extracorporeal treatment for theophylline poisoning: systematic review and recommendations from the EXTRIP workgroup. Clin Toxicol (Phila). 2015;53(4):215–29.
60. Ma YJ, et al. Theophylline: a review of population pharmacokinetic analyses. J Clin Pharm Ther. 2016;41(6):594–601.
61. Yaman A, et al. Severe theophylline poisoning treated with continuous venovenous hemodialysis in a child. Turk J Pediatr. 2016;58(3):297–300.
62. Mactier R, et al. Extracorporeal treatment for barbiturate poisoning: recommendations from the EXTRIP workgroup. Am J Kidney Dis. 2014;64(3):347–58.
63. Söylemezoğlu O, et al. Haemodialysis treatment in phenobarbital intoxication in infancy. Int Urol Nephrol. 1993;25(1):111–3.
64. Kihtir HS, et al. Single-pass albumin dialysis in a child aged six months with phenobarbital poisoning. Turk Pediatri Ars. 2016;51(4):228–30.
65. Goktas U, Kati I, Yuce HH. Management of a severe carbamazepine overdose with continuous venovenous hemodiafiltration. Am J Emerg Med. 2010;28(2):260.e1–2.
66. Ghannoum M, et al. Extracorporeal treatment for carbamazepine poisoning: systematic review and recommendations from the EXTRIP workgroup. Clin Toxicol (Phila). 2014;52(10):993–1004.
67. Yildiz TS, et al. Continuous venovenous hemodiafiltration to treat controlled-release carbamazepine overdose in a pediatric patient. Paediatr Anaesth. 2006;16(11):1176–8.
68. Anseeuw K, et al. Extracorporeal treatment in phenytoin poisoning: systematic review and recommendations from the EXTRIP (extracorporeal treatments in poisoning) workgroup. Am J Kidney Dis. 2016;67(2):187–97.
69. Fischer JH, Patel TV, Fischer PA. Fosphenytoin clinical pharmacokinetics and comparative advantages in the acute treatment of seizures. Clin Pharmacokinet. 2003;42:33–58.

70. Singh S, Rathore S, Verma DK, Kumar P, Bhatia BD. Tandem plasmapheresis with hemodialysis in phenytoin intoxication: a case report. Int J Adv Med. 2015;2(3):269–71.
71. Dönmez O, Cetinkaya M, Canbek R. Hemoperfusion in a child with amitriptyline intoxication. Pediatr Nephrol. 2005;20(1):105–7.
72. Presley JD, Chyka PA. Intravenous lipid emulsion to reverse acute drug toxicity in pediatric patients. Ann Pharmacother. 2013;47(5):735–43.
73. Mutlu M, et al. Charcoal hemoperfusion in an infant with supraventricular tachycardia and seizures secondary to amitriptyline intoxication. Hum Exp Toxicol. 2011;30(3):254–6.
74. Bek K, et al. Charcoal haemoperfusion in amitriptyline poisoning: experience in 20 children. Nephrology (Carlton). 2008;13(3):193–7.
75. Karaci M, et al. Severe childhood amitriptyline intoxication and plasmapheresis: a case report. Turk J Pediatr. 2013;55(6):645–7.
76. Kolsal E, Tekin I, Cumhur A, Akyuz M, Cabuk H, Eldes N, Numanoglu V. Treatment of severe amitriptyline intoxication with plasmapheresis. J Clin Apher. 2009;24:21–4.
77. Ghannoum M, et al. Extracorporeal treatment for valproic acid poisoning: systematic review and recommendations from the EXTRIP workgroup. Clin Toxicol (Phila). 2015;53(5):454–65.
78. Thanacoody RH. Extracorporeal elimination in acute valproic acid poisoning. Clin Toxicol (Phila). 2009;47(7):609–16.
79. Mock CM, Schwetschenau KH. Levocarnitine for valproic-acid-induced hyperammonemic encephalopathy. Am J Health Syst Pharm. 2012;69(1):35–9.
80. Tsai MF, Chen CY. Valproate-induced hyperammonemic encephalopathy treated by hemodialysis. Ren Fail. 2008;30(8):822–4.
81. Dharnidharka VR, Fennell RS, Richard GA. Extracorporeal removal of toxic valproic acid levels in children. Pediatr Nephrol. 2002;17(5):312–5.

22 RRT in Liver Failure

Vimal Chadha and Bradley A. Warady

22.1 Case Presentation

A 5-year-old boy was seen in the outpatient clinic for evaluation of yellow discoloration of his eyes and skin for the past 2–3 days. His parents reported that his appetite has decreased over the past 1 week and he had been complaining of generalized abdominal discomfort. On examination, he had scleral and cutaneous icterus. His abdomen was distended, and his liver was palpable 3 cm below the costal margin; it was firm and mildly tender. His blood tests revealed hemoglobin 10.7 g/dL, WBC count 6560/mm^3, platelet count 168,000/mm^3, sodium 140 mEq/L, potassium 4.1 mEq/L, chloride 105 mEq/L, bicarbonate 23 mEq/L, urea nitrogen 4 mg/dL, creatinine 0.37 mg/dL, calcium 9.5 mg/dL, glucose 93 mg/dL, albumin 4 g/dL, bilirubin 13.1 (conjugated 11.7) mg/dL, AST 4410 U/L, ALT 2858 U/L, GGT 155 U/L, and alkaline phosphatase 435 U/L. Imaging studies (ultrasound and MRCP) confirmed hepatosplenomegaly and showed a thickened gall bladder and a normal caliber common bile duct, in addition to mild to moderate ascites. He was hospitalized for a day and then followed as an outpatient. Tests for viral studies and alpha-1 antitrypsin came back negative.

A week later, his serum bilirubin had increased to 19.5 (conjugated 17.1) mg/dL; and the remainder of the liver function tests revealed AST 3990 U/L, ALT 2291 U/L, GGT 88 U/L, and alkaline phosphatase 291 U/L. He was hospitalized for further evaluation. Over the next 4 days, his serum bilirubin increased to 21.6 (conjugated 19.1) mg/dL, while AST and ALT levels decreased to 1674 and 1258 U/L, respectively; the serum albumin also decreased to 2.9 g/dL. A coagulation profile revealed

V. Chadha · B. A. Warady (✉)
Department of Pediatrics, University of Missouri–Kansas City School of Medicine, Kansas City, MO, USA

Division of Pediatric Nephrology, Children's Mercy Kansas City, Kansas City, MO, USA
e-mail: bwarady@cmh.edu

S. K. Sethi et al. (eds.), *Critical Care Pediatric Nephrology and Dialysis: A Practical Handbook*, https://doi.org/10.1007/978-981-13-2276-1_22

prothrombin time (PT) 44.7 s, international normalized ratio (INR) 4.5, and fibrinogen 65 mg/dL. At this time, he started exhibiting changes in his mental status, and a serum ammonia was 63 μmol/L. Six hours later, his mental status worsened (lethargy and confusion), and a repeat serum ammonia level was 90 μmol/L. He was diagnosed with fulminant acute liver failure with hepatic encephalopathy (grade II) and transferred to the intensive care unit (ICU). By the next day, the serum ammonia had increased to 126 μmol/L. He was evaluated by the liver transplant team and listed for emergent liver transplant. During his ICU stay, his blood pressure and respiratory status remained stable. He did receive three units of fresh frozen plasma and a unit of cryoprecipitate.

The nephrology service was consulted to provide supportive therapy until a liver transplant could be performed. He had no significant acid-base or electrolyte abnormalities, his renal function was normal (urea nitrogen <2 mg/dL, creatinine 0.32 mg/dL), and his urine output was adequate. A plan was made to initiate continuous renal replacement therapy (CRRT) with single pass albumin dialysis (SPAD). CRRT was initiated with a total clearance of 2 L/h/1.73 m^2 (70% of the clearance was provided as diffusive clearance). Four hundred milliliters of 25% albumin was added to a 5 L dialysate bag for a final albumin concentration of 1.85%. In view of the prolonged PT and thrombocytopenia (66,000/mm^3), CRRT was performed without anticoagulation. Over the next 36 h, the serum ammonia and bilirubin level decreased to 86 μmol/L and 10.6 (conjugated 8.9) mg/dL, respectively, and a liver became available from an ABO-incompatible donor. The orthotopic liver transplant took place without any complications, and the postoperative course was uneventful. He is currently a 1-year post-liver transplant patient with normal liver and renal function.

22.2 Introduction

Acute liver failure (ALF) in children is a devastating condition with reported mortality rates as high as 70% without liver transplant [1, 2]. While one third of the children with ALF might recover spontaneously [3], ALF is commonly a rapidly progressive disease and leads to multiple organ failure and death in the rest. These patients are, therefore, always managed in the intensive care setting by a multidisciplinary team including a hepatologist, intensivist, liver transplant surgeon, nephrologist, hematologist, toxicologist, and infectious disease specialist. In the absence of any definitive determinants that can differentiate patients who might recover spontaneously from those who will rapidly deteriorate, several supportive therapies utilizing different extracorporeal modalities have been provided to stabilize the patient until spontaneous recovery or as a bridge to liver transplant. However, because of a low number of pediatric ALF patients seen in most tertiary care hospitals, there are no adequately powered studies to provide specific management algorithms for optimal outcomes. Accordingly, delineating and standardizing the supportive therapies that are employed in the management of pediatric ALF is an area of growing importance [4–6]. Specific liver support systems such as Molecular Adsorbents Recirculating System (MARS), which consists of hemodialysis against a closed albumin circuit with additional toxin absorbers, and Prometheus dialysis (fractionated plasma separation and adsorption) are not available in many centers, and a detailed discussion of these techniques is beyond the scope of this chapter. In contrast, as many patients with ALF develop acute kidney injury (AKI) and associated complications such as fluid overload, acid-base disorders, and electrolyte abnormalities, renal support with continuous renal replacement therapy (CRRT) is commonly prescribed as an important component of the treatment regimen for these critically ill patients. In fact, a recent single-center study demonstrated the beneficial effect of CRRT on the outcome of pediatric patients with ALF and raised the question of whether the use of CRRT should be extended to nonrenal indications in children with ALF as a detoxification mechanism [7]. Given the paucity of proven treatment modalities, many centers use a combination of extracorporeal therapies such as CRRT with therapeutic plasma exchange (TPE) and single pass albumin dialysis (SPAD) [8]. Accordingly, nephrologists are increasingly playing an important role in the management of patients with ALF.

22.3 Common Causes of ALF

The spectrum of ALF etiologies varies with age. While metabolic disorders predominate in infants, viral hepatitis (40%) and drug intoxication (10%) are the most common causes in older children. It is important to note that the etiology of ALF remains obscure in up to 50% of cases [3, 9]. Some of the ALF causes such as acetaminophen ingestion, herpes simplex virus hepatitis, autoimmune hepatitis, Wilson's disease, and certain inborn errors of metabolism are amenable to specific treatments. These treatable causes, therefore, should be carefully looked for.

22.4 Comorbidities Associated with ALF

The various comorbidities associated with ALF result from the loss of myriads of functions (homeostasis, detoxification, excretion, synthetic) performed by normal liver and often influence the selection and performance of extracorporeal therapy. Hepatic encephalopathy (HE), cerebral edema, coagulopathy, AKI, acid-base, metabolic (hypoglycemia), and electrolyte disorders and eventually multi-organ dysfunction syndrome (MODS) may all occur.

22.4.1 Hepatic Encephalopathy (HE) and Cerebral Edema

While the exact pathophysiology of HE and cerebral edema is not completely understood, there is substantial evidence that hyperammonemia plays a significant role in the development of both HE and cerebral edema. High levels of ammonia are detoxified to glutamine in the brain, a product which is osmotically active and is believed to be responsible for the cytotoxic edema seen in ALF [10]. According to the position paper by the American Association for the Study of Liver Diseases, a serum ammonia concentration of >100 μmol/L represents an independent risk factor for the development of high-grade HE, and a level of >200 μmol/L is highly predictive of intracranial hypertension (ICH) [11]. In addition, the presence of hyponatremia and volume overload can increase the severity of cerebral edema and HE. The risk of developing ICH is decreased by raising the serum sodium to 144–155 mEq/L with hypertonic saline [12].

22.4.2 Acute Kidney Injury (AKI)

Acute kidney injury frequently complicates ALF and is seen in approximately 55% of all cases [13]. In a retrospective review of the US Acute Liver Failure Study Group database, the highest incidence of AKI was observed in those patients with acetaminophen-induced liver injury and ALF resulting from ischemic shock [14]. While AKI in ALF is usually multifactorial, it can develop secondary to fluid restriction (prerenal azotemia), systemic hypotension due to sepsis or hemorrhage, and nephrotoxic medications. Hepatorenal syndrome, which is commonly seen in chronic liver disease but can also occur in ALF, should be suspected when other causes of AKI have been ruled out. In this condition, the urine sodium is very low, and the condition can be rapidly progressive and reversible only after liver transplant.

The presence of AKI requiring renal replacement therapy (RRT) in patients with ALF is associated with decreased transplant-free survival (37%) in contrast to those patients without AKI (64%), regardless of etiology of ALF [14]. Furthermore, those with AKI have a lower chance of spontaneous hepatic recovery [14]. In the prospective pediatric CRRT registry, children with AKI due to liver disease had the lowest survival (31%) compared to the average (58%) for all other causes of AKI [15]. It is important to note that the presence of AKI before liver transplant in patients with ALF influences the degree of kidney dysfunction after transplantation.

22.4.3 Coagulopathy

Coagulopathy is a constant feature of ALF. Prothrombin time (PT) and international normalization ratio (INR) are the commonly used tests to assess the synthetic liver function and help characterize the severity of ALF. These tests assess the production of clotting factors, particularly factors V and VII, which have the shortest half-lives. However, it is important to note that PT and INR are not good markers for the risk of bleeding in patients with ALF as there is a balanced reduction in both procoagulant (factor V, VII, X, and fibrinogen) and anticoagulant proteins (antithrombin, protein C, and protein S) [16]. The coagulation dysregulation in hepatic failure is complex, and the underlying abnormalities can only be elucidated with viscoelastic tests such as thromboelastography (TEG®) or rotational thromboelastometry (ROTEM®). Correction of the coagulopathy with plasma products should be avoided unless the patient is actively bleeding or requires a surgical procedure as these products further add to the protein load and can worsen hyperammonemia.

22.5 Extracorporeal Therapies in ALF

The primary goal of an ideal extracorporeal support system in ALF should be detoxification of blood (removal of both water-soluble and protein-bound toxins); correction of fluid, acid-base, and electrolyte disorders; and management of synthetic and coagulation perturbations. While hemodialysis or CRRT can correct the fluid, acid-base, and electrolyte abnormalities and remove water-soluble toxins, these therapies are inefficient in terms of their capacity to remove protein-bound toxins. Combining dialysis therapy with MARS (when available) or with SPAD is, however, effective in removing protein-bound toxins. In addition, TPE can correct the coagulation abnormalities without adding an extra protein load to the system. Accordingly, many centers use a combination (hybrid) of the above therapies in patients with ALF until spontaneous recovery of liver function or liver transplant occurs. Arikan et al. recently reported their experience with hybrid extracorporeal therapies combining high-flux CRRT for hyperammonemia, TPE for coagulopathy, and albumin-assisted dialysis (MARS) for hepatic encephalopathy [8].

22.6 Indications for Extracorporeal Therapies

While one third of children recover with supportive management [3], the other two thirds require emergency liver transplant. Due to scarcity of organs, the wait time to transplant can be considerably long, and extracorporeal therapies are required as a bridge until an organ becomes available. It is important to note that extracorporeal therapies to support patients with ALF should be started only if a curative therapy, i.e., usually liver transplantation, or significant recovery of liver function can be expected (Table 22.1). The timing of initiation and choice of extracorporeal therapies vary markedly among treatment centers as no one therapy has shown superiority over the other. The criteria that help make the decision regarding the initiation of extracorporeal therapy are listed in Table 22.2. Because of the high risk of

Table 22.1 Indications for liver replacement therapy

Acute liver failure
• Bridging to liver transplantation
• Post-liver transplant in case of primary dysfunction
• Liver dysfunction after hepatobiliary surgery
• Acute intoxication
• Acute hepatitis
Secondary liver dysfunction
• Multi-organ dysfunction syndrome (MODS)
• Sepsis
• Systemic inflammatory response syndrome (SIRS)
Acute-on-chronic liver failure
• Biliary atresia
• Progressive familial intrahepatic cholestasis

Table 22.2 Criteria for initiating support with extracorporeal device

• Hepatic encephalopathy stage 2 or higher
• Increased intracranial pressure
• Acute kidney injury
• Fluid overload
• Hemodynamic instability
• Coagulopathy
• Severe hyperbilirubinemia
• Hyperammonemia

life-threatening complications of ALF and the usually excellent tolerability of the procedures, an early initiation is most often justified, particularly in patients exhibiting rapid disease progression.

22.7 Dialysis Therapies

In addition to the AKI that occurs in more than half of the ALF patients (vide supra), fluid overload and acid-base and electrolyte disorders are common in these critically ill patients, and dialysis therapy is often required. CRRT is the preferred dialysis modality as hemodynamic instability and fluid shifts that accompany ALF result in poor tolerance of intermittent modes of dialysis therapy [17]. Furthermore, intermittent modalities are associated with an increased risk of significant increases in intracranial pressure [18]. Successful usage of sustained low-efficiency dialysis (SLED) in place of CRRT has also been reported. It is important to note that while CRRT can control fluid balance, correct metabolic abnormalities, and remove some of the water-soluble toxins such as ammonia and lactate, it does not remove protein-bound toxins (such as bile acids, bilirubin, aromatic amino acids, endogenous benzodiazepines, and phenols) that accumulate in ALF and which likely determine patient outcome. To enhance the removal of protein-bound toxins, dialysis therapies are usually combined with albumin-assisted dialysis (MARS or SPAD). However, in a recent retrospective analysis, Deep et al. reported improved survival in ALF patients using CRRT with high clearance rates (90 mL/kg/h); the survival advantage was seen only in the group that showed a decline in the serum ammonia level with CRRT [7]. A similar experience which supports the use of high-volume CRRT was reported in 22 children with liver failure listed for high-urgency OLT in a single unit in France [19].

22.8 Albumin-Assisted Dialysis

MARS is one of the well-known systems utilized for the removal of protein-bound toxins in which the patient's blood is dialyzed through a high-flux dialyzer against albumin-containing dialysate (usually 20% albumin). In this system, albumin acts as an acceptor for protein-bound toxins. The albumin-containing dialysate runs in a closed circuit, and albumin is regenerated by including an ion exchanger and charcoal absorber in the closed circuit. However, as mentioned previously, MARS is not available in many pediatric hospitals, and the use of the system requires special training for the dialysis staff.

On the other hand, single pass albumin dialysis (SPAD) is a simple method of albumin dialysis, which uses standard CRRT machines. Albumin is added to the dialysis solution, and most of the clearance is provided as diffusive clearance. The albumin solution is discarded with the effluent after it passes through the filter. Sauer et al. showed SPAD to be superior to MARS in its ability to remove bilirubin in in vitro studies [20]. While many of the studies have used dialysate with ~5% albumin concentration, Chawla et al. did not show any clinically significant increase in bilirubin removal by using 5% albumin dialysate compared with 1.85% [21]. We too have effectively used 1.85% albumin solution while performing SPAD at our center. This albumin concentration is achieved by adding 400 mL of 25% albumin to a 5 L bag of dialysate. The use of the decreased concentration of albumin decreases cost without compromising efficacy. While once daily sessions of 6–12 h duration have been reported to attenuate hepatic intoxication, continuous SPAD may be performed to achieve higher clearance rates in children with severe hepatic failure, but at the expense of higher costs.

22.9 Total Plasma Exchange (TPE)

Patients with ALF frequently require blood products such as fresh frozen plasma (FFP) and cryoprecipitate to correct the various coagulopathies that are common in these patients. Infusion of these products adds to the risk of volume overload and provides an additional protein load that can worsen hepatic encephalopathy. In contrast, TPE treats the coagulopathy effectively, avoids an exogenous protein load, and has the added benefit of being fluid neutral. The high citrate load that accompanies the large volumes of FFP used for replacement can cause hypocalcemia and often prohibits this therapy as a stand-alone treatment in ALF, typically requiring the addition of dialytic therapy such as hemodialysis or CRRT.

22.10 Choice of Anticoagulation Therapy

Anticoagulation therapy is needed in about 40% of patients with ALF and should be administered if the activated clotting time (ACT) is below 160 s to maintain patency of the extracorporeal circuit. As ALF patients have reductions in both procoagulant and anticoagulant proteins, measurement of PT and INR is an unreliable measure of coagulopathy, and tests such as TEG® and ROTEM® are often needed to determine the underlying coagulation abnormalities (vide supra). As these patients can be deficient in antithrombin III (substrate upon which heparin acts), heparin can be ineffective in them. Heparin usage is further complicated because of the dynamic nature of the coagulation dysfunction seen in patients with ALF. While some centers [7] have reported successful usage of prostacyclin (an antiplatelet agent), widespread usage of this agent is uncommon.

Historically, most centers have avoided using regional citrate anticoagulation (RCA) in patients with ALF due to concerns for impaired citrate metabolism and fear of citrate accumulation. However, several recent publications have reported on the safety and efficacy of RCA in ALF patients [22] when the citrate infusion rate is decreased by ~33% from the normal recommended rate (see Chap. 10 for details on RCA). When citrate is used in this manner, the calcium infusion rate is kept similar to that used in the standard protocol as these patients receive an extra citrate load from the blood products they commonly receive. The occurrence of citrate accumulation (citrate lock) can be avoided by increasing the monitoring frequency for ionized calcium.

Key Points

1. ALF is a rapidly progressive disease that can lead to MODS.
2. AKI, which is seen in more than half of ALF cases, decreases the odds of spontaneous hepatic recovery while increasing the overall mortality risk.
3. The use of CRRT, even in the absence of AKI, can help improve the outcome of patients with ALF by optimizing fluid balance, correcting electrolyte abnormalities, and clearing ammonia and lactate.
4. Anticoagulation of the extracorporeal circuits as part of the treatment of ALF is usually required despite a prolonged PT and INR, as these tests do not accurately reflect the bleeding risk.
5. Hybrid extracorporeal therapies such as SPAD with TPE are more effective than any individual therapy.
6. Extracorporeal therapies to support patients with ALF should be started only if a curative therapy, i.e., usually liver transplantation, or significant recovery of liver function can be expected.

References

1. Squires RH Jr, Shneider BL, Bucuvalas J, et al. Acute liver failure in children: the first 348 patients in the pediatric acute liver failure study group. J Pediatr. 2006;148:652–8.
2. Bansal S, Dhawan A. Acute liver failure. Indian J Pediatr. 2006;73:931–4.
3. Lee WS, McKiernan P, Kelly DA. Etiology, outcome and prognostic indicators of childhood fulminant hepatic failure in the United Kingdom. J Pediatr Gastroenterol Nutr. 2005;40:575–81.
4. Stadbauer V, Jalan R. Acute liver failure: liver support therapies. Curr Opin Crit Care. 2007;13:215–21.
5. Phua J, Lee KH. Liver support devices. Curr Opin Crit Care. 2008;14:208–15.
6. Hoste EA, Dhondt A. Clinical review: use of renal replacement therapies in special groups of ICU patients. Crit Care. 2012;16:201.
7. Deep A, Stewart CE, Dhawan A, et al. Effect of continuous renal replacement therapy on outcome in pediatric acute liver failure. Crit Care Med. 2016;44:1910–9.

8. Arikan AA, Srivaths P, Himes RH, et al. Hybrid extracorporeal therapies as a bridge to pediatric liver transplantation. Pediatr Crit Care Med. 2018;19(7):e342–9.
9. Cochran JB, Losek JD. Acute liver failure in children. Pediatr Emerg Care. 2007;23(2):129–35.
10. Desjardins P, Du T, Jiang W, et al. Pathogenesis of hepatic encephalopathy and brain edema in acute liver failure: role of glutamine redefined. Neurochem Int. 2012;60:690–6.
11. Lee WM, Stravitz RT, Larson AM. Introduction to the revised American association for the study of liver diseases position paper on acute liver failure 2011. Hepatology. 2012;55:965–7.
12. Murphy N, Auzinger G, Bernal W, et al. The effect of hypertonic sodium chloride on intracranial pressure in patients with acute liver failure. Hepatology. 2002;39:464–70.
13. Mohan N, Ragunathan V, Dhaliwal M, et al. Prevalence of acute kidney injury network (AKIN) in pediatric non acetaminophen acute liver failure (pNA-ALF) & addition of AKIN staging to King's college criteria (Kcc) in pNAALF improves prognostic value. J Clin Exp Hepatol. 2013;3:S17.
14. Tujios SR, Hynan SL, Vazquez MA, et al. Risk factor and outcomes of acute kidney injury in patients with acute liver failure. Clin Gastroenterol Hepatol. 2015;13(2):352–9.
15. Symons JM, Chua AN, Somers MJ, et al. Demographic characteristics of pediatric continuous renal replacement therapy: a report of the prospective pediatric continuous renal replacement therapy registry. Clin J Am Soc Nephrol. 2007;2:732–8.
16. Squires RH Jr. Acute liver failure in children. Semin Liver Dis. 2008;28:153.
17. Davenport A, Will EJ, Davidson AM. Improved cardiovascular stability during continuous modes of renal replacement therapy in critically ill patients with acute hepatic and renal failure. Crit Care Med. 1993;21:328–38.
18. Davenport A, Will EJ, Davison AM. Early changes in intracranial pressure during hemofiltration treatment in patients with grade 4 hepatic encephalopathy and acute oliguric renal failure. Nephrol Dial Transplant. 1990;5(3):192–8.
19. Chevret L, Durand P, Lambert J, et al. High-volume hemofiltration in children with acute liver failure. Pediatr Crit Care Med. 2014;15:e300–5.
20. Sauer IM, Goetz M, Steffen I, et al. In vitro comparison of the molecular adsorbent recirculation system (MARS) and single-pass albumin dialysis (SPAD). Hepatology. 2004;39:1408–14.
21. Chawla LS, Georgescu F, Abell B, et al. Modification of continuous venovenous hemodiafiltration with single-pass albumin dialysate allows for removal of serum bilirubin. Am J Kidney Dis. 2005;3:e51–6.
22. Rodriguez K, Srivaths PR, Tal L, et al. Regional citrate anticoagulation for continuous renal replacement therapy in pediatric patients with liver failure. PLoS One. 2017;12:e0182134.

Advances in Liver Failure and Management

23

Moreshwar Desai and Ayse Akcan-Arikan

23.1 Introduction

Liver failures in children, whether acute (ALF) or acute-on-chronic (ACLF), are devastating clinical conditions, which despite current advancements in science and technology have a transplant-free survival of only 55–60%. The current consensus definitions of ALF and ACLF are depicted in Table 23.1 [1–5].

Both ALF and ACLF pose significant challenges to bedside care providers, as hepatocyte destruction leads to rapid release of toxins and inflammatory mediators. Multiple known and unknown water-soluble and protein-soluble toxins, along with circulating mediators, induce extrahepatic organ failure, in the form of hepatic encephalopathy, hepatic cardiomyopathy, hepato-pulmonary syndrome, and acute kidney injury (AKI) which includes hepatorenal syndrome [6]. This chapter will focus primarily on pathophysiology of AKI in liver failure and discuss the available modalities to support the kidneys until successful liver transplantation or recovery.

M. Desai
Department of Pediatrics, Section of Pediatric Critical Care,
Baylor College of Medicine, Texas Children's Hospital, Houston, TX, USA

Liver Intensive Care Unit, Texas Children's Hospital, Houston, TX, USA
e-mail: mdesai@bcm.edu

A. Akcan-Arikan (✉)
Department of Pediatrics, Sections of Critical Care and Nephrology,
Baylor College of Medicine, Texas Children's Hospital, Houston, TX, USA

Extracorporeal Liver Support, Texas Children's Hospital, Houston, TX, USA

Critical Care Nephrology, Texas Children's Hospital, Houston, TX, USA
e-mail: aysea@bcm.edu

S. K. Sethi et al. (eds.), *Critical Care Pediatric Nephrology and Dialysis: A Practical Handbook*, https://doi.org/10.1007/978-981-13-2276-1_23

Table 23.1 Consensus definitions of acute liver failure (ALF) and acute-on-chronic liver failure (ACLF)

ALF	
Consensus from the Pediatric Acute Liver Failure Study Group	Coagulopathy with INR ≥1.5 with encephalopathy not correctable by intravenous vitamin K, with biochemical evidence of acute liver injury INR ≥2 without encephalopathy not correctable by intravenous vitamin K, with biochemical evidence of acute liver injury In a child with no evidence of chronic liver disease
ACLF	
Consensus from the American Association for the Study of Liver Diseases, European Association for the Study of Liver Diseases and Asian Pacific Association of the Study of Liver Diseases	Acute deterioration of a pre-existing, chronic liver disease, usually related to a precipitating event and associated with increased mortality at 3 months due to multi-system organ failure if not transplanted Acute hepatic insult manifesting as jaundice and coagulopathy, complicated within 4 weeks by ascites and/or encephalopathy in a patient with previously diagnosed or undiagnosed chronic liver disease

23.2 Renal Involvement in Liver Failure

The causes of AKI in liver failure can be further classified into (a) functional (prerenal) causes, (b) intrinsic causes including acute tubular necrosis, and (c) hepatorenal syndrome—an independent disease entity [7–10]. Additionally, bile cast nephropathy might be observed in patients with long-standing cholestasis and severe hyperbilirubinemia.

23.2.1 Functional (Prerenal) Causes

Children with cirrhosis have reduced central blood volume at baseline due to splanchnic vasodilatation and frequent diuretic treatment used for accompanying ascites. Gastrointestinal bleeds, sepsis, infections, vomiting, diarrhea, excessive use of diuretics, excessive use of laxatives like lactulose, and inappropriate fluid management during large-volume paracentesis can further compromise the intravascular volume status and cause hypotension and functional AKI. Additionally, accumulation of ascites in advanced liver failure, especially diuretic-resistant ascites, could lead to increased intra-abdominal pressure and abdominal compartment physiology, compounding the prerenal azotemia.

23.2.2 Intrinsic (Renal) Causes

Tubular, glomerular, and interstitial injury can occur from use of broad-spectrum antibiotics like vancomycin, aminoglycosides, diuretics, contrast agents, and anesthetics or coexisting infections like urinary tract infections, central line infections, or peritonitis. Septic AKI, largely inflammatory in nature, can be seen in the case of cholangitis or peritonitis. Bile cast nephropathy is likely underreported in children.

23.2.3 Hepatorenal Syndrome (HRS)

This unique form of functional failure is a direct consequence and a complication of a failing liver which results in severely decreased GFR that is unresponsive to volume expansion or diuretics, with minimal histologic injury to renal parenchyma, induced as a direct result of vascular changes in a patient with advanced liver failure and cirrhosis, in the absence of shock or nephrotoxic drugs, and above all only reversible with resolution of liver dysfunction (liver transplantation).

Though well characterized in adults, HRS is not widely studied in children. In adults, HRS is subdivided into two types, Type-1 and Type-2. Type-1 HRS (acute decline in renal function in a patient with liver failure) is the most common form of HRS, where serum creatinine doubles in <2 weeks and is rapidly fatal unless treated. In Type-2 HRS (chronic decline in renal function in a patient with liver failure), the deterioration is gradual, is associated with refractory ascites, and has a median survival of ~6 months without transplantation [11].

23.2.4 Conditions that Involve Simultaneous Liver and Kidney Dysfunction

These are rare genetic and metabolic conditions that are more common in pediatrics and often require a combined liver-kidney transplantation. They include primary hyperoxaluria Type-1, methylmalonic acidemia, autosomal recessive polycystic kidney disease (genetic cause of dual organ failure), and miscellaneous ciliopathies. Children with these conditions often require a combined liver-kidney transplantation [7].

23.3 Epidemiology

Most data on prevalence of AKI in liver failure comes from adults. The overall incidence of AKI in adults with liver failure is as high as 70%, with ~30% requiring dialysis and more specifically continuous renal replacement therapy (CRRT). The incidence varies with etiology of the liver dysfunction. The incidence of AKI, as well as need for CRRT, is higher in acetaminophen toxicity compared with other etiologies. AKI has an estimated prevalence of approximately 20–50% among hospitalized patients with liver failure. The total incidence of HRS is reported at 8–12%, and probability of diagnosing HRS in patients with cirrhosis and ascites at 1 and 5 years is reported to be 18 and 39%, respectively. Overall, AKI is likely much more common than actually reported in both adults and pediatrics due to falsely low serum creatinine levels in patients with advanced liver disease secondary to decreased synthesis of creatinine in the liver and loss of muscle mass due to chronic malnutrition [9, 12, 13].

23.4 Pathophysiology of Renal Dysfunction and Hepatorenal Syndrome in Liver Failure

In acute liver failure, sudden accumulation of toxic metabolites, cytokines, toxins released from dying hepatocytes, systemic infections/ingested poisons, can cause AKI directly or indirectly as a part of multi-system organ failure.

Renal dysfunction in chronic advanced cirrhosis and portal hypertension is far more nuanced. A cirrhotic patient has total body fluid overload with significant ascites but has a decreased effective arterial blood volume and intravascular fluid status. Advanced cirrhosis and portal hypertension lead to profound abnormalities in systemic and splanchnic circulatory physiology with systemic and splanchnic vasodilation as a result of mediators such as nitric oxide, carbon monoxide, bile acids, and other circulating vasodilator peptides. Compensation for arterial underfilling via the renin-angiotensin-aldosterone axis (RAAS), sympathetic nervous system, and arginine vasopressin leads to water retention, hyponatremia, and severe vasoconstriction of the renal vasculature, thereby leading to HRS. Abnormalities in vascular tone and splanchnic pooling are further compounded by bacterial translocation from the gut and release of pro-inflammatory cytokines such as TNFα and IL-6 in the circulation. Cirrhotic cardiomyopathy, now a well-recognized distinct comorbid consequence of end-stage cirrhosis in both adults and children, further impairs the splanchnic and renal blood flow and reduces renal perfusion ("cardiorenal link") [14, 15]. Patients with ascites and portal hypertension are at higher risk of development of subacute bacterial peritonitis. All of the abnormalities cumulatively lead to HRS. Additional tertiary insults, often iatrogenic, such as large-volume paracentesis-associated fluid shifts, aggressive use of diuretics, use of aminoglycosides, and some non-iatrogenic events like hemorrhagic shock and systemic bacteremia can lead to further damage of the kidneys leading to renal failure [16] (Fig. 23.1).

23.5 Diagnosing Renal Failure in Liver Disease

Determining whether a child/adult with liver failure has renal dysfunction is a challenge to bedside clinicians. The traditionally used lab tests are often misleading in liver failure. Inability of the liver to produce proteins, low albumin level-related fluid overload, presence of ascites secondary to portal hypertension, and lack of muscle mass because of malnutrition make interpretation of urea, creatinine, and urine output difficult. Under- and missed diagnosis of mild renal impairment is of particular concern. This was addressed in 2015 by the International Ascites Club (IAC) and the Acute Dialysis Quality Initiative (ADQI) who redefined AKI in adult cirrhotic patients; the definition is now easy to follow, accommodates the realities and confounders inherent to advanced stages of liver disease, and tries to include HRS and non-HRS-mediated renal dysfunction (see Table 23.2) [10]. Serial measurements of serum cystatin C, a protein produced constantly by all nucleated cells, and not altered by confounders such as age, muscle mass, degree of cholestasis, or use of diuretics or dialysis (intermittent or continuous), is being increasingly used to aid in the diagnosis of renal dysfunction and prognostication in this patient

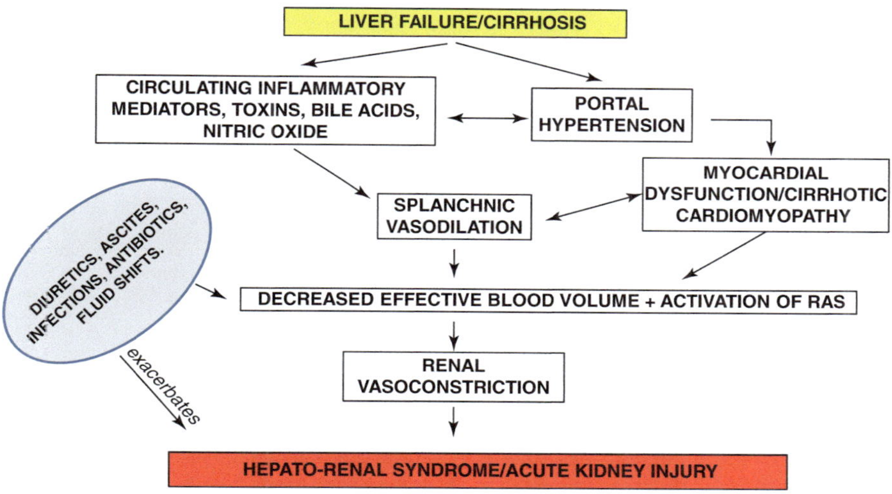

Fig. 23.1 Pathophysiology of AKI/HRS in liver failure

Table 23.2 New diagnostic criteria for AKI and HRS

	Diagnostic criteria
Stages of AKI	
Stage 1	↑ in SCr ≥0.3 mg/dL (or 26.5 μmol/L) ≤48 h ↑ in SCr ≥1.5–2× from baseline ≤48 h
Stage 2	↑ in SCr ≥2–3× from baseline
Stage 3	↑ in SCr >3× from baseline or need for CRRT
Types of HRS	
Type-1	All criteria for stage 2 AKI+ 1. No response (in serum creatinine) after 2 consecutive days of withdrawal from diuretics and 1 g/kg albumin infusion 2. Absence of shock or use of nephrotoxic agents 3. No evidence of macroscopic/structural kidney injury
Type-2	Chronic increase in SCr+ 1. Refractory ascites 2. Death within 6 months without transplant

population. Other novel biomarkers such as neutrophil gelatinase-associated lipocalin (NGAL), interleukin 18 (IL-18), kidney injury marker-1 (KIM-1), and liver-associated fatty acid-binding protein (L-FABP) are still being studied [17].

23.6 Treatment of AKI Associated with Liver Failure

23.6.1 Early Recognition and Prevention

Early identification and rapid correction of precipitating factors are keys to successful management of AKI. Prompt attention should be given toward maintaining intravascular volume status of the patient. Intravascular depletion in a child with liver failure is often missed because of their overall edematous appearance and falsely lower BUN and creatinine. Random and aggressive diuresis should be avoided, as it can rapidly precipitate further kidney injury and HRS. Excessive gastrointestinal losses secondary to use of lactulose should be prevented with appropriate fluid replacement. Nephrotoxic antibiotics, NSAIDs, and use of contrast in radiologic procedures should be avoided as much as possible. Infections should be identified and treated aggressively using appropriate antibiotics, with a careful monitoring of pharmacodynamics and drug levels.

23.6.2 Pharmacologic Options

Cirrhosis and portal hypertension cause ascites. Excessive accumulation of ascetic fluid increases intra-abdominal pressures, which leads to compromised renal blood flow. Use of aldosterone antagonists such as spironolactone has been shown to be effective in management of mild to moderate ascites. Albumin serves as a very effective plasma volume expander in children with liver failure by increasing the plasma oncotic pressure and serving to pull extravascular fluid into the intravascular space and improve renal perfusion, urine output, and ascites; it should be the replacement solution of choice after large-volume abdominal paracentesis. Albumin also may act as an antioxidant, an anti-inflammatory, and an immune-modulator agent. Vasoconstrictors like vasopressin, terlipressin, ornipressin, midodrine, octreotide, and norepinephrine are often used along with plasma expansion to reverse splanchnic vasodilation, reverse HRS, and improve renal perfusion and urine output. In fact, typical treatment of HRS involves withdrawal of diuretic, plasma expansion with albumin in conjunction with vasoconstrictors, and careful reintroduction of diuretics.

23.6.3 Abdominal Paracentesis and Shunts

Abdominal paracentesis is indicated in patients with ascites refractory to diuretics, vasoconstrictors, and volume expansion to relieve intra-abdominal pressure, which in turn improves renal perfusion and alleviates respiratory compromise caused by elevations of diaphragm and low lung volumes. Paracentesis has to be done judiciously to avoid massive fluid shifts and intravascular depletion with prompt replacement with albumin. Trans-jugular intrahepatic portosystemic shunts (TIPSs) are also effective in severe cirrhosis and refractory ascites to maintain renal hemodynamics and rapid progression into HRS. These procedures, though common in adults, are infrequent in children. These shunts increase the risk for hepatic encephalopathy due to increase in blood levels of ammonia and other gut-derived toxic mediators shunted to systemic circulation.

23.6.4 Renal Replacement Therapy

In advanced stages of AKI, renal replacement therapies are instituted in the form of continuous renal replacement therapy (CRRT). In addition to providing renal support in AKI, CRRT potentially assists in detoxification by removing water-bound toxins; allows safe administration of nutrition, blood products, and plasma; and corrects electrolyte and acid-base imbalances. Conventional dialysis effectively removes water-soluble substances of small molecular weight such as urea, creatinine, and ammonia through diffusion. Addition of convective clearance with hemodiafiltration enhances middle-molecule clearance. However, highly protein-bound substances cannot be removed effectively even with hemodiafiltration, and CRRT often has to be combined with other extracorporeal clearance systems, such as tandem use of total plasma exchange (for coagulopathy) [18, 19] and albumin dialysis (for encephalopathy) [12, 20–22].

23.7 Indications for CRRT in Liver Failure

CRRT is indicated in critically ill children with liver failure for standard indications such as electrolyte imbalance (hyperkalemia and hyperphosphatemia), fluid overloaded state with respiratory or cardiac compromise, inability to administer nutrition and blood products secondary to fluid overload or relative oliguria, symptomatic uremia, intractable metabolic acidosis, and lactic acidosis.

Ammonia, a weak base derived from protein metabolism, is central to the pathogenesis of hepatic encephalopathy, cerebral edema, and intracranial hypertension. Ammonia is extremely toxic to the host and needs to be detoxified and eliminated. Most of the ammonia is generated in the intestines by the breakdown of proteins by the intestinal bacteria and brought into the liver via the portal circulation and detoxified into urea in hepatocytes and eliminated through urine. Ammonia is also cleared through conversion to glutamine in the brain, the skeletal muscles, and the liver. Glutamine is then taken up by the kidneys, split into glutamate and ammonia by glutaminase, and subsequently excreted in urine. Ammonia production from glutamine and excretion in urine predominantly occurs in the proximal tubule and is regulated by acid-base status, potassium levels, mineralocorticoids, glucocorticoids, and the overall health of the kidneys.

Ammonia rises to toxic levels when the hepatocytes are unable to convert intestinally derived ammonia into urea (in hepatocyte destruction) or to metabolically detoxify ammonia to urea (in inborn errors of metabolism—like propionic acidemia, methylmalonic acidemia, or urea cycle defects). Ammonia also rises when it bypasses the liver and spills into the circulation (seen in portosystemic shunts—either surgical or endogenous secondary to collaterals from severe portal hypertension). When rate of generation of ammonia is higher than the capacity of the hepatocytes to detoxify it to urea, peripheral conversion of ammonia to glutamine that occurs in the brain and skeletal muscles takes predominance. In malnourished children with cirrhosis and inborn errors of metabolism, when muscle mass is insufficient, the brain and especially the astrocytes bear the brunt of peripheral metabolism of ammonia which then leads to hepatic encephalopathy and increased intracranial pressures—the most feared and fatal complication of liver failure irrespective of etiology.

Hepatic encephalopathy is a spectrum of neuropsychiatric disturbances, which can range from mere confusion, incoherence, and irritability to stupor and coma. Hepatic encephalopathy is an amalgamation of multiple processes that occur within the brain cells that lead to inflammatory, oxidative, and osmotic injuries that are rapid and fatal. In the presence of hyperammonemia, extracellular glutamate activates the N-methyl-D-aspartate (NMDA) receptors. Hyperammonemia also causes increases in tryptophan and its by-products, which stimulate the NMDA receptors. This triggers alterations in nitric oxide metabolism; depletion of ATP; influx of sodium, potassium, and calcium; and accumulation of reactive oxygen species which leads to a cascade of inflammatory of events, which culminate into cell swelling and death. Unlike ammonia, glutamine, the precursor of glutamate, is osmotically active. Accumulation of glutamine leads to increased intracellular osmolarity and draws extracellular water leading to astrocyte swelling and destruction of the blood-brain barrier, influx of toxic mediators, and increased intracranial pressures. Ongoing infections, systemic inflammatory response, and sepsis potentiate the effects of hyperammonemia and exacerbate HE. Pro-inflammatory cytokines, such as IL-1β, IL-6, and TNFα, correlated to the severity of brain edema, injury, and encephalopathy. Circulating and locally produced pro-inflammatory cytokines disrupt the brain microvascular endothelial cells, alter the blood-brain barrier, and induce vasogenic edema. Hyponatremia, a frequent occurrence in end-stage liver disease, thought to be dilutional and secondary to diuretic use, also exacerbates HE. Sodium is a key determinant of serum osmolarity. Low sodium levels decrease the osmotic pressure resulting in astrocyte edema, intracranial hypertension, and worsening of HE [20, 23, 24].

Peak levels, rapidity of rise, as well as persistence and duration of hyperammonemia correlate with development of cerebral edema (CE) and intracranial hypertension (ICH) and have to be avoided at all costs. There is no consensus on what level of ammonia is dangerous. Coexisting inflammation, electrolyte (sodium) imbalance, acid-base status, hemodynamic status, vasopressor use, and presence/absence of extrahepatic organ failure determine the degree and rapidity with which an elevated ammonia level will induce brain injury. A level >100 μmol/L predicts the onset of severe HE with 70% accuracy, while ammonia levels >200 μmol/L are associated with development of cerebral edema and intracranial hypertension [25]. Individuals who have persistence of hyperammonemia are more likely to progress to advanced HE and have higher incidence of renal failure and infections. Persistently elevated ammonia over 3 days of hospital stay is associated with complications and death in patients with ALF [20, 23, 24].

The main goals of management are (1) urgent reduction in ammonia levels, (2) avoiding rapid swings in the levels, and (3) keeping circulating levels where they are least likely to cause cellular damage while awaiting recovery or transplant. Additionally, factors that potentiate encephalopathy and brain injury such as electrolyte and acid-base imbalance have to be avoided at all costs. CRRT thus forms an essential pillar of the support system that is needed to stabilize and manage a critically ill child or adult who has hepatic encephalopathy, hyperammonemia, cardiovascular instability, and significant coagulopathy needing large amounts of plasma and blood products [26]. These indications are over and above the routine indications for AKI in liver failure. In the intensive care unit, CCRT is preferred over peritoneal dialysis (PD) or intermittent hemodialysis (HD). The advantages of CRRT over PD and HD are detailed in Table 23.3.

Deployment of CRRT specifically for acute liver failure can be further modified by adjusting the "dose" of CRRT (based on effluent flow rate [ultrafiltrate + dialysate]) depending on the severity of hyperammonemia and encephalopathy. Typical CRRT dose is 25–35 mL/kg/h but can be augmented to filtration volume rates as 80–90 mL/kg/h, called high-volume hemodiafiltration (HVHDF). Though there are no conclusive randomized trials, a 2014 single-center French study suggested a beneficial effect of HVHDF over conventional dose CRRT on hemodynamics, renal function, degree of encephalopathy, and survival to transplant within 48 h [27]. Though extrapolation of this data to the USA is difficult due to longer wait times for pediatric liver organs, hemodynamic and neurologic benefits may be postulated to result from high-dose CRRT-removing cytokines such as TNFalpha and IL-1beta, which often exacerbate circulatory failure and HE. Electrolyte imbalance, more specifically hyponatremia, hypokalemia, and hypophosphatemia, should be actively monitored and corrected in HVHDF.

Table 23.3 Benefits of CRRT over HD and PD in ALF and ACLF

Advantages of CRRT over PD or HD
1. Fewer treatment interruptions
2. Steady continuous clearance in face of continuous production of ammonia, which prevents rebound spikes which are often deleterious to the brain
3. Less fluid shift and steady hemodynamics
4. Maintaining sodium, pH, acid-base, and electrolyte balance
5. Better control of body temperature as hyperthermia is to be avoided at all costs, and controlled hypothermia is desired
6. Not dependent on splanchnic perfusion like PD

23.7.1 Intraoperative CRRT

In liver transplantation, intraoperative CRRT is indicated to better control metabolic acidosis during anhepatic phase and hyperkalemia during the reperfusion phase, for management of large-volume fluid shifts, and if massive blood loss and blood transfusions are anticipated (redo surgeries) in children with pre-existing severe AKI already on CRRT preoperatively. In our institution, we have used intraoperative CRRT in two children of over ~250 liver transplants since 2010. Both of them were on hybrid extracorporeal therapies prior to liver transplantation. Neither recovered renal function posttransplant and remained hemodialysis-dependent.

23.7.2 Postoperative Indications for CRRT

AKI, fluid overload, electrolyte abnormalities, and acid-base imbalance are the common indications why CRRT may be used in the postoperative period. In adults, the incidence of AKI is ~40% to as high as 70% of patients with 15% needing CRRT. In adults, patients with hepatic encephalopathy, HRS, deceased donor liver donations, high MELD, intraoperative blood loss, perioperative hypovolemia, and hepatocellular carcinoma as an indication for transplant increase the odds for needing postoperative CRRT [28]. No such data exists in children, but in our experience, AKI needing CRRT prior to transplantation, intraoperative blood loss and need for massive transfusions, early ischemic liver insult, acute graft dysfunction, acute graft failure, persistence of ascites and increased intra-abdominal pressure, and hemodynamic instability needing inotropic support are all observed risk factors for post-transplant CRRT.

23.7.3 Role of Dialysis in Metabolic Liver Failure

Inborn errors of metabolism, which cause hyperammonemia, are broadly categorized into two subgroups, the urea cycle disorders and organic acidemias. Initial therapy focuses on controlling the rise of blood ammonia levels, by minimizing nitrogen/protein intake, decreasing endogenous protein breakdown by early recognition and treatment of infection, preventing dehydration and hypermetabolic states, and promptly replacing deficient enzymes. Nitrogen scavengers like sodium benzoate and arginine are administered to patients with urea cycle defects to provide alternative pathways for ammonia excretion. Carnitine, hydroxycobalamin, biotin, and a combination of intravenous phenylacetate and benzoate can be used prior to hemodialysis. If ammonia continues to rise despite the pharmacological therapies, dialysis should not be delayed or withheld despite the fact that these metabolic cocktails may be dialyzed along with the ammonia [29, 30].

Ammonia is water-soluble, and its clearance is dependent on blood flow rate (Q_b) and dialyzer membrane surface area (mL/min). The highest rate of reduction of blood ammonia levels can be achieved by intermittent hemodialysis, when compared to peritoneal dialysis or even CRRT. Hence, if the goal is only to rapidly reduce ammonia and restart the pharmacotherapies, intermittent HD could be used in select cases of metabolic liver failure. The level of serum ammonia when dialysis can be considered as a therapy may vary with degree of encephalopathy and hemodynamics of the child. Higher ammonias are typically tolerated in patients with metabolic liver failure as opposed to other forms of liver failure because these children may not have other comorbidities such as electrolyte imbalance, inflammation, cytokine surges, or other circulating inflammatory mediators. In our institution ammonia of 400 is used as a trigger to initiate dialysis as opposed to 150 in other forms of liver failure. The current standard of care in a critically ill neonate, infant, or child who presents with hyperammonemia secondary to metabolic liver failure entails rapid correction of dehydration and establishing euvolemia, treating underlying infection if any, preventing further catabolism and ammonia production, use of nitrogen scavengers, and high-volume CRRT [29, 30].

23.7.4 Emerging Uses for Combination Therapy

CRRT also allows for the safe implementation of extracorporeal support in the form of albumin-assisted blood purification system and therapeutic plasma exchange, all of which are often needed in managing these children as a bridge to recovery or transplant. A failing liver is unable to detoxify ammonia. Along with ammonia, it also fails to clear many known toxins such as bile acids, aromatic amino acids, GABA substances, tryptophans, vasoactive and vasodilatory mediators, and many unknown protein-bound substances that exacerbate encephalopathy and cardiovascular instability. Extracorporeal support in liver failure has been a topic of interest for decades. Published literature however is sparse, and randomized trials comparing the various modalities are nonexistent in pediatrics. Though there is debate over what the best mode of extracorporeal system to support the liver is, there is no controversy over the need for blood detoxification. Highly protein-bound substances need albumin-based dialysis systems or plasma filtration/adsorption where the colloid rich plasma is separated from the cellular elements of the blood and either replaced with fresh plasma or "cleansed" via adsorption/hemoperfusion.

Many albumin-based systems have been used over past three decades. These are:

(a) Single-pass albumin dialysis (SPAD) where albumin is added to the dialysate to enhance removal of protein-bound substances. Single pass refers to the fact that albumin containing spent dialysate is discarded after it flows countercurrent to the blood and is not reused.
(b) Molecular adsorbent recirculating system (MARS), where blood is dialyzed across a high flux membrane. MARS combines traditional continuous renal replacement therapy (CRRT) technology with protein-bound substance removal via albumin dialysis. It removes ammonia, bilirubin, bile acids, aromatic amino acids, nitric oxide, tryptophan, and other unknown and unmeasured

protein-bound substances along with ammonia, creatinine, and urea. The albumin dialysate is regenerated online by passage through a second dialyzer and two adsorbable columns containing charcoal and anion exchanger.

(c) The Prometheus system, where plasma filtration treatment is coupled with adsorption and hemodialysis. CRRT can also be combined with TPE, a nonselective form of blood purification, where patient's plasma is replaced by fresh banked plasma [31–37].

In our institution, hybrid extracorporeal therapy (HET) is used in children with acute liver failure or acute-on-chronic liver failure, as a bridge to transplant or recovery. HET includes MARS (8 h/day for 3–5 days) + total plasma exchange + continuous CRRT. Indications for HET are (1) Grade 3 or 4 hepatic encephalopathy—irrespective of ammonia levels—(2) ammonia of 150 μmol/L and climbing despite conventional medical therapy, (3) malignant coagulopathy (need for more than 30 cc/kg/day of plasma products), (4) clinical bleeding irrespective of INR levels, and (5) vasodilatory shock needing vasopressors in a child with hyperbilirubinemia [38]. These indications, though distinct, often coexist together. HET is resource intensive but has been proven safe and beneficial in our hands [38]. Protocols for CRRT and HET at TCH are listed in Tables 23.4 and 23.5.

Table 23.4 Protocol for HET at TCH

Therapy	Indications	Dose	Duration	Monitoring
CRRT (in CVVHDF mode)	Hyperammonemia[a] Oliguric AKI Fluid overload	3000 mL/1.73 m2/h	Continuous	Keep total Ca/iCal <10 (mg/dL)
TPE (centrifugal)	Medically refractory coagulopathy[b] Clinical life-threatening bleeding	1.3–1.5× plasma volume exchange volume with all FFP replacement	As indicated	Q 15 min calcium monitoring, increased rate of calcium infusion
MARS (in series with CVVHDF and ± TPE)	HE grade 3 or higher HE grade 2 +MODS[c]	3000 mL/1.73 m2/h	ACLF: minimum 8 h session, at least 5 consecutive days, and then as needed ALF: daily minimum 8 h treatments until recovery/transplant	Keep platelets >50,000; fibrinogen >150

[a]>75 mmol/L or rapidly rising while on maximum medical therapy
[b]>30 mL/kg of fresh frozen plasma in 24 h
[c]Two or more failing organ systems

Table 23.5 CRRT in ALF/ACLF at TCH

Weight	<5 kg	5–15 kg	15–30 kg	>30 kg
Catheter size	7–8 Fr	8–10 Fr	11–12 F	12–13 F
Anticoagulation	RCA	RCA	RCA	RCA
Blood flow rate	3–10 mL/kg/min			
Clearance/dose	2000–8000 mL/1.73 m²/h depending of the degree of hyperammonemia. Dose titrated to keep ammonia levels below 100 μmol/L			

23.8 Anticoagulants Used During CRRT

In patients with ALF, there is a deficiency of both pro- and anticoagulant factors, balancing the coagulation profile [39]. Hence despite high INR, children with ALF do not have a higher propensity for bleeding. In acute-on-chronic liver failure, on the other hand, coexisting thrombocytopenia and impaired platelet function secondary to portal hypertension and hypersplenism may put a child at higher risk for bleeding. In addition, infection and inflammation related to disseminated intravascular coagulation if present further add to the dysregulated homeostasis. Keeping a CRRT circuit and filter from clotting is a challenge in patients with liver failure, and some form of anticoagulation is essential for optimizing filter and circuit life in these situations [40]. The common options for anticoagulation are systemic heparin, regional citrate, or antiplatelet agent prostacyclin [41–43]. For over a decade, our institution (Table 23.5) has used regional citrate anticoagulation (RCA) regardless of the etiology or severity of liver failure or the coagulation status [44]. Citrate induces anticoagulation by chelating ionized calcium, a cofactor for multiple steps in the coagulation cascade. Citrate is more advantageous to heparin especially in LF, as it avoids the need for systemic anticoagulation, lengthens filter life, and has fewer incidences of bleeding and clotting compared to heparin. A residual amount of citrate spills over into the circulation and leads to citrate toxicity, especially since citrate metabolism is impaired in liver dysfunction. Accumulation of systemic citrate chelates ionized calcium in vivo and induces metabolic acidosis and may compromise the hemodynamics. The RCA protocol is modified in LF patients to lower citrate flow rates and higher circuit calcium (up to 0.6) with 30–50% higher clearance dose that is adjusted for concerns of citrate accumulation. Citrate accumulation is closely monitored by keeping total calcium/ionized calcium ratio <2.5 (in mmol/L) or <10 (in mg/dL) [41, 42, 44].

23.9 Complications of CRRT

As with any mode of extracorporeal support, the complications vary with age, weight, hemodynamic status, and other coexisting comorbidities [45]. Complications can be subdivided into:

(a) *Complications associated with the catheter and its placement*: Risk of bleeding, infections, thrombosis, and injury to the major vessel during catheter placements.
(b) *Complications associated with the CRRT run*: Systemic citrate accumulation causes citrate toxicity and results in low ionized calcium, high-serum total calcium, and metabolic acidosis and symptomatic hypocalcemia, hypotension, shock, and cardiac arrest. Other complications include hypothermia, air embolism, consumptive coagulopathy, electrolyte imbalance, and hypovolemia.

23.10 Long-Term Outcomes in Patients on CRRT in the Perioperative Period

Literature regarding the survival benefits of CRRT in patients with liver failure is sparse. In both adults and children, need for CRRT in the perioperative period negatively impacts outcomes. In adults, in a meta-analysis that included 464 patients with end-stage liver disease with renal failure who received either pre- or posttransplantation CRRT, Thorat et al. found that 1- and 3-year survival of patients with pre-LT CRRT were comparable with those of liver transplant recipients without renal failure; however, patients who needed hemodialysis post-liver transplant for prolonged periods showed poor 3-year survival of under 40% [46]. In a single-center study in pediatrics, conducted by Deep et al., authors found that of all the children admitted to their ICU with acute liver failure, ~33% received continuous renal replacement therapy prior to transplantation or recovery. Of those who needed CRRT, 58% survived to either transplant or spontaneous recovery. They further showed that early recognition of AKI and prompt initiation of high-dose CRRT led to increased survival, with maximal effect visible within first 2 weeks of initiation. The ability to reduce hyperammonemia within 48 h increased the likelihood for survival to transplant/spontaneous recovery [20].

23.11 Conclusions

Continuous renal replacement therapy can be used successfully in critically ill children with pediatric acute liver failure, acute-on-chronic liver failure, and children with metabolic liver failure either while awaiting a liver transplant or while awaiting spontaneous recovery. Overall, despite the higher morbidity and mortality in children with liver failure who develop AKI, it is universally advisable to diagnose AKI and start CRRT alone or as a hybrid extracorporeal therapy early, as risk of mortality is unacceptably higher without any intervention.

References

1. Arroyo V, Jalan R. Acute-on-chronic liver failure: definition, diagnosis, and clinical characteristics. Semin Liver Dis. 2016;36(2):109–16.
2. Sarin SK, Choudhury A. Acute-on-chronic liver failure: terminology, mechanisms and management. Nat Rev Gastroenterol Hepatol. 2016;13(3):131–49.
3. Squires RH. End-stage liver disease in children. Curr Treat Options Gastroenterol. 2001;4(5):409–21.
4. Squires RH Jr, Shneider BL, Bucuvalas J, Alonso E, Sokol RJ, Narkewicz MR, et al. Acute liver failure in children: the first 348 patients in the pediatric acute liver failure study group. J Pediatr. 2006;148(5):652–8.
5. Miloh T, Desai MS. Chapter 419: acute liver failure. In: Rudolph's pediatrics. 23rd ed. New York: McGraw Hill; 2018.
6. Bernal W, Wendon J. Acute liver failure. N Engl J Med. 2013;369(26):2525–34.
7. Bacchetta J, Mekahli D, Rivet C, Demede D, Leclerc AL. Pediatric combined liver-kidney transplantation: a 2015 update. Curr Opin Organ Transplant. 2015;20(5):543–9.
8. Cheng XS, Tan JC, Kim WR. Management of renal failure in end-stage liver disease: a critical appraisal. Liver Transpl. 2016;22(12):1710–9.
9. Maiwall R, Sarin SK, Moreau R. Acute kidney injury in acute on chronic liver failure. Hepatol Int. 2016;10(2):245–57.
10. Wong F. Acute kidney injury in liver cirrhosis: new definition and application. Clin Mol Hepatol. 2016;22(4):415–22.
11. Bucsics T, Krones E. Renal dysfunction in cirrhosis: acute kidney injury and the hepatorenal syndrome. Gastroenterol Rep (Oxf). 2017;5(2):127–37.
12. Davenport A. Continuous renal replacement therapy for liver disease. Hemodial Int. 2003;7(4):348–52.
13. Deep A, Saxena R, Jose B. Acute kidney injury in children with chronic liver disease. Pediatr Nephrol. 2018. https://doi.org/10.1007/s00467-018-3893-7.
14. Krag A, Bendtsen F, Henriksen JH, Moller S. Low cardiac output predicts development of hepatorenal syndrome and survival in patients with cirrhosis and ascites. Gut. 2010;59(1):105–10.
15. Krag A, Bendtsen F, Burroughs AK, Moller S. The cardiorenal link in advanced cirrhosis. Med Hypotheses. 2012;79(1):53–5.
16. Durand F, Graupera I, Gines P, Olson JC, Nadim MK. Pathogenesis of hepatorenal syndrome: implications for therapy. Am J Kidney Dis. 2016;67(2):318–28.
17. Francoz C, Nadim MK, Durand F. Kidney biomarkers in cirrhosis. J Hepatol. 2016;65(4):809–24.
18. Schaefer B, Ujszaszi A, Schaefer S, Heckert KH, Schaefer F, Schmitt CP. Safety and efficacy of tandem hemodialysis and plasma exchange in children. Clin J Am Soc Nephrol. 2014;9(9):1563–70.
19. Singer AL, Olthoff KM, Kim H, Rand E, Zamir G, Shaked A. Role of plasmapheresis in the management of acute hepatic failure in children. Ann Surg. 2001;234(3):418–24.
20. Deep A, Stewart CE, Dhawan A, Douiri A. Effect of continuous renal replacement therapy on outcome in pediatric acute liver failure. Crit Care Med. 2016;44(10):1910–9.
21. Durand F, Olson JC, Nadim MK. Renal dysfunction and cirrhosis. Curr Opin Crit Care. 2017;23(6):457–62.
22. Karvellas CJ, Durand F, Nadim MK. Acute kidney injury in cirrhosis. Crit Care Clin. 2015;31(4):737–50.
23. Hadjihambi A, Arias N, Sheikh M, Jalan R. Hepatic encephalopathy: a critical current review. Hepatol Int. 2018;12(Suppl 1):135–47.

24. Romero-Gomez M, Montagnese S, Jalan R. Hepatic encephalopathy in patients with acute decompensation of cirrhosis and acute-on-chronic liver failure. J Hepatol. 2015;62(2):437–47.
25. Polson J, Lee WM. AASLD position paper: the management of acute liver failure. Hepatology. 2005;41(5):1179–97.
26. Cardoso FS, Gottfried M, Tujios S, Olson JC, Karvellas CJ. Continuous renal replacement therapy is associated with reduced serum ammonia levels and mortality in acute liver failure. Hepatology. 2017;67(2):711–20.
27. Chevret L, Durand P, Lambert J, Essouri S, Balu L, Devictor D, et al. High-volume hemofiltration in children with acute liver failure*. Pediatr Crit Care Med. 2014;15(7):e300–5.
28. Kim JM, Jo YY, Na SW, Kim SI, Choi YS, Kim NO, et al. The predictors for continuous renal replacement therapy in liver transplant recipients. Transplant Proc. 2014;46(1):184–91.
29. Alam S, Lal BB. Metabolic liver diseases presenting as acute liver failure in children. Indian Pediatr. 2016;53(8):695–701.
30. Gupta S, Fenves AZ, Hootkins R. The role of RRT in hyperammonemic patients. Clin J Am Soc Nephrol. 2016;11(10):1872–8.
31. Banares R, Nevens F, Larsen FS, Jalan R, Albillos A, Dollinger M, et al. Extracorporeal albumin dialysis with the molecular adsorbent recirculating system in acute-on-chronic liver failure: the RELIEF trial. Hepatology. 2013;57(3):1153–62.
32. Saliba F, Samuel D. Artificial liver support: a real step forward. Minerva Med. 2015;106(1):35–43.
33. Saliba F, Camus C, Durand F, Mathurin P, Letierce A, Delafosse B, et al. Albumin dialysis with a noncell artificial liver support device in patients with acute liver failure: a randomized, controlled trial. Ann Intern Med. 2013;159(8):522–31.
34. Saliba F. The molecular adsorbent recirculating system (MARS) in the intensive care unit: a rescue therapy for patients with hepatic failure. Crit Care. 2006;10(1):118.
35. Schaefer B, Schaefer F, Engelmann G, Meyburg J, Heckert KH, Zorn M, et al. Comparison of molecular adsorbents recirculating system (MARS) dialysis with combined plasma exchange and haemodialysis in children with acute liver failure. Nephrol Dial Transplant. 2011;26(11):3633–9.
36. Schaefer B, Schmitt CP. The role of molecular adsorbent recirculating system dialysis for extracorporeal liver support in children. Pediatr Nephrol. 2013;28(9):1763–9.
37. Lexmond WS, Van Dael CM, Scheenstra R, Goorhuis JF, Sieders E, Verkade HJ, et al. Experience with molecular adsorbent recirculating system treatment in 20 children listed for high-urgency liver transplantation. Liver Transpl. 2015;21(3):369–80.
38. Akcan AA, Srivaths P, Himes RW, Tufan PN, Lam F, Nguyen T, et al. Hybrid extracorporeal therapies as a bridge to pediatric liver transplantation. Pediatr Crit Care Med. 2018;19(7):e342–9.
39. Habib M, Roberts LN, Patel RK, Wendon J, Bernal W, Arya R. Evidence of rebalanced coagulation in acute liver injury and acute liver failure as measured by thrombin generation. Liver Int. 2014;34(5):672–8.
40. Goonasekera CD, Wang J, Bunchman TE, Deep A. Factors affecting circuit life during continuous renal replacement therapy in children with liver failure. Ther Apher Dial. 2015;19(1):16–22.
41. Chadha V, Garg U, Warady BA, Alon US. Citrate clearance in children receiving continuous venovenous renal replacement therapy. Pediatr Nephrol. 2002;17(10):819–24.
42. Elhanan N, Skippen P, Nuthall G, Krahn G, Seear M. Citrate anticoagulation in pediatric continuous venovenous hemofiltration. Pediatr Nephrol. 2004;19(2):208–12.
43. Brophy PD, Somers MJ, Baum MA, Symons JM, McAfee N, Fortenberry JD, et al. Multicentre evaluation of anticoagulation in patients receiving continuous renal replacement therapy (CRRT). Nephrol Dial Transplant. 2005;20(7):1416–21.
44. Rodriguez K, Srivaths PR, Tal L, Watson MN, Riley AA, Himes RW, et al. Regional citrate anticoagulation for continuous renal replacement therapy in pediatric patients with liver failure. PLoS One. 2017;12(8):e0182134.
45. Santiago MJ, Lopez-Herce J, Urbano J, Solana MJ, Del CJ, Ballestero Y, et al. Complications of continuous renal replacement therapy in critically ill children: a prospective observational evaluation study. Crit Care. 2009;13(6):R184.
46. Thorat A, Jeng LB. Management of renal dysfunction in patients with liver cirrhosis: role of pretransplantation hemodialysis and outcomes after liver transplantation. Semin Vasc Surg. 2016;29(4):227–35.

Hyperammonemia and Metabolic Diseases

24

Stefano Picca and Carlo Dionisi-Vici

24.1 Clinical Case

A 5-day-old newborn boy is admitted at the emergency department of our hospital with cardiorespiratory failure and coma.

The patient is a second-born from a healthy mother by vaginal delivery, gestational age 35 weeks, birth weight 3.140 kg, and 1-min and 5-min Apgar scores of 8 and 9, respectively. The boy is discharged to home within 24 h of birth. The elder sibling is a healthy 3-year-old boy. In the first 2 days of life, poor feeding and recurrent vomiting are noted. On day 3, feeding is refused, and the boy is noted as "sleeping too long." On day 5, mother is not able to awaken him and takes him to our hospital.

At admittance, the patient shows moderate dehydration, moderate subcostal retractions, shallow respirations, and stage IV neurologic coma. Body weight is 2.650 kg, blood pressure 58/31 mmHg, HR 175 bpm, pCO_2 19 mmHg, and pO_2 62 mmHg. Lab investigation shows plasma glucose 58 mg/dL, pH 7.15, bicarbonate 19 mEq/L, BE +2, creatinine 0.78 mg/dL, sodium 134 mEq/L, potassium 5.9 mEq/L, chloride 91 mEq/L, lactate 4.1 mEq/L, CRP 0.7 mg/dL, and ammonium levels 1650 μmol/L. A second-level metabolic screening including plasma amino acids, blood acylcarnitines, urinary organic acids, and orotic acid is performed.

S. Picca (✉)
Pediatric Dialysis Unit, Department of Pediatrics, "Bambino Gesù" Children's Research Hospital, IRCCS, Rome, Italy

C. Dionisi-Vici
Metabolic Unit, Department of Pediatrics, "Bambino Gesù" Children's Research Hospital, IRCCS, Rome, Italy

S. K. Sethi et al. (eds.), *Critical Care Pediatric Nephrology and Dialysis: A Practical Handbook*, https://doi.org/10.1007/978-981-13-2276-1_24

Urine output is 2.7 mL/kg/h. Patient is intubated after muscle relaxant drug administration and starts pressure-controlled ventilation. A 3F central catheter is placed in the right jugular vein, and fluid administration with glucose 10% solution and normal saline is started at 18 mL/h. Blood cultures for bacteria and viruses are collected. Echocardiography shows EF of 45%.

In the hypothesis of a metabolic decompensation due to an inborn error of metabolism, therapy with arginine (1500 mg iv per day), sodium benzoate (1500 mg iv per day), carnitine (300 mg iv per day), hydroxocobalamin (1 mg per day), carbamylglutamate (300 mg via nasogastric tube per day), and biotin (10 mg per day) is started. Energy is supplied as parenteral at the rate of 100 kcal/kg/24 h. Insulin is added to maintain blood glucose levels between 100 and 200 mg/dL. A urea cycle defect is suspected, and the dialysis unit team is alerted in case of a metabolic crisis not responding to medical treatment.

After 4 h, BP is 67/32, HR 151 bpm, pCO_2 38 mmHg, pO_2 94 mmHg, pH 7.31, bicarbonate 21 mEq/L, and BE +3. Despite pharmacological treatment, unvaried severe clinical conditions and hyperammonemia (1410 μmol/L) persist. A 6.5 F, 7.5 cm double-lumen venous catheter is placed in the right internal jugular vein after rewiring of the 3F catheter. Another 3F catheter is placed in the left jugular vein to continue infusions. In the meanwhile, a Prismaflex™ CRRT monitor equipped with a HF20™ pediatric circuit (Baxter-Gambro™) is prepared. The priming volume of the circuit is 61 mL. The circuit is pre-primed with 50% packed red blood cells and 50% saline pre-warmed at 37 °C before CRRT start. CVVHD with blood flow of 30 mL/min, dialysate flow of 2500 mL/h, and no body weight loss is started. Dialysis fluid is Phoxilium™ (Baxter-Gambro™) (Ca^{2+}1.25, Mg^{2+} 0.6, Na^+ 140, Cl^- 115.9, $HPO4^{2-}$ 1.2, $HCO3^-$ 30, K^+ 4 mmol/L). Dialysis bags are pre-warmed at 38 °C, and the neonate is placed on a convective warming system (Bair Hugger™, 3 M). After 4 h of CVVHD, cardiovascular conditions remain stable, and plasma ammonium decreases at 462 μmol/L. After 24 h of CVVHD, neurological improvement occurs with reprise of spontaneous movements, improvement of mydriasis, and response to painful stimuli. CVVHD is discontinued after 42 h with an ammonium level of 98 μmol/L, BP 69/41 mmHg, HR 175 bpm, pCO_2 39 mmHg, pO_2 99 mmHg, plasma glucose 169 mg/dL, pH 7.41, bicarbonate 27 mEq/L, BE +1, creatinine 0.24 mg/dL, sodium 139 mEq/L, potassium 4.7 mEq/L, chloride 109 mEq/L, and lactate 1.8 mEq/L. The boy is successfully extubated. During the whole CVVHD treatment, parenteral support is continued unvaried. Two days later, enteral nutrition is started with breast milk (10 mL × 5/24 h) and is well tolerated. From day 3 after extubation, enteral nutrition is progressively increased, while parenteral support is progressively tapered. At day 6 after extubation, neurologic examination and EEG are normal.

The boy is now 11-month-old and shows borderline neurological development with modest mild abnormal hypersignal of the periventricular white matter at brain MRI.

Metabolic investigation shows massive elevation of plasma glutamine and citrulline and increased urinary excretion of orotic acid, a profile consistent with the diagnosis of citrullinemia type I.

Table 24.1 Bedside diagnostic orientation of hyperammonemia based on first-level investigations in a critical child (modified from [2])

	UCDs	OAs	β-OX	HI-HA	TMEM70	CAVA	PC (type B)
↑ NH_3	++	++	+	+	+	+	+
Acidosis	–	+	–	–	+	+	+
Hypoglycemia	–	±	++	++	±	±	+
↑ lactate	–	+	–	–	++	+	++
↑ transaminases	+	–	++			–	±
↑ CK	–	–	++			–	–
↑ uric acid	–	+	+	–	++	–	–
↓ WBC/plt	–	+	–	–	–	–	–
Ketonuria	–	++	–	–	±	–	++
Heart disease	–		CMP Arrhythmias	–	CMP Pulmonary hypertension	–	–

UCDs urea cycle defects, *OAs* organic acidurias, *β-OX* beta-oxidation defects, *HI-HA* hyperinsulinism-hyperammonemia syndrome, *CAVA* carbonic anhydrase type Va, *PC* pyruvate carboxylase deficiency, *CMP* cardiomyopathy

24.2 Causes of Hyperammonemia

The most frequent causes of hyperammonemia (HA) in children with inborn errors of metabolism (IEM) are urea cycle defects (UCDs) and organic acidurias (OAs). Both UCDs and OAs are recessively transmitted diseases, except for OTC deficiency, an X-linked disorder. In UCDs, partial or complete failure of activity of key enzymes/transporter of the urea cycle (carbamoyl phosphate synthetase 1 [CPS1], ornithine transcarbamylase [OTC], argininosuccinate synthetase [ASS], argininosuccinate lyase [ASL], arginase 1 [ARG1], N-acetylglutamate [NAG], ornithine/citrulline antiporter [ORNT1]) induces primary accumulation of ammonium. In OAs, HA is caused by accumulation of propionyl-CoA which decreases the synthesis of N-acetylglutamate, the natural activator of CPS1, thus inducing a secondary block of urea cycle enzymes and leading to HA. Other inherited disorders causing HA are listed in Table 24.1.

24.3 Ammonium Toxicity

IEM are rare diseases (1:9000 live births) [1], and HA defined as >350 μmol/L [2] is one of the most frequent causes of metabolic decompensation in IEM. Ammonium (NH_4) is a small molecule (molecular weight, 17d) derived from ammonia gas (NH_3) hydration and its subsequent dissociation. NH_3/NH_4 ratio equilibrium is dependent on blood pH, and in physiologic conditions (pH 7,4), 98% is represented by NH_4. Increase from 7.1 to 7.5 in pH value induces a fourfold increase of NH_3 that freely diffuses into the cell, resulting in increased neurotoxicity. HA exerts a direct toxic effect on CNS by altering intracellular pH, by raising the membrane potential and by depolarizing both neurons and astrocytes [3]. Moreover, the intracellular conversion of glutamate to glutamine catalyzed by the enzyme glutamine synthetase is primed by the excess of ammonium. This reaction, which represents an endogenous buffer for accumulated ammonium, becomes an uncontrolled source of glutamine, a highly osmotic molecule that accumulates in astrocytes, determining intracellular swelling and brain edema [4].

24.4 The Clinical Course of the Critical Hyperammonemic Child

24.4.1 Supportive Care

The hyperammonemic child with metabolic decompensation is a severe patient needing urgent supportive care. The following must be rapidly guaranteed:

- Stabilize patient.
- Circulatory support.
- Respiratory support (when needed).
- Rehydration.
- Electrolyte correction.
- Investigations for infection → antibiotic.

24.4.2 Diagnostic Approach

- *Clinical History*: HA first symptoms can occur at any age, but neonatal onset is typical in the most severe cases of UCDs and OAs. Disease manifestation beyond 28 days is classified as late onset [2]. Clinical history must ascertain if older siblings are healthy or if there are cases of not established death in the same sibling line. In comatose children, a valuable information is coma duration. This information is often unavailable, or the duration definition is inaccurate, but, if available, it is a useful tool for prognosis, given the relation of this time with the outcome [5–8].
- *Physical Examination*: neurologic deterioration is the hallmark of a critical hyperammonemic child. Altered level of consciousness (from somnolence and lethargy to coma) mimicking encephalitis or drug intoxication, seizures, multiorgan failure, and peripheral circulatory failure are typical signs of acute HA. In neonates, sepsis-like picture, temperature instability, respiratory distress, hyperventilation, and stage III (unconsciousness, decerebrate posture with reduced response to painful stimuli) or stage IV (flaccid tone with dilated pupils and no response to painful stimuli) coma are most frequent presentations [4].

Table 24.2 Diagnostic orientation: "two-step" levels of laboratory investigations in a child with hyperammonemia

Routine laboratory analyses	• Routine clinical chemistry (blood count, liver and kidney function, CRP, electrolytes, anion gap, blood gases, urinalysis) • Glucose • Lactate • Ammonia • CK • Uric acid • Urinary ketones • Blood cultures • ECG, US, CT, MRI, etc.
Second-level metabolic investigations	• Plasma amino acids • Blood acylcarnitines • Urinary organic acids • Urinary orotic acid

- *Laboratory Investigation*: for practical purposes can be divided into two steps: routine laboratory testing, useful for diagnostic orientation, and second-level metabolic analyses (see Table 24.2).
- *Differential Diagnosis*: a practical approach to differentiate between the different causes of HA based on routine laboratory testing is shown in Table 24.2.

24.4.3 Treatment

After the stabilization of the patient, the treatment must be continued through the following interventions:

24.4.3.1 Nutrition

The three hallmarks of nutrition treatment are the following:

- Stop protein.
- Provide calories.
- Promote anabolism.

Protein intake must be stopped with any grade of HA, but this cannot be prolonged for more than 2 days. In the first phase of the treatment, energy must be provided with iv/peroral glucose at the rate of 80–100 kcal/kg/day (glucose 6–8 mg/kg/min, 10 mg/kg/min in neonates). Lipids can be added after FAODs are excluded. Insulin can be added to control possible hyperglycemia and promote anabolism according to blood glucose levels. During this phase, ammonium levels should be measured every 3–4 h [2].

24.4.3.2 Specific Therapies

The critical child with an undiagnosed HA needs a multipurpose therapeutic approach waiting for a causal diagnosis. The "metabolic cocktail" is aimed to

Table 24.3 Medical treatment of acute hyperammonemia: drugs, mechanism of action, dosages, and administration route [2, 9]

	Mechanism of action	Dosages	Administration route
Energy	Contrasting catabolism	80–100 kcal/kg/day [glucose 6–8 mg/kg/min + lipids]	iv/peroral
Insulin	Promoting energy utilization	According to blood glucose	iv
Arginine	Priming the arginine-ornithine passage in the urea cycle to maximize urea formation and nitrogen elimination	250 (up to 400) mg/kg in 2 h >250 mg/kg/day	iv
Carnitine	Preventing secondary carnitine deficiency in methylmalonic and propionic acidemias [14]	100 mg/kg bolus >100 mg/kg/day	iv
Vitamins	Cofactors of enzymes potentially involved in HA	B_{12} 1 mg, biotin 10 mg, thiamine 100 mg	iv
Carbamylglutamate	Replacing the CPS1 activator *N*-acetylglutamate	100 mg/kg	Peroral
Benzoate	Conjugating with glycine to form hippuric acid, rapidly excreted by the kidneys	250 mg/kg in 2 h > 250 (up to 500) mg/kg/day	iv

provide the initial therapy for UCDs and OAs and is based on scavenger drugs promoting alternative ammonium elimination pathways, primers of metabolic pathways to maximize ammonium excretion in UCDs, and cofactor supplementation in OAs [2, 9]. Table 24.3 shows drugs, mechanism of action, dosages, and administration route.

24.4.3.3 Extracorporeal Procedures for Toxin Removal

In healthy subjects, ammonium excretion is regulated by glutamine metabolism and by renal excretion. Approximately 20% of the daily generated ammonia load is excreted by normally functioning kidneys. In the neonate, this quote is supposed to be lesser, due to immature tubular mechanisms. In HA due to IEM, these elimination routes become largely insufficient, and an artificial clearance must be added in HA nonresponsive to medical treatment. Although the space of distribution of the NH_3/NH_4 system in body fluids is not exactly defined, both gaseous and ionic components are able to cross the cell membrane rapidly [3]. Consequently, when dialyzing ammonium, one must refer to a distribution space like that of total body water (see Fig. 24.1). In acute HA, ammonium generation rate may be extremely high and hardly predictable, depending also on often associated catabolism, infections, and multiple organ failure. Ammonium is a small, nonprotein-bound molecule. As such, it diffuses freely through artificial and biological membranes while it is removed in a lesser extent by convection [10].

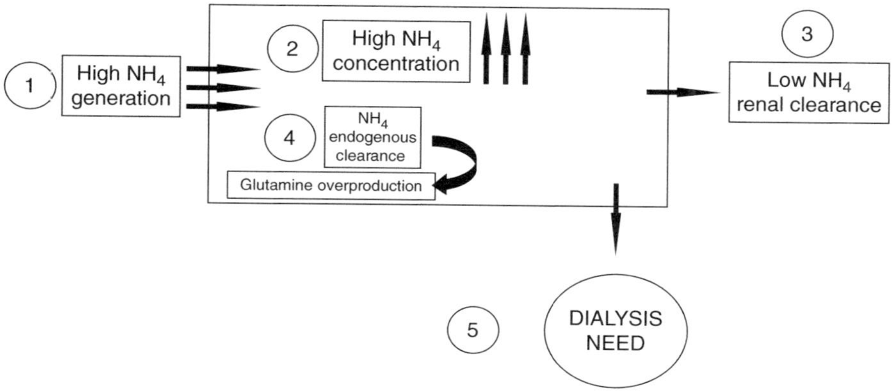

Fig. 24.1 Events leading to dialysis need in acute hyperammonemia. (1) Uncontrolled ammonium production generation. (2) High ammonium concentration. (3) Saturation of renal ammonium excretion capacity. (4) Excessive glutamine generation catalyzed by glutamine synthetase enzyme. (5) Need for dialysis

When to Start

There are basically three possible scenarios determining the decision-making for dialysis in HA.

(a) *Untreated patient (usually coming from home)*: the time passing from diagnosis of HA >500 μmol/L to the start of dialysis is usually 2–4 h, including admission, lab determination, transferring to NICU, patient intubation and stabilization, placement of blood lines, start of medical therapy, dialysis access creation, alerting dialysis unit, dialysis setting up, blood units availability, etc. A second ammonium determination can address to dialysis according to the plasma ammonium course. We have shown that patients responding in 4 h to medical therapy did not need dialysis and had generally a good outcome, excluding those with initial ammonium levels >1000 μmol/L (see Fig. 24.2). This interval being inevitable, we suggest to recheck ammonium levels and to consider this together with the clinical conditions in making decision about dialysis start.

(b) *Patient already on medical treatment (usually transferred from another hospital)*: if a medical treatment has been started, it is essential to ascertain if the treatment has been appropriate and the duration of this treatment before dialysis start.

(c) *Patient with unfavorable prognosis*: prognosis and expected neurodevelopmental outcome are related to:
   - Coma lasting for more than 2 days
   - Increase of intracranial pressure
   - Peak ammonium level >1000 μmol/L [7, 11]

We have found an association between coma duration and outcome in ten neonates treated with extracorporeal dialysis. All neonates having experienced a coma

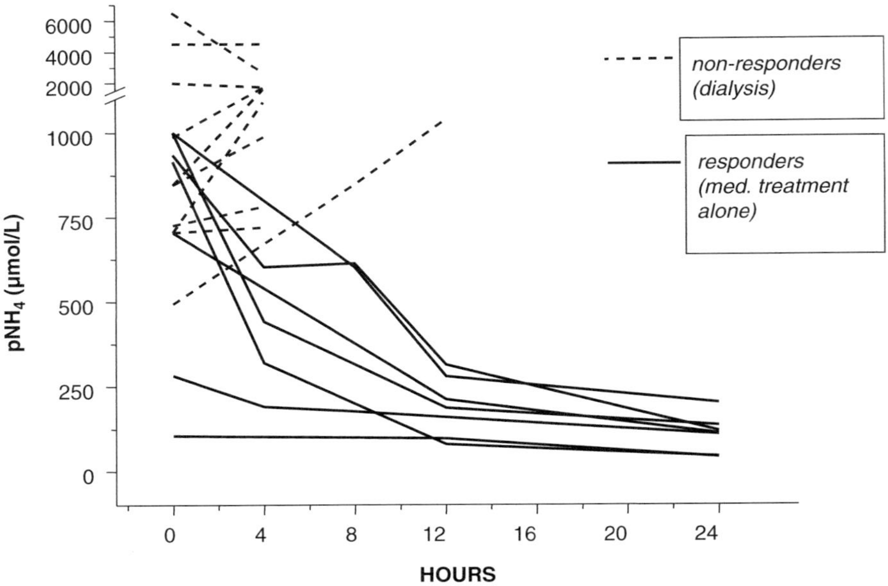

Fig. 24.2 First 0–4 h medical treatment in neonatal hyperammonemia. Early response was followed by a further reduction of ammonium plasma levels in all cases below 1000 μmol/L [6]

Table 24.4 Ammonium clearances and filtration fractions in CVVHD, HD, and PD

Patients	Dialysis	Qb (mL/min)	Qd (mL/min)	NH_4 clearance (mL/min/kg)	NH_4 filtration fraction (%)
3	CVVHD [6]	20–40	33.3–83.3 (2–5 L/h)	2.65–3.80	53–58
2	HD [6]	10–15	500	3.95–5.37	95–96
4	PD [12]	–	–	0.48–2.70 (1.4 ± 1.1, about 0.48 mL/min/kg)	–

PD was performed with 10–25 mL/kg body weight fill volume and dwell time of 60 min

duration >33 h showed an unfavorable outcome [6]. Although associations between ammonium peak levels and outcome have been described [5–7, 11], there are cases of good outcome in children having experienced ammonium peak levels >1000 μmol/L [6, 8], so in our opinion very high ammonium levels per se do not represent criteria of exclusion from dialysis treatment. In very severe children, these data must be considered together with all clinical aspects before starting dialysis or limiting the assistance to supportive care.

All three acute dialysis modalities have been used in HA (see Table 24.4):

Peritoneal Dialysis (PD)

Peritoneal dialysis (PD) provides the lowest ammonium clearance [6, 12]. It is easily performed by a peritoneal catheter even in smallest children and does not require anticoagulation nor highly specialized training. PD prescription in HA includes:

- Filling volume: 10 mL/kg BW. If no leakage from the catheter exit site: increase up to 25 mL/kg BW. Heparin 125 IU/L and an antibiotic (we use ceftazidime 250 mg/L) are added to PD fluid.
- Dwell time: 30–45 min.

Continuous Venovenous Hemodialysis (CVVHD)

Continuous venovenous hemodialysis (CVVHD) provides higher ammonium clearance than PD. It requires a vascular access, specific equipment, and highly specialized staff. CVVHD prescription in HA includes:

- Access: 6.5 F, 7 cm, dual-lumen catheter in the right internal jugular vein (RIJV) or two 4–5F single lumen catheters in jugular or femoral veins, according to local expertise and available vessels. RIJV gives best results on catheter survival and performance [13].
- CRRT monitor is equipped with low priming volume circuits, and the circuit is pre-primed with warmed packed red blood cells and saline (50% proportion) to minimize the impact of extracorporeal circulation on cardiovascular stability.
- Filter surface must be adapted to patient size. In neonates, a 0.2–0.3 m^2 device is suitable to provide a good ammonium clearance.
- Blood flow rate is set at 10 mL/kg BW/min in neonates and at 5 mL/kg BW/min in older children, according to the catheter performance.
- Dialysis fluid flow rate is set at highest possible rate, according to the machine limits (2.5–5 L/h, in neonates) with close control of patient temperature in neonates to avoid hypothermia induced by heat loss and maximizing patient's heating.
- Electrolyte concentration of dialysis bags should be adjusted according to patient's needs.

There are no data on ammonium dialysis efficiency with the last generation of neonatal CRRT machines like Nidus® [14], Carpediem® [15], or Aquadex® (adapted for neonatal CRRT) [16]. However, it is presumable that ammonium clearance is inferior to that of machines providing higher dialysate flow. Studies are needed on this issue.

Hemodialysis (HD)

Hemodialysis (HD) provides the highest ammonium clearance and most rapid plasma ammonium reduction (see Table 24.4). HD has been therefore recommended as gold dialytic standard in HA due to IEM in some guidelines [17]. However, in neonates HD may induce cardiovascular instability, hypotension, and reduced ammonium clearance [6]. HD prescription in HA includes:

- Access: as for CRRT.
- HD monitor should be equipped with low priming volume circuits and neonatal lines in neonates. Preparation of the circuit like in CRRT.
- Filters and blood flows resemble those used in CRRT.
- Dialysate flow is set at 500 mL/min, maximizing small molecule clearance, what makes the difference in efficiency between HD and CRRT.

During dialysis, medical therapy remains unchanged. Drug dosage should be adapted to dialysis in children [18], taking into account that high dialysate flows increase drug clearance and consequently higher dosages compared to those recommended are probably required. It is therefore recommended to use antimicrobials, the plasma level of which is available. Plasma ammonium levels should be measured every 4 h.

When to Stop

When ammonium levels are below 100 μmol/L [2], we suggest to continue dialysis for at least two consecutive controls at 4 h distance after refeeding.

An algorithm providing a practical approach to medical and dialytic treatment to HA in IEM is shown in Fig. 24.3.

Which Dialysis Modality?

While the fastest reduction of ammonium levels is mandatory [2], there is no clear evidence that either short- or long-term outcome is related to dialysis modality [2, 6, 7]. The reason for this apparent contradiction probably relies on the following issues.

1. Both peak ammonium levels and duration of HA are related to the outcome [5–8].
2. Studies suggesting a relation between dialysis modality (and/or detoxification rapidity) and the outcome are probably biased by lack of randomization or by unavailability of pre-dialysis coma length [12, 19, 20].
3. HD provides higher ammonium clearance than PD and CVVHD, but good outcome results were obtained also with the latter two modalities [7, 8].

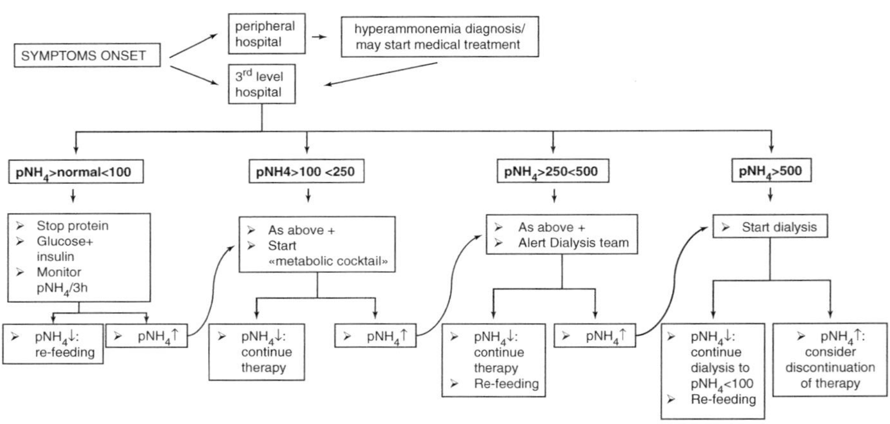

Fig. 24.3 Algorithm for acute hyperammonemia in metabolic decompensation: (1) In the algorithm, it is considered that the initial referral is often to a peripheral hospital, (2) hyperammonemia is expressed in μmol/L, and (3) dialysis preparation by the dialysis team usually takes 2–4 h. Data are partially taken from [2]

4. In most studies, dialysis efficiency has been evaluated by ammonium 50% decay time, an easy parameter to extrapolate from retrospective data, but not entirely reflecting dialysis efficiency. High ammonium levels in neonatal HA are the combined result of limited renal clearance and increased ammonium generation rate. Likewise, decreased ammonium levels during dialysis reflect increased clearance, but also slower generation after initiation of medical treatment. In the largest published series of hyperammonemic neonates, we reported no significant difference in ammonium decay time between PD and CVVHD [7]. Possible explanations are the following: (a) late referral of patients inducing extremely high ammonium generation, thus affecting the plasma reduction even during dialysis with a more effective modality (i.e., CRRT); (b) in patients treated with PD, dialysis could be initiated more rapidly due to the larger diffusion and the easy performance of PD compared to extracorporeal dialysis; (c) utilization of glucose of PD fluid improving energy supply and anabolism; and (d) negative nitrogen balance induced by PD and lesser ammonium production [21].

24.4.3.4 Protein Refeeding

It is suggested to start the protein refeeding during dialysis to control possible HA rebound. Reintroduction of protein/essential amino acids should not be delayed beyond 48 h from their stop. If the patient cannot be fed enterally, IV amino acids should be started, increasing daily to the required amount and replacing the quote lost with dialysis that can reach 25% of intake [22].

24.5 In Summary

Very rare patients provide uncertain results. However, we believe that dialysis must be regarded as a means of accelerating the effects of medical treatment by removing excesses of ammonium that accumulated during a metabolic decompensation. Under these circumstances, delaying initiation of dialysis in order to transfer patients to centers with expertise in pediatric or neonatal extracorporeal dialysis must be discussed. Early referral for diagnosis and initiation of medical and dialysis treatment remain the major determinants of the outcome of infants and children with acute HA.

Take-Home Messages

- In children and infants, acute hyperammonemia is a life-threatening condition involving elevated risk of death and of neurological permanent sequelae in survivors.
- Early response to medical and dialysis treatment is associated with good outcome and should be started as early as possible.
- Once HA is established, early treatment start is more important than dialysis modality or efficiency.

- HD and CVVHD are the gold standard of dialysis in hyperammonemia.
- PD can be used when local facilities do not allow extracorporeal dialysis or waiting for patient's transferring to a center providing extracorporeal dialysis.

References

1. Dionisi-Vici C, Rizzo C, Burlina AB, Caruso U, Sabetta G, Uziel G, Abeni D. Inborn errors of metabolism in the Italian pediatric population: a national retrospective survey. J Pediatr. 2002;140(3):321–7.
2. Häberle J, Boddaert N, Burlina A, Chakrapani A, Dixon M, Huemer M, Karall D, Martinelli D, Crespo PS, Santer R, Servais A, Valayannopoulos V, Lindner M, Rubio V, Dionisi-Vici C. Suggested guidelines for the diagnosis and management of urea cycle disorders. Orphanet J Rare Dis. 2012;7:32.
3. Bosoi CR, Rose CF. Identifying the direct effects of ammonia on the brain. Metab Brain Dis. 2009;24(1):95–102.
4. Brusilow SW, Horwich AL. Urea cycle enzymes. In: Scriver CR, Beaudet AL, Sly WS, Valle D, editors. The metabolic and molecular bases of inherited disease. 7th ed. New York: McGraw-Hill; 1995. p. 1187–232.
5. Msall M, Batshaw ML, Suss R, Brusilow SW, Mellits ED. Neurologic outcome in children with inborn errors of urea synthesis. N Engl J Med. 1984;310:1500–5.
6. Picca S, Dionisi-Vici C, Abeni D, Pastore A, Rizzo C, Orzalesi M, Sabetta G, Rizzoni G, Bartuli A. Extracorporeal dialysis in neonatal hyperammonemia: modalities and prognostic indicators. Pediatr Nephrol. 2001;16:862–7.
7. Picca S, Dionisi-Vici C, Bartuli A, De Palo T, Papadia F, Montini G, Materassi M, Donati MA, Verrina E, Schiaffino MC, Pecoraro C, Iaccarino E, Vidal E, Burlina A, Emma F. Short-term survival of hyperammonemic neonates treated with dialysis. Pediatr Nephrol. 2015;30(5):839–47.
8. Pela I, Seracini D, Donati MA, Lavoratti G, Pasquini E, Materassi M. Peritoneal dialysis in neonates with inborn errors of metabolism: is it really out of date? Pediatr Nephrol. 2008;23:163–8.
9. Fraser JL, Venditti CP. Methylmalonic and propionic acidemias: clinical management update. Curr Opin Pediatr. 2016;28(6):682–93.
10. Semama DS, Huet F, Gouyon JB, Lallemant C, Desgres J. Use of peritoneal dialysis, continuous arteriovenous hemofiltration, and continuous arteriovenous hemodiafiltration for removal of ammonium chloride and glutamine in rabbits. J Pediatr. 1995;126(5 Pt 1):742–6.
11. Bachmann C. Outcome and survival of 88 patients with urea cycle disorders: a retrospective evaluation. Eur J Pediatr. 2003;162:410–6.
12. Arbeiter AK, Kranz B, Wingen AM, Bonzel KE, Dohna-Schwake C, Hanssler L, Neudorf U, Hoyer PF, Büscher R. Continuous venovenous haemodialysis (CVVHD) and continuous peritoneal dialysis (CPD) in the acute management of 21 children with inborn errors of metabolism. Nephrol Dial Transplant. 2010;25:1257–65.
13. Hackbarth R, Bunchman TE, Chua AN, Somers MJ, Baum M, Symons JM, Brophy PD, Blowey D, Fortenberry JD, Chand D, Flores FX, Alexander SR, Mahan JD, McBryde KD, Benfield MR, Goldstein SL. The effect of vascular access location and size on circuit survival in pediatric continuous renal replacement therapy: a report from the PPCRRT registry. Int J Artif Organs. 2007;30(12):1116–21.
14. Coulthard MG, Crosier J, Griffiths C, Smith J, Drinnan M, Whitaker M, Beckwith R, Matthews JN, Flecknell P, Lambert HJ. Haemodialysing babies weighing <8 kg with the Newcastle infant dialysis and ultrafiltration system (Nidus): comparison with peritoneal and conventional haemodialysis. Pediatr Nephrol. 2014;29(10):1873–81.

15. Ronco C, Garzotto F, Ricci Z. CA.R.PE.DI.E.M. (cardio–renal Pediatric Dialysis emergency machine): evolution of continuous renal replacement therapies in infants. A personal journey. Pediatr Nephrol. 2012;27:1203–11.
16. Askenazi D, Ingram D, White S, Cramer M, Borasino S, Coghill C, Dill L, Tenney F, Feig D, Fathallah-Shaykh S. Smaller circuits for smaller patients: improving renal support therapy with Aquadex™. Pediatr Nephrol. 2016;31(5):853–60.
17. Summar M. Current strategies for the management of neonatal urea cycle disorders. J Pediatr. 2001;138:S30–9.
18. Pediatric Drug Book. https://kdpnet.kdp.louisville.edu/drugbook/pediatric/.
19. McBryde KD, Kershaw DB, Bunchman TE, Maxvold NJ, Mottes TA, Kudelka TL, Brophy PD. Renal replacement therapy in the treatment of confirmed or suspected inborn errors of metabolism. J Pediatr. 2006;148(6):770–8.
20. Schaefer F, Straube E, Oh J, Mehls O, Mayatepek E. Dialysis in neonates with inborn errors of metabolism. Nephrol Dial Transplant. 1999;14:910–8.
21. Bunchman TE. The complexity of dialytic therapy in hyperammonemic neonates. Pediatr Nephrol. 2015;30:701–2.
22. Btaiche IF, Mohammad RA, Alaniz C, Mueller BA. Amino acid requirements in critically ill patients with acute kidney injury treated with continuous renal replacement therapy. Pharmacotherapy. 2008;28(5):600–13.

Anticoagulation During RRT in the ICU 25

Vimal Chadha and Bradley A. Warady

25.1 Case Presentation

A 10-year-old boy presented to the Emergency Department with a history of fever and abdominal pain of 2 days' duration. His parents reported that his condition worsened over the past few hours as he became lethargic and looked pale, and his abdomen was distended. On examination, he was lethargic and febrile (39.5 °C; 103 °F) with a heart rate of 140/min and blood pressure 90/50 mmHg, and his respirations were slow with minimal movement of the abdominal wall. His abdomen was distended, and there was guarding and tenderness on palpation. He received two 0.9% saline (20 mL/kg) fluid boluses, and he was taken to the operating room for evaluation of a presumed surgical abdomen. During surgery, he was found to have a perforated appendix and purulent peritoneal fluid. He was subsequently admitted to the PICU where he was on mechanical ventilation and received vasopressors (epinephrine and norepinephrine) for blood pressure support. He also received broad-spectrum antibiotics with coverage for anaerobic organisms. Over the next 24 h, he became 15% fluid overloaded as his urine output progressively decreased to anuria over 12 h. His serum chemistries revealed sodium 143 mEq/L, potassium 5.6 mEq/L, chloride 98 mEq/L, bicarbonate 17 mEq/L, urea nitrogen 48 mg/dL, creatinine 2.4 mg/dL, and calcium 8.9 mg/dL. Hematology labs revealed hemoglobin 8.6 g/dL and WBC count 22,000 with platelet count of 66,000/mm^3. A nephrology consult was obtained for management of acute kidney injury (AKI).

V. Chadha · B. A. Warady (✉)
Department of Pediatrics, University of Missouri – Kansas City School of Medicine, Kansas City, MO, USA

Division of Pediatric Nephrology, Children's Mercy Kansas City, Kansas City, MO, USA
e-mail: bwarady@cmh.edu

S. K. Sethi et al. (eds.), *Critical Care Pediatric Nephrology and Dialysis: A Practical Handbook*, https://doi.org/10.1007/978-981-13-2276-1_25

Peritoneal dialysis was not possible because of his recent abdominal surgery, and he was considered too unstable to tolerate hemodialysis. A plan was made to initiate continuous renal replacement therapy (CRRT) without anticoagulation, as he had recently undergone major abdominal surgery and he had thrombocytopenia. The CRRT circuit clotted 4 h after therapy initiation, and two more circuits were lost because of clotting over the subsequent 12 h despite frequent flushing with 0.9% saline. Anticoagulation was then provided by regional citrate anticoagulation (RCA). Four days later, he started passing urine with a steady decline in serum urea nitrogen and creatinine. On day six, he was transferred from the PICU to the floor.

25.2 Introduction

Acute kidney injury (AKI) is a common problem in critically ill children and is associated with increased morbidity and mortality [1]. In a recently completed multinational, prospective study involving patients admitted to pediatric intensive care units (PICU), AKI was seen in one-quarter of the patients; 40% of the AKI episodes were severe and 10–15% of patients with severe AKI required renal replacement therapy [1]. In the absence of specific treatment for most cases of AKI, renal replacement therapy in addition to other supportive measures such as maintaining adequate renal perfusion, avoiding nephrotoxic medications, providing adequate nutritional support, and managing comorbidities becomes the mainstay of managing severe AKI. While any of the three available dialysis modalities, namely, hemodialysis, peritoneal dialysis, and continuous renal replacement therapy (CRRT), may be used to help address electrolyte imbalance and/or fluid overload in critically ill patients, CRRT (if available) has become the most common dialysis modality used for managing these patients in many centers. More recently, modification of the hemodialysis prescription to provide sustained low-efficiency dialysis (SLED) has gained popularity as an alternative to CRRT and can be used when the latter therapy is unavailable [2]. The purpose of this chapter is to provide general guidelines for effective anticoagulation during dialysis therapies involving extracorporeal circuits.

25.3 Rationale for Anticoagulation

It is a natural tendency for blood to clot upon contact with extracorporeal surfaces such as tubing or a dialysis filter. Anticoagulation is therefore required to prevent clotting for the majority of procedures involving extracorporeal circulation. In contrast to hemodialysis therapy (conventional or SLED) where anticoagulation is usually required for the specified duration of the therapy, continuous anticoagulation is required during CRRT. The clotting risks are high during CRRT in most patients because of the relatively low blood flow rates and prolonged exposure to extracorporeal surfaces that is characteristic of this modality. Most important is the fact that the unexpected loss of an extracorporeal circuit due to clotting results in an interruption of therapy leading to a decrease in the delivered clearance, loss of blood, and possible patient exposure to blood products resulting from the need to prime a new extracorporeal circuit. As critically sick patients have both increased bleeding and clotting risks, the provision of ongoing efficient and safe anticoagulation for the extracorporeal circuit can become a challenge for even the experienced nephrologist or intensivist.

25.4 Extracorporeal Anticoagulation

The three approaches to anticoagulation for patients on dialysis are either none (anticoagulation-free), systemic, or regional (anticoagulation limited to extracorporeal circuit).

25.4.1 Anticoagulation-Free Therapy

Anticoagulation therapy is unsafe in patients with ongoing active bleeding in association with events such as recent trauma, intracranial hemorrhage, and during the immediate postoperative period. While regional anticoagulation therapy (*vide infra*) is preferred under these conditions, anticoagulation-free dialysis can be performed if the former technique is unavailable or not feasible due to lack of expertise. Dialysis therapy without anticoagulation is likely to succeed when the prothrombin time/international normalized ratio (PT-INR) and activated partial thromboplastin time (APTT) are prolonged, with associated thrombocytopenia. During anticoagulation-free therapy, it is prudent to use higher blood flow rates and perform frequent flushing with normal saline to maintain the circuit patency. Anticoagulation-free dialysis is commonly performed during shorter dialysis sessions but has also been used with SLED [2] and CRRT [3, 4]. Increasing the delivery of prefilter replacement fluids as the main mode of clearance in the setting of CRRT can also help prevent filter clotting. The extracorporeal circuit should be closely observed for any signs of clotting and changed preemptively to prevent unnecessary blood loss. One of the drawbacks of anticoagulation-free therapy with CRRT can be a shorter filter life either due to frequent clotting or preemptive change of circuits, both of which incur additional costs.

25.4.2 Systemic Anticoagulation Therapy

25.4.2.1 Unfractionated Heparin

Because of long-standing familiarity, convenience, and low cost, unfractionated heparin is the most widely used anticoagulant worldwide. However, active bleeding and a high risk for bleeding, especially in the postsurgical setting, are considered contraindications to heparin usage as the incidence of heparin-induced major bleeding complications can be as high as 50% [5, 6]. Even when heparin is used selectively for patients at low risk for bleeding, the risk of hemorrhagic events remains high (26%) [7]. Additionally, heparin may not be a suitable anticoagulant in bone marrow transplant patients with thrombocytopenia and in patients with low levels of antithrombin III, as heparin acts by activating antithrombin anticoagulant function; antithrombin levels of >80% of normal are required for effective anticoagulation. Heparin-induced thrombocytopenia (HIT) is a rare but severe complication and is a contraindication for further heparin usage.

Dose requirements for unfractionated heparin show marked inter- and intrapatient variability. The heparin dosage is titrated based on the degree of anticoagulation as measured by the bedside whole blood activated clotting time (ACT). An initial heparin bolus (20–50 U/kg) is given if the baseline ACT is <150 s, and the ACT is rechecked after 5 min. Heparin boluses can be repeated until the ACT is >150 s, followed by a continuous heparin infusion which is started at a rate of 20 U/kg/h if the ACT is between 150–200 s. The goal is to achieve and maintain an ACT of 180–220 s in patients with a low risk of bleeding and between 150 and 180 s in patients with a higher risk of bleeding. However, if the initial ACT is >200 s and anticoagulation is to be provided, the heparin infusion should be started at 10 U/kg/h. In addition, we routinely flush the extracorporeal circuit with heparinized saline (5000 IU/L) to reduce the thrombogenicity of the circuit before initiating dialysis therapy.

The anticoagulant effect of heparin can be reversed with protamine (1–1.5 mg for every 100 U of heparin; maximum protamine dose 50 mg). This combination has been used to create a regional anticoagulation (*vide infra*) protocol for both hemodialysis [8] and CRRT in which heparin is infused prefilter and protamine is given post-filter [9, 10].

25.4.2.2 Low-Molecular-Weight Heparin (LMWH)

LMWH (3000–7000 Da) are heparin derivatives which primarily inhibit factor Xa. LMWH has a half-life that is characteristically about twice that of unfractionated heparin (2–4 h) and even more prolonged in patients with renal failure [11]. While LMWH has been used successfully in patients receiving maintenance hemodialysis for ESRD, its use in patients with AKI is scarcely reported. Therapeutic monitoring is achieved by checking the anti-factor Xa activity, which should be between 0.4 and 0.8 IU/mL 2 h after initial loading [12]. In addition, LMWH is much more expensive than standard heparin.

25.4.2.3 Additional Anticoagulants

Direct thrombin inhibitors such as argatroban and bivalirudin [13–15], the prostaglandin prostacyclin that acts by platelet inhibition [16], and the serine protease inhibitor nafamostat which blocks factor Xa, XIIa, and thrombin [17] have been used for anticoagulation during extracorporeal therapies. These agents are expensive and are not available in many countries. As a result, these approaches have not been widely used which has limited the published experience in pediatrics.

25.4.3 Regional Anticoagulation Therapy

This approach to anticoagulation, in which the treatment is limited to the extracorporeal circuit only, is particularly beneficial because of the avoidance of the systemic complications/side effects of anticoagulation.

25.4.3.1 Regional Anticoagulation with Protamine Reversal

This is one of the earliest methods described to provide regional anticoagulation, in which heparin is infused pre-dialyzer and protamine is infused post-dialyzer before the blood is returned to the patient (*vide supra*) [8–10]. Protamine reversal has been largely abandoned due to its technical difficulties, issues with dose titration, and problems with rebound bleeding 2–4 h after the end of dialysis when the reticuloendothelial system releases free heparin from the protamine-heparin complex back into the circulation.

25.4.3.2 Regional Citrate Anticoagulation (RCA)

Since its first description by Mehta et al. [18] in the early 1990s, RCA has replaced heparin anticoagulation, especially during CRRT, at many centers in developed countries. RCA has repeatedly been reported to be associated with the lowest risk of bleeding complications and comparable or better circuit survival compared to heparin [19]. However, the perceived complexity of RCA and the resultant lack of experience with its use have unfortunately prompted many nephrologists to avoid using RCA.

Citrate acts as an anticoagulant by chelating ionized calcium (iCa), an essential co-factor of several steps in the clotting cascade. Accordingly, this property of citrate has been used by blood banks for storing blood since the early 1900s. During RCA, anticoagulation is limited to the extracorporeal circuit by infusing the citrate solution into the arterial limb of the circuit, while systemic anticoagulation is avoided by restoring iCa in the systemic circulation by infusing a calcium solution through (preferably) a separate central line. Despite the simplicity of this basic principle, the availability of numerous protocols with variations in the concentration of citrate solutions and rates of infusion has caused unnecessary confusion for novice users.

A basic understanding of the practical chemical facts that are at the core of citrate anticoagulation can help the reader use any of the previously described protocols or make one of their own based on the local availability of citrate and calcium solutions. However, it is strongly suggested that a uniform protocol be established for each center, making sure that all of the team members are familiar with it, thus avoiding unnecessary complications.

Citrate works as an effective anticoagulant when the iCa is decreased to <0.5 mmol/L. As there is a dose-effect relationship, a citrate level of 4–6 mmol/L is consistently associated with an iCa of <0.5 mmol/L. This level is easily achieved in the extracorporeal circuit by infusing 3–4 mmol of citrate for every liter of blood flow. It is important to note that 1–2 mmol/L of citrate is already present in the patient's blood entering the extracorporeal circuit, a result of the unmetabolized citrate fraction which increases from <0.15 mmol/L (pre-RCA initiation) to an average of 1–2 mmol/L in the systemic circulation during RCA anticoagulation. The variations in citrate protocols such as flow rate in mL/h for any citrate solution depend on the composition and concentration of citrate solution. The various citrate solutions reported in the literature are either customized, hospital pharmacy formulated, or commercially available. Examples of different solutions with their associated citrate concentrations and projected flow rates are provided in Table 25.1. Replacement fluids containing low concentrations of citrate are commercially available, thus avoiding the need for a separate citrate infusion. These products have been used in adult patients. Detailed discussion of these fluids is beyond the scope of this chapter.

Approximately 20–30% of the calcium citrate complex is lost in the effluent with the standard 2 L/h/1.73 m^2 clearance with CRRT without any difference between convective or diffusive clearance techniques [21]. The unfiltered portion of the calcium citrate complex enters the systemic circulation, and the majority of it is metabolized primarily by the liver, with additional contributions by the kidney and skeletal muscle. One millimole of citrate is converted to 3 mmol of bicarbonate that can result in alkalosis (*vide infra*). The calcium that is released from the calcium citrate complex enters the systemic circulation, but additional calcium is required to replenish the calcium that is lost as part of the calcium citrate complex in the effluent.

The calcium that is infused during CRRT can be either calcium chloride or calcium gluconate and preferably should be infused through a separate central line to avoid thrombosis of the venous limb of the dialysis catheter; the third lumen of a triple lumen catheter can be used in the situation where a separate line is not available. The usual amount of calcium required to achieve a systemic iCa of 1.0–1.2 mmol/L is 0.15–0.3 mmol for every mmol of infused citrate.

Calcium-free replacement and dialysis fluids are used during RCA to prevent chelation of a portion of the infused citrate that will lead to a higher citrate

Table 25.1 Composition of various citrate solutions and projected infusion rate per liter of blood flow rate

Citrate solution	Trisodium citrate (mmol/L)	Citric acid (mmol/L)	Sodium (mmol/L)	Glucose (mmol/L)	Projected flow rate[a] mL/L of blood
4% Tri-Na citrate	136	0	408	0	20
2% Tri-Na citrate[b]	68	0	204	138	40
ACD-A	75	38	224	124	25
Prismocitrate® 10/2[c]	10	2	136	0	233
Prismocitrate® 18/0[c]	18	0	140	0	156

[a]Approximate citrate solution flow rate for every L of blood flow to achieve citrate concentration of 4–6 mmol/L in extracorporeal circuit
[b]Two percent trisodium citrate was made by 1:1 dilution with 5% dextrose [20]
[c]Prismocitrate® is a commercially produced citrate solution used as prefilter replacement fluid (it is currently not available in the United States)

Table 25.2 Standard citrate and calcium titration protocol

Circuit iCa level (mmol/L)	Change in citrate (ACD) infusion rate	Systemic iCa level (mmol/L)	Change in calcium infusion rate
<0.25	↓ by 10 mL/h	>1.2	↓ by 5 mL/h
0.25–0.5	No change	1.0–1.2	No change
>0.5	↑ by 10 mL/h	0.9–1.0	↑ by 5 mL/h
		<0.9	↑ by 10 mL/h

The changes shown in the table are for acid citrate dextrose (ACD) and 0.8% calcium chloride solution
The rate of change should be lower when absolute rates of citrate or calcium infusion are low when dialyzing infants or toddlers
The suggested degree of change will differ for citrate and calcium solutions based on the solution concentration and will be different for another calcium salt such as gluconate

requirement. Calcium is also removed from any intravenous fluids and/or total parenteral nutrition to avoid interference with the calcium infusion protocol. Supplemental phosphate is added to the replacement fluid and dialysis bags, and the sodium and bicarbonate content of the fluids is adjusted as required (*vide infra*).

While using RCA, systemic and circuit (post-filter) iCa are checked within 30–60 min of therapy initiation, change in citrate or calcium infusion rate, and every 30–60 min thereafter until they are in the desired range; systemic 1.0–1.2 and circuit <0.5 mmol/L (preferably ≤0.4). Once in the desired range, the iCa levels are checked every 6 h. The iCa level is also checked more frequently if the patient receives blood products or there are early signs of filter clotting such as increasing transmembrane pressure or filter pressure drop. The titration protocol that we use is provided in Table 25.2.

25.5 RCA-Associated Complications

RCA can be associated with several metabolic complications that need to be monitored closely. Hypo- and hypercalcemia are avoided by titration of citrate and calcium infusion rates as shown in Table 25.2. As reversal of access and return lines during dialysis therapy is not uncommon to maintain treatment efficacy, attention to the route of citrate infusion is critical. Failure to switch the citrate infusion line simultaneously during line reversal can result in systemic (vs. regional) citrate infusion with life-threatening hypocalcemia. In situations when CRRT is interrupted either due to clotting or because the patient is taken off therapy for another medical procedure (e.g., visit to radiology or operating room) and the citrate infusion has been discontinued, failure to modify or discontinue the calcium infusion can result in hypercalcemia. Although citrate has a higher affinity for calcium, it can also bind other divalent cations such as magnesium and lead to a decrease in the ionized magnesium level. Magnesium levels therefore should be monitored at least once daily.

As sodium citrate metabolism results in the production of three mmols of bicarbonate per mmol of citrate, alkalosis is a common complication associated with RCA. The risk of alkalosis is increased in patients who receive frequent blood products because of the extra citrate load they receive from the blood products. This can be avoided by using low-bicarbonate (22 mEq/L instead of regular 32 mEq/L) replacement and dialysis fluids. The incidence of alkalosis is reduced when a portion of total citrate comes from citric acid as in an acid citrate dextrose (ACD) solution. In addition, alkalosis is more common in patients who are also receiving mechanical ventilation as respiratory compensation for the alkalosis is not possible.

Trisodium citrate also has a very high sodium content (Table 25.1) and a concentrated solution such as 4% TSC can result in hypernatremia requiring adjustment of the sodium content in both the replacement and dialysis fluids.

Finally, citrate metabolism can be significantly reduced in patients with severe liver failure or mitochondrial dysfunction leading to progressive citrate accumulation. While citrate itself is not toxic, the metabolic consequences resulting from this can be life-threatening. This condition is commonly labeled as "citrate lock" and is characterized by an increasing requirement for the systemic calcium infusion to maintain a normal iCa, while the total serum calcium is elevated. This occurs because the total serum calcium measurement includes the calcium that is bound to citrate. As a result, the ratio of total to iCa increases; a ratio of >2.5 is diagnostic of citrate lock [22]. In addition, these patients develop an increased anion gap acidosis as citrate is an "unmeasured anion." Young infants and children are at greatest risk for citrate lock since they have the highest blood flow rates on a per kilogram basis and the citrate infusion is directly proportional to the blood flow rate (Table 25.3). Citrate lock can be managed by one or more of the following interventions:

1. Decreasing the blood flow rate (if possible), thereby decreasing the citrate infusion
2. Decreasing the citrate infusion rate and accepting a slightly higher circuit iCa level (e.g., 0.45 instead of 0.35 mmol/L)
3. Increasing the dialysis and/or convective clearance (usually by 50%) to increase citrate losses
4. Replacing the bicarbonate containing dialysate with 0.9% saline and adjusting the dialysate rate based on degree of alkalosis
5. Holding citrate infusion until systemic iCa is >1.0 mmol/L and then reinitiating the citrate infusion at 50–70% of the initial rate

Table 25.3 Comparison of citrate load exposure for a child and an adult

	10 kg child	80 kg adult
Blood flow (mL/min)	50 (5 mL/kg)	180 (2.3 mL/kg)
ACD infusion rate (mL/h)[a]	75 (7.5 mL/kg)	270 (3.4 mL/kg)

[a]The citrate infusion rate is proportional to blood flow rate. The typical ACD infusion rate (mL/h) is 1.5 * blood flow rate (mL/min); see text under section 25.5 for details

25.6 RCA Protocol Used at Author's Center

The citrate anticoagulation protocol utilized at our center is described below. The authors have used this protocol for nearly 20 years with excellent efficacy and without any major complications.

Commercially available ACD-A solution (Baxter Healthcare Corp., Deerfield, IL) is used for the citrate infusion. This solution contains 113 mmol/L of citrate with one-third of the citrate from citric acid (Table 25.1). This solution is infused into the arterial limb of the vascular access by way of a three-way stopcock placed as close to the patient (proximal) as possible. The ACD solution is infused at a rate in mL/h which is 1.5 times the blood flow rate measured as mL/min (see the example below). A citrate infusion at this rate provides 2.8 mmol of citrate for every liter of blood flow and results in an extracorporeal circuit citrate level between 4–6 mmol/L with a resultant iCa of <0.5 mmol/L. CRRT clearance (CVVH, CVVHD, or CVVHDF) is provided at a rate of 2 L/h/1.73m^2.

The calcium infusion is a 0.8% calcium chloride solution that contains 54 mmol/L of calcium. This solution is infused into a separate central line at one-third the rate of the ACD infusion and provides ~0.2 mmol of calcium for every mmol of citrate infusion and maintains the systemic iCa between 1.0 and 1.2 mmol/L. The CRRT replacement fluid and the dialysate are calcium-free, and calcium is also removed from other parenteral fluids including TPN. The bicarbonate concentration of the replacement and dialysis fluids is based on the patient's acid-base status, and phosphate (as potassium or sodium salt) is usually added to both the replacement fluid and the dialysate to maintain a normal serum phosphorus level.

Example Typical CRRT prescription with RCA for a 6-year-old boy (weight 21 kg, height 110 cm, BSA 0.8 m^2). Blood flow, 100 mL/min (~5 mL/kg/min); clearance, 900 mL/h (~2 L/h/1.73 m^2). ACD infusion rate 150 mL/h (1.5 * blood flow rate in mL/min) and $CaCl_2$ infusion rate of 50 mL/h (one-third of the ACD infusion rate)

Key Points

1. CRRT has become a frequently used dialysis modality for the management of critically ill patients with acute kidney injury.
2. While anticoagulation-free extracorporeal therapy is feasible, the majority of patients require some form of anticoagulation for uninterrupted and efficient dialysis therapy.
3. Regional anticoagulation is preferred when systemic anticoagulation is likely to lead to bleeding complications.
4. Regional citrate anticoagulation (RCA) has become one of the most popular approaches to anticoagulation therapy in children receiving CRRT.
5. A uniform center-specific protocol for RCA that is followed consistently is highly desirable to achieve success and avoid complications.

References

1. Kaddourah A, Basu RK, Bagshaw SM, Goldstein SL, for the AWARE Investigators. Epidemiology of acute kidney injury in critically ill children and young adults. NEJM. 2017;376:11–20.
2. Sethi SK, Sinha R, Jha P, et al. Feasibility of sustained low efficiency dialysis in critically sick pediatric patients: a multicentric retrospective study. Hemodial Int. 2018;22(20):228–34.
3. Tan HK, Baldwin I, Bellomo R. Continuous veno-venous hemofiltration without anticoagulation in high-risk patients. Intensive Care Med. 2000;26:1652–7.
4. The VA/NIH Acute Renal Failure Trial Network. Intensity of renal support in critically ill patients with acute kidney injury. NEJM. 2008;26:1652–7.
5. van de Wetering J, Westendrop RG, ven der Hoeven JG, et al. Heparin use in continuous renal replacement procedures: the struggle between filter coagulation and patient hemorrhage. J Am Soc Nephrol. 1996;7:145–50.
6. Oudemans-Van Straaten HM, Wester JP, et al. Anticoagulation strategies in continuous renal replacement therapy: can the choice be evidence based? Intensive Care Med. 2006;32:188–202.
7. Ward DM, Mehta RL. Extracorporeal management of acute renal failure patients at high-risk of bleeding. Kidney Int. 1993;43(Suppl 41):237–44.
8. Maher JF, Lapierre L, Schreiner GE, et al. Regional heparinization for hemodialysis. N Engl J Med. 1963;268:451.
9. Uchino S, Fealy N, Baldwin I, et al. Continuous venovenous hemofiltration without anticoagulation. ASAIO J. 2004;50:76–80.
10. Gattas DJ, Rajbhandari D, Bradford C, et al. A randomized controlled trial of regional citrate versus regional heparin anticoagulation for continuous renal replacement therapy in critically ill adults. Crit Care Med. 2015;43(8):1622–9.
11. Hetzel GR, Sucker C. The heparins: all a nephrologist should know. Nephrol Dial Transplant. 2005;20:2036–42.
12. Schrader J, Stibbe W, Kandt M, et al. Low molecular weight heparin versus standard heparin. A long-term study in hemodialysis and hemofiltration patients. ASAIO Trans. 1990;36:28–32.
13. Murray PT, Reddy BV, Grossman EJ, et al. A prospective comparison of three argatroban treatment regimens during hemodialysis in end-stage renal disease. Kidney Int. 2004;66:2446.
14. Link A, Girndt M, Selejan S, et al. Argatroban for anticoagulation in continuous renal replacement therapy. Crit Care Med. 2009;37:105.
15. Kiser TH, MacLaren R, Fish DN, et al. Bivalirudin versus unfractionated heparin for prevention of hemofilter occlusion during continuous renal replacement therapy. Pharmacotherapy. 2010;30:1117.
16. Langenecker SA, Felfernig M, Werba A, et al. Anticoagulation with prostacyclin and heparin during continuous venovenous hemofiltration. Crit Care Med. 1994;22:1774.
17. Nakae H, Tajimi K. Pharmacokinetics of nafamostat mesilate during continuous hemodiafiltration with a polyacrylonitrile membrane. Ther Apher Dial. 2003;7:483.
18. Mehta RL, McDonald BR, Aguilar MM, et al. Regional citrate anticoagulation for continuous arteriovenous hemodialysis in critically ill patients. Kidney Int. 1990;38:976–81.
19. Bai M, Zhou M, He L, et al. Citrate versus heparin anticoagulation for continuous renal replacement therapy: an updated meta-analysis of RCTs. Intensive Care Med. 2015;41:2098.
20. Tolwani AJ, Campbell RC, Schenk MB, et al. Simplified citrate anticoagulation for continuous renal replacement therapy. Kidney Int. 2001;60:370–4.
21. Chadha V, Garg U, Warady BA, et al. Citrate clearance in children receiving continuous venovenous replacement therapy. Pediatr Nephrol. 2002;17:819–24.
22. Meier-Kriesche HU, Gitomer J, Finkel K, et al. Increased total to ionized calcium ratio during continuous venovenous hemodialysis with regional citrate anticoagulation. Crit Care Med. 2001;29:748–52.

Toxic Nephropathy: Uric Acid, Rhabdomyolysis, and Tumor Lysis Syndrome

26

Timothy E. Bunchman

In this chapter we will discuss the relative risk of toxic (pigment) nephropathy in certain disease states. We will discuss the specific complication associated with uric acid, rhabdomyolysis, as well as that associated with tumor lysis syndrome. This section will also discuss the relative approaches to prevention and intervention if necessary.

26.1 Uric Acid

Uric acid is the end product of purine degradations and is excreted via the kidney. Decades ago uric acid was a hot topic in nephrology that has gone away. In the last decade though emerging data on uric acid has a complication of chronic renal disease (CKD) and involved in acute renal failure (AKI) has emerged [1, 2].

Uric acid is seen in a number of states but usually as part of tumor lysis syndrome. In the setting of massive tissue destruction, uric acid may result in AKI that in turn causes worsening of AKI. The hematology-oncology literature has demonstrated an improvement in renal function with the use of uric acid-lowering agents (in the setting of elevated uric acid and malignancy), and perhaps this date could be used in other disease states [3].

In patients with tumor lysis syndrome (TLS) where there is a risk for elevated uric acid, often the drug allopurinol has been used to help lower the uric acid. Allopurinol has shown to decrease uric acid but increase the risk of xanthine stones. Allopurinol may take days to be effective. In a study, allopurinol was compared to rasburicase as an intervention in patients at risk for uric acid nephropathy. What is

T. E. Bunchman (✉)
Children's Hospital of Richmond at Virginia Commonwealth University, Richmond, VA, USA
e-mail: timothy.bunchman@vcuhealth.org

S. K. Sethi et al. (eds.), *Critical Care Pediatric Nephrology and Dialysis: A Practical Handbook*, https://doi.org/10.1007/978-981-13-2276-1_26

demonstrated is that rasburicase will diminish the uric acid immediately, whereas the allopurinol may take days [3]. Therefore this is considered the standard occur in the Pediatric hematology-oncology literature that if someone is at risk for uric acid nephropathy to prevent of AKI. In these studies, those leukemic children who received rasburicase had a lower serum creatinine when compared to those who received allopurinol.

Work by Hobbs and colleagues demonstrated use of rasburicase in neonatal AKI [4]. These children had AKI secondary to a hypoxia ischemia event in the newborn period. In this small series of infants with a mean creatinine 3.1 mg/dL with an average uric acid of 13 mg/dL, rasburicase was given as a single dose (0.2 mg/kg/dose × 1). Within 24 h of rasburicase treatment, the uric acid decreased from an average of 13 mg/dL down to 0.9 mg/dL, and the creatinine improved from an average of 3.1 mg/dL down to 2 mg/dL. None of these infants require renal replacement therapy (RRT) during this period of time.

Other studies have demonstrated in single-case series the same outcome, but also deaths have been associated with the use of rasburicase. In the setting of patients with G6PD deficiency, the use of rasburicase has resulted in acute hemolysis and death. Therefore if one will intervene with uric acid with the use of rasburicase, then screening for G6PD would be in order.

Uric acid elevation is also seen in volume depletion and CKD. The treatment of volume depletion correct elevation of urinc acid. In cases of adequate volume repletion with persistent elevation of uric acid, the use of a uric acid-lowering agent should be considered.

The CKIDs study demonstrated that uric acid is elevated in CKD, and our center (personal communication from Dr. Cristin Kaspar) has demonstrated uric acid elevation in sickle cell disease [2]. The use of uric acid-lowering agents in these disease states effecting outcome are in process.

Lastly many medications may elevate uric acid including most diuretics, calcineurin inhibitors, and some antihypertensive (e.g., ACE inhibitors), while others such as ARBs (specifically Losartan) may lower uric acid in some conditions. The latter findings are best seen in patients with metabolic syndrome that is associated with elevated uric acid and hypertension that when the uric acid is lowered in some (but not all), the hypertension improves [5].

26.2 Rhabdomyolysis

Rhabdomyolysis can occur from crush injury, compartment syndromes, underlying myopathies, burns, and vasculitis as well as from a number of (usually viral) infections [6]. Rhabdomyolysis can result in pigment nephropathy causing AKI. The pigment (free myoglobin) nephropathy then causes a disruption of tubular integrity and a decrease in GFR [7]. This rhabdomyolysis can result in myoglobinuria (as seen clinically as gross hematuria) as a sign and symptom that a patient will seek out. They often will see pink-colored urine or blood in urine that shows positivity for urine dipstick for blood, yet no red cells are seen.

The treatment of rhabdomyolysis is to remove the offending cause while avoiding other potential nephrotoxins (e.g., NSAIDs). In situations of crush injury, burns, viral illness, or compartment syndromes, avoidance or treatment of the underlying cause may be obvious, but in the cases of mitochondrial diseases, then the intervention with a "mitochondrial cocktail" may be in order.

Regardless of the etiology, the first treatment of choice for AKI prevention from rhabdomyolysis is hydration. Studies using bicarbonate as well as other scavenger medications including mannitol have not been found to be superior to its normal saline alone [8]. The difficulty with continuous saline infusion of these patients is the acidosis that will occur because of chloride excess. Therefore it is not unusual that bicarbonate is added to quarter normal and half normal and the intravenous fluids are given at least twice maintenance in order to "flush out the kidneys" to prevent toxin nephropathy. The use of IV bicarbonate can be a problem because it can lower the calcium and potassium level causing complications due to electrolyte imbalance. Therefore if bicarbonate is necessary, then monitoring calcium (ionized) and potassium levels is needed.

If loss of kidney function occurs, then intervention with renal replacement therapy (RRT) may be in order. The RRT will not effectively remove the myoglobin because the myoglobin in a large molecular, large protein substance that is poorly cleared either in convection or diffusive mode of RRT [9]. Therefore the use of RRT is to support the physiological consequence of the rhabdomyolysis-induced AKI until recovery of renal function should be considered. When these patients recover renal function, there may be a residual mild tubulopathy that may take weeks to fully resolve. The rhabdomyolysis in the sports injury which can occur often in the fall during the preseason for football and other tryouts often exacerbated by the use of NSAIDs, therefor avoiding these and other potentially nephrotoxic drugs should be considered.

26.3 Tumor Lysis Syndrome

Tumor lysis syndrome (TLS) is often associated with B-cell lymphoma or leukemia. At the initiation of chemotherapy, rapid lysis of the cells could occur [10]. This can result in elevated uric acid, elevated potassium, elevated or diminished calcium, as well as elevated phosphorus. This can cause AKI due to hemolyzed cells deposited in the kidney (often uric acid) with perturbation of electrolytes. Tumor lysis syndrome patients are at risk if they have a tumor that is very responsive to chemotherapy with a large tumor load. This can be demonstrated by an elevated white count with or without organomegaly. Many programs track the lactate dehydrogenase (LDH) during the acute time of chemotherapy to use as a marker of tissue destruction.

The use of high fluid intake may minimize the AKI risk and abnormal electrolyte risk seen in tumor lysis syndrome. The use of rasburicase, as noted in the uric acid section, may result in a rapid decrease in the uric acid lessening the risk of TLS nephropathy. The use of rasburicase will not change potassium, phosphorus, or calcium but may improve renal function which may improve electrolyte excretion.

Therefore the use of high fluid intake to cause electrolyte wasting with or without the use of rasburicase is considered common practice.

The use of potassium and phosphorus restricted diet in patients at risk may be in order, but the major source of the potassium and phosphorous is not the diet but is the tumor so the impact of oral restriction would be minimal.

The use of potassium binders (e.g., Kayexalate) is considered, but these meds have been associated with bowel necrosis; therefore use should be minimalized [11]. Use of phosphonate binders using calcium carbonate or aluminum hydroxide has been ordered. Aluminum hydroxide is contraindicated with elevated phosphorus in end-stage renal disease and in CKD because of the absorption and then the deposition of aluminum in the bone as well as the brain [12]. Therefore the long-term use of aluminum hydroxide should not be considered as a frontline drug.

Calcium can be rapidly lowered due to acute hyperphosphatemia but also can be raised due to the TLS itself. Therefore attention to the ionized calcium during this high-risk time should be considered.

Those patients at risk of complications of severe tissue breakdown associated with chemotherapy with TLS should be considered for early intervention of RRT. The choice or RRT should be decided in part by the duration of anticipated TLS. Whether it hemodialysis (HD) or peritoneal dialysis or SLED or continuous renal replacement therapy (CRRT) is a style of practice [13]. CRRT is often reserve for patients with hemodynamic instability. The use of peritoneal dialysis is probably the least favorable because PD is the least efficient form of RRT. Hemodialysis and SLED are short timed treatment options and are very effective for the time that the child is on therapy, but once discontinued, and if the TLS is ongoing, reinstitution of HD or SLED would be needed. Therefore in the majority of the time, the use of CRRT is the preferred modality of RRT due to the continuous clearance of solute that it provides [14].

If RRT is utilized at the time of chemotherapy, this question often arises: Does the RRT itself remove the chemotherapy agents limiting the effectiveness of the chemotherapy? This is best analyzed based on the molecular weight and the protein binding of these drugs. Small-molecular-weight and low protein-binding medications are easily cleared on most forms of RRT. Often one will have to look at the impact of tissue breakdown as a true indicator of whether the drugs have been removed or not.

The dialysate bath in TLS needs to be low to no potassium initially until one can assess the true risk of hyperkalemia from the tumor burden itself.

RRT could be used in the absence of AKI (due to concern of high tumor burden) and in this case would be seen as an adjunct to the native renal function. It can also be used associated with AKI, in this case replacing native renal function. Regardless of the native renal function, frequent monitoring of calcium, phosphorous, potassium, and uric acid levels is in order.

In essence uric acid, rhabdomyolysis, and complications of TLS all result in the classic form of toxic (pigment) nephropathy. The first therapy of choice to remove offending cause, the next therapy choices hydration, the use of uric acid-lowering agents and RRT may be needed. This author would use this order to assess and minimize or treat AKI (Table 26.1).

Table 26.1 Algorithm of treatment of toxic nephropathies

Uric acid
Evaluation for etiology
Consider volume expansion unless contraindicated
Remove medications that may be nephrotoxic
Remove medications that may promote elevation of uric acid
Consider use of uric acid-lowering agent (e.g., allopurinol, rasburicase)
Rhabdomyolysis
Evaluation for etiology
Consider volume expansion unless contraindicated
Remove medications that may be nephrotoxic
Consider
1. Metabolic cocktail use (e.g., coenzyme Q, B complex vitamins, carnitine) if mitochondrial disease exists
2. Fasciotomy if compartment syndrome is present
3. Treatment of viral or bacterial if that is the etiology
4. Dialysis is indicated if conditions of solute excess, fluid overload, or inadequate "room" for nutrition or medication exist
Tumor lysis syndrome
Evaluation for etiology
Consider volume expansion unless contraindicated
Remove medications that may be nephrotoxic
Remove medications that may promote elevation of uric acid
Consider use of uric acid-lowering agent (e.g., allopurinol, rasburicase)
Cytopheresis with or without dialysis should be considered if WBC > 100,000
Dialysis should be considered early if evidence of
1. Excessive solute (e.g., potassium) levels that cannot be medically managed
2. Large tumor load with high risk of rapid lysis as determined by total white blood count, LDH, and organomegaly

References

1. Tsuji T, Ohishi K, Takeda A, et al. The impact of serum uric acid reduction on renal function and blood pressure in chronic kidney disease patients with hyperuricemia. Clin Exp Neprhol. 2018. https://doi.org/10.1007/s10157-018-1580-4.
2. Xu X, Hu J, Song N, et al. Hyperuricemia increases the risk of acute kidney injury: a systematic review and meta-analysis. BMC Nephrol. 2017;18:27.
3. Goldman SC, Holcenberg JS, Finklestein JZ, et al. A randomized comparison between rasburicase and allopurinol in children with lymphoma or leukemia at high risk for tumor lysis. Blood. 2001;97:2998–3003.
4. Hobbs DJ, Steinke J, Chung J, et al. Rasburicase improves hyperuricemia in infants with acute kidney injury. Pediatr Nephrol. 2010;25:305–9.
5. Feig DI. Serum uric acid and the risk of hypertension and chronic kidney disease. Curr Opin Rheumatol. 2014;26(2):176–85.
6. Al-Ismaili Z, Piccioni M, Zappitelli M. Rhabdomyolysis: pathogenesis of renal injury and management. Pediatr Nephrol. 2011;26:1781–8.
7. Mannix R, Tan ML, Wright R, et al. Acute pediatric rhabdomyolysis: cause and rates of renal failure. Pediatrics. 2006;118:2119–25.

8. Eneas JF, Schoenfeld PY, Humphreys MH. The effect of infusion of mannitol-sodium bicarbonate on the clinical course of myoglobinuria. Arch Intern Med. 1979;139:801–5.
9. Naka T, Jones D, Baldwin I, et al. Myoglobin clearance by super high-flux hemofiltration in a case of severe rhabdomyolysis: a case report. Crit Care. 2005;9:R90–5.
10. Prusakowski MK, Cannone D. Pediatric oncologic emergencies. Hematol Oncol Clin N Am. 2017;31:959–80.
11. Nguyen T, Ondrik D, Zhufyak O, et al. Hyperkalemia and potential pitfalls of sodium polystyrene sulfonate. JAAPA. 2015;28(3):41–5.
12. Bakir AA. The fatal interplay of aluminum and citrate in chronic renal failure: a lesson from three decades ago. Artif Organs. 2015;39(2):87–9.
13. Sinha R, Sethi SK, Bunchman T, et al. Prolonged intermittent renal replacement therapy in children. Pediatr Nephrol. 2018;33(8):1283–96.
14. Sakarcan A, Quigley R. Hyperphosphatemia in tumor lysis syndrome: the role of hemodialysis and continuous veno-venous hemofiltration. Pediatr Nephrol. 1994;8(3):351–3.

Part V

Outcomes

27 Outcomes of Pediatric Acute Kidney Injury

Hui-Kim Yap and Lourdes Paula R. Resontoc

27.1 Case

JJ is the first child of non-consanguineous parents. He was born full term to a 26-year-old mother via normal delivery with birth weight of 3.10 kg. His APGAR scores were 8 and 9 at 1 and 5 min respectively. At birth he had features of Down syndrome which was confirmed by karyotyping (trisomy 21). He had episodes of non-bilious vomiting since birth and was admitted to the neonatal intensive care unit for further work-up. He was sent home allegedly well. After discharge, he had episodes of recurrent non-bilious vomiting. At 8 months of age, he was hospitalized for severe dehydration secondary to intractable vomiting secondary to duodenal stenosis and complicated by poor urine output, rising creatinine to a peak of 201 μmol/L, hyponatremia, and hypokalemia. Following rehydration, his renal function slowly recovered over the course of 1 week, improving to a baseline of 40 μmol/L. However, on follow-up over the next 10 years, JJ was noted to have intermittently raised creatinine to 128 μmol/L during febrile illnesses. With rehydration, his creatinine returned to a baseline of 46 μmol/L or estimated glomerular filtration rate of 70 mL/min/1.73m^2. In addition, he was noted to have renal tubular acidosis type 2 which required supplementation with sodium citrate to maintain the serum bicarbonate above 20 mmol/L. At the age of 10 years, he developed mild proteinuria of 0.06 g/mmol and was started on treatment with losartan. His estimated glomerular filtration rate also showed a decline to 56 mL/min/1.73m^2, accompanied by mild

H.-K. Yap (✉) · L. P. R. Resontoc
Department of Paediatrics, Yong Loo Lin School of Medicine, National University of Singapore, Singapore, Singapore

Khoo Teck Puat-National University Children's Medical Institute, National University Health System, Singapore, Singapore
e-mail: hui_kim_yap@nuhs.edu.sg

S. K. Sethi et al. (eds.), *Critical Care Pediatric Nephrology and Dialysis: A Practical Handbook*, https://doi.org/10.1007/978-981-13-2276-1_27

hyperparathyroidism with serum intact parathyroid hormone levels ranging between 10 and 17 pmol/L.

27.2 Introduction

Acute kidney injury (AKI) was earlier thought of as transient, often reversible and therefore full recovery as the endpoint. However, epidemiologic evidence point out that proteinuria, hypertension, chronic kidney disease (CKD), and end-stage kidney disease (ESKD) have been observed to occur years after the acute insult among adult and pediatric survivors of AKI. In addition, cardiovascular events are higher among adult survivors of AKI compared to those who had no AKI. This excess mortality risk had been shown to persist months to years after hospital discharge especially in those who had a severe and prolonged AKI episode requiring various renal replacement therapies (RRT).

Long-term studies on the outcome of AKI among adult and pediatric patients have been categorized into community- or hospital-acquired AKI. Community-acquired AKI (CA-AKI) is defined as a condition which involves patients presenting to the hospital with reduced urine output and/or glomerular filtration rate [1]. Hospital-acquired AKI (HA-AKI) is considered when AKI occurs within 48 h of hospital stay. HA-AKI has been shown to have a more ominous outcome, while CA-AKI has a much better prognosis. In pediatric patients, severity and duration of AKI, the presence of existing CKD and other comorbidities such as congenital heart disease and hematological and oncological problems, and those who required renal replacement therapies (RRT) during the acute stage have been identified to play a role in the long-term sequelae of AKI. Table 27.1 summarizes the studies that described the long-term outcomes following an episode of pediatric AKI.

27.3 Patient Survival

Geographical, etiological, cultural, and socioeconomic differences account for variations in short- and long-term survival outcomes for community-acquired AKI (CA-AKI) and hospital-acquired AKI (HA-AKI). CA-AKI etiologies from the developing countries include diarrhea secondary to preventable infectious etiologies, post-infectious glomerulonephritis, leptospirosis, tetanus and malaria, ingestion of toxic herbs or chemicals, envenomations, and obstetric complications [2–4]. In developed countries, CA-AKI have been reported to occur among children and adolescents with pre-existing CKD, in those with congenital anomalies, and with exposure to nephrotoxic agents, malignancies, recent hospitalizations, and cardiac diseases [5]. Limitations in availability, accessibility, and affordability of therapeutic options contribute to the high burden of morbidity and mortality in children after an episode of AKI in low-income regions. For instance, infectious diarrhea that initially causes volume-responsive AKI can lead to full recovery if treated promptly. However, in patients who present late in the course of the disease, it can

Table 27.1 Long-term outcomes of pediatric acute kidney injury (AKI)

Author/year	Aki definition	No. of patients with AKI	No. of patients with follow-up	Follow-up (mean) (years)	Outcomes (n)[a]				
					Mortality	Abnormal GFR	ESKD	Proteinuria	Hypertension
Sinha et al. 2009 [4]	Acute rise of SCr ≥2× the upper limit of normal range for age and sex	37	16	10	35	5	1	3	3
Garg et al. 2003 [13]	Patients who had diarrhea associated HUS	3476	3476	4.4	0–23% (pooled average: 9%)	0–64% (pooled average: 25%)	0–17% (pooled average: 3%)	0–40 (pooled average: 15%)	0–26 (pooled average: 10%)
Greenberg et al. 2014 [15]	Six different definitions of AKI	346	346	2–16 (6.5)	9–68 (in-hospital) 3.7 per 100 person years (long-term)	6.3 per 100 person years	0.9 per 100 person years	3.1 per 100 person years	1.4 per 100 person years
Scharer et al. 1999 [17]	GFR was determined by single-injection ^{51}chromium EDTA clearance or inulin clearance, taking 40 mL/min/1.73 m^2 as the upper limit for the definition of renal failure	17	17	1–23	1	3	9	4	4
Abitbol et al. 2003 [20]	(SCr) >176.8 μmol/l) >48 h and/or oliguria <0.5 mL/kg/h urine flow for >24 h during the neonatal course after the third day of life	20	20	18 (3)	49	8	4	9	2
Askenazi et al. 2006 [22]	eGFR <75 mL/min/1.73 m^2	174	29	3–5	20	14	9	28	21

SCr serum creatinine, *HUS* hemolytic uremic syndrome, *eGFR* estimated glomerular filtration rate

[a]Expressed as absolute number unless otherwise stated as % and/or per 100 person years

subsequently evolve into severe acute tubular necrosis requiring renal replacement therapy (RRT), with a higher chance of dying during the acute course of RRT or subsequently developing ESKD in the long term. In developing countries, envenomations have a high mortality rate of more than 50% during the acute stage, with progression to ESKD in the survivors because of late presentation and late initiation of antivenom therapy [4, 6]. Cultural and socioeconomic discrimination in countries with big gender inequities leads to high mortality from obstetric complications such as septic abortion and puerperal sepsis associated with AKI, seen also in adolescent girls due to early age of marriage, conditions that are rarely observed among developed countries that do not espouse gender discrimination.

Data on pediatric HA-AKI are mostly centered around critically ill patients or from some specific sub-groups of medical and surgical patients such as patients with congenital heart disease who had undergone surgical repair or following bone marrow transplantation. AKI is a frequent complication of critically ill pediatric patients admitted to the neonatal and pediatric intensive care unit. In this subset of patients, HA-AKI usually occurs as part of multi-organ involvement, often following surgical or diagnostic interventions or iatrogenic factors. AKI often develops in critically sick children as a result of systemic illness or its treatment and not from primary kidney etiology [7]. Studies in both adult and pediatric populations have shown that mortality for HA-AKI in the acute setting is high compared to CA-AKI. Moreover, HA-AKI is an independent risk factor for death and prolonged hospital stay [8–10].

With regard to long-term data on mortality, studies in adult patients revealed that among those who sustained in-hospital AKI, 34% died in hospital, and 42% were dead at 90 days and 48% at 1 year post discharge, compared to 12% 1-year mortality in patients without AKI [11]. The mortality rate in HA-AKI remained high in the years after hospital discharge, and even when the AKI is mild, it is a well-known contributor to increased mortality and morbidity in hospitalized patients compared to the general population [12–14]. Although pediatric patients do not have similar comorbidities that may influence long-term mortality as seen in adult cohorts, Askenazi et al. described a cohort of pediatric survivors of AKI followed up for 3–5 years and found patient survival to be 56.8%, with the majority of deaths occurring within 2 years after the AKI episode.

27.4 Renal Survival

Three patterns have been described by which patients with AKI who have normal baseline kidney function might progress to CKD. Firstly, the initial insult to the kidney can result in permanent kidney failure, and the patient remains dependent on dialysis (AKI to ESKD). Secondly, the initial episode of AKI may lead to incomplete recovery resulting in CKD (AKI to CKD). Lastly, the kidney function initially returns close to baseline after AKI, and later the patient progresses to CKD (AKI to "subclinical CKD") [7]. A systematic review and meta-analysis among pediatric patients following an episode of AKI demonstrated a threefold higher risk of developing proteinuria, almost twofold risk of hypertension, and eightfold risk of de novo CKD and ESKD [15]. In a similar meta-analysis among adult survivors of AKI, the long-term risk for CKD and ESRD is eightfold higher than patients without AKI [12]. Studies revealed that the presence of normal glomerular and tubular functions after hospital discharge is not an indication of permanent full renal recovery. Survivors of AKI during and after cardiac surgery, those with hemolytic uremic syndrome and Henoch-Schonlein purpura nephritis, and preterm neonates have been shown to have long-term renal injury [16–20]. An important observation among preterms revealed that progressive renal disease was not due to loss of renal mass (as a consequence of prematurity) or nephrocalcinosis (from diuretic use) but persistence of proteinuria after an episode of AKI [20]. A study done on adults evaluated the long-term risks of de novo CKD following reversible AKI. These adults had no clinically evident renal disease both before and after the insult. The study demonstrated that despite rapid recovery of renal function, mild episodes of AKI involving modest increases in serum creatinine were associated with a 90% increased risk of developing CKD on longitudinal follow-up [21]. CKD progression was already evident as early as the third month after hospital discharge in adults, and over 50% of children from various causes of AKI had at least one sign of CKD 3–5 years after the initial event [22, 23].

A 10-year follow-up of survivors of CA-AKI in a developing region found that almost 25% of the AKI survivors had either of the following: abnormal creatinine, hypertension, hematuria, or proteinuria [4]. For those who received RRT, 34–40% of patients had renal dysfunction (decreased glomerular filtration rate, hypertension, hematuria, or proteinuria) or remain dialysis dependent at discharge. In addition, children with primary kidney disease-associated AKI had a higher kidney dysfunction at hospital discharge [24, 25].

The causative relationship between AKI and the risk of developing CKD remains unknown. Animal studies demonstrated that AKI causes permanent damage to the peritubular capillaries [26]. It also triggers molecular pathways leading to prolonged inflammation and eventually induces renal fibrosis even after renal recovery as per serum creatinine [27–29]. Studies blocking fibrogenic signaling cascades in animal models of AKI demonstrated a reduced rate of subsequent tubulointerstitial fibrosis [30]. Through these inflammatory and fibrotic signaling pathways, the residual kidney damage can lead to progressive functional and structural kidney damage, leading to increased predisposition of worsening hypertension, proteinuria, and rapid decline in glomerular filtration rate. It is important to emphasize that subclinical renal and extrarenal damage persists despite clinical resolution of AKI as per serum creatinine criteria.

27.5 Long-Term Follow-Up

With technological and pharmacological advances that provide effective treatment for life-threatening events among neonates and children, survival from AKI has significantly improved. Despite the epidemiological evidence demonstrating an association between AKI and adverse long-term consequences, long-term follow-up of survivors of either mild or severe episodes remains low. Askenazi proposed that after an episode of AKI, children should be followed within 1 month of discharge, quarterly for two visits, and then annually for at least 2 years [22]. In order to standardize and to establish an organized system of long-term follow-up, the Assessment, Serial Evaluation, and Subsequent Sequelae of Acute Kidney Injury (ASSESS-AKI) study was established. To address the current knowledge gap on the causative relationship between AKI and long-term outcomes, ASSESS-AKI aims to characterize the short- and long-term natural history of AKI, to evaluate the incremental utility of novel blood and urine biomarkers to refine the diagnosis and prognosis of AKI, and to identify high-risk patients who could be targeted for future clinical trials to improve outcomes [31]. We propose that a follow-up of AKI survivors by

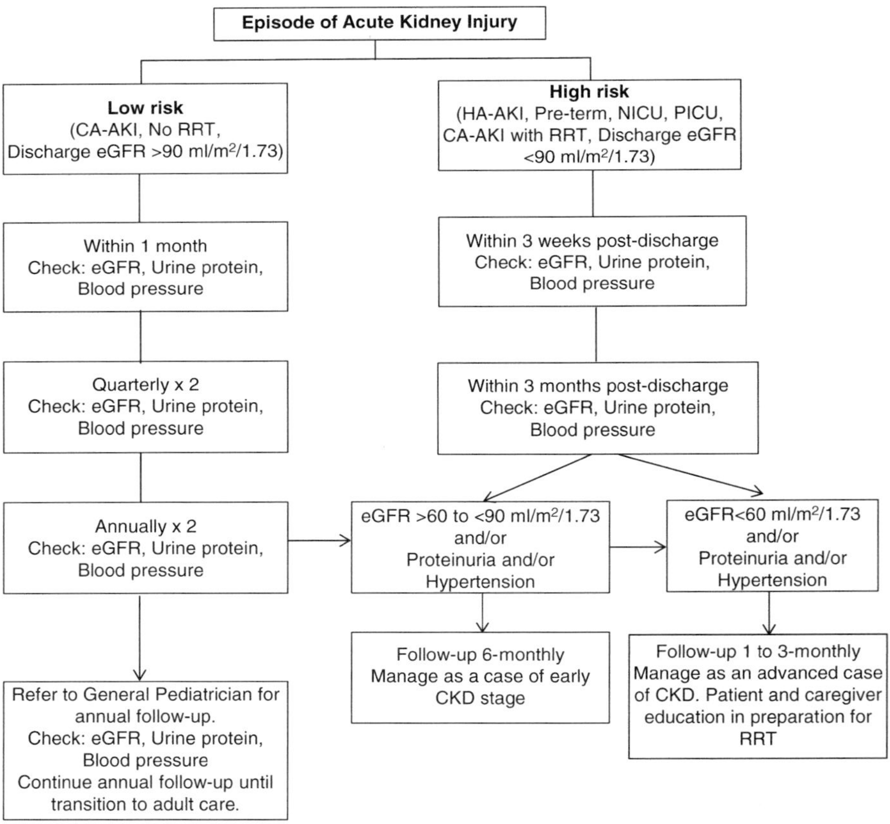

Fig. 27.1 Proposed algorithm for renal follow-up after an episode of AKI in infants and children. *NICU* neonatal intensive care unit, *PICU* pediatric intensive care unit, *CA-AKI* community-acquired AKI, *HA-AKI* hospital-acquired AKI, *eGFR* estimated glomerular filtration rate, *RRT* renal replacement therapy

general pediatricians and pediatric nephrologists should be done in a systematic manner following risk stratification, with closer monitoring of kidney function, blood pressure, and proteinuria, management of CKD complications including blood pressure control, and, most importantly, patient and caregiver education (Fig. 27.1).

27.6 Conclusion

- Survivors of AKI are at persistent risk of mortality and long-term adverse renal outcomes including the development of ESKD.
- Compared with CA-AKI, HA-AKI is characterized by high in-hospital and long-term mortality especially for those with pre-existing CKD, malignancies, congenital anomalies, and other systemic medical or surgical conditions.
- It is believed that AKI triggers molecular pathways that lead to cellular inflammation that contributes to renal fibrosis and eventual structural and functional renal abnormalities.
- All survivors of AKI should be closely monitored and evaluated for resolution or new onset or worsening of pre-existing CKD.

References

1. Kaufman J, Dhakal M, Patel B, Hamburger R. Community-acquired acute renal failure. Am J Kidney Dis. 1991;17:191–8.
2. Jha V, Parameswaran S. Community-acquired acute kidney injury in tropical countries. Nat Rev Nephrol. 2013;9:278–90.
3. Cerda J, Bagga A, Kher V, Chakravarthi RM. The contrasting characteristics of acute kidney injury in developed and developing countries. Nat Clin Pract Nephrol. 2008;4:138–53.
4. Sinha R, Nandi M, Tullus K, Marks SD, Taraphder A. Ten-year follow-up of children after acute renal failure from a developing country. Nephrol Dial Transplant. 2009;24(3):829–33.
5. Hsu CN, Chen HL, Tain YL. Epidemiology and outcomes of community-acquired and hospital-acquired acute kidney injury in children and adolescents. Pediatr Res. 2018;83(3):622–9.
6. Skolnik AB, Ewald MB. Pediatric scorpion envenomation in the United States: morbidity, mortality, and therapeutic innovations. Pediatr Emerg Care. 2013;29(1):98–103.
7. Goldstein SL. Acute kidney injury in children and its potential consequences in adulthood. Blood Purif. 2012;33:131–7.
8. Uchino S, et al. Beginning and ending supportive therapy for the kidney (BEST kidney) investigators: acute renal failure in critically ill patients: a multinational, multicenter study. JAMA. 2005;294:813–8.
9. Chertow GM, Levy EM, Hammermeister KE, Grover F, Daley J. Independent association between acute renal failure and mortality following cardiac surgery. Am J Med. 1998;104:343–8.
10. Price JF, et al. Worsening renal function in children hospitalized with decompensated heart failure: evidence for a pediatric cardiorenal syndrome? Pediatr Crit Care Med. 2008;9:279–84.
11. Jurawan N, Pankhurst T, Ferro C, Nightingale P, Coleman J, Rosser D, Ball S. Hospital acquired acute kidney injury is associated with increased mortality but not increased readmission rates in a UK acute hospital. BMC Nephrol. 2017;18(1):317.

12. Coca SG, Yusuf B, Shlipak MG, Garg AX, Parikh CR. Long-term risk of mortality and other adverse outcomes after acute kidney injury: a systematic review and meta-analysis. Am J Kidney Dis. 2009;53(6):961–73.
13. Garg AX, et al. Long-term renal prognosis of diarrhea-associated hemolytic uremic syndrome: a systematic review, meta-analysis, and meta-regression. JAMA. 2003;290:1360–70.
14. White SL, et al. Is low birth weight an antecedent of CKD in later life? A systematic review of observational studies. Am J Kidney Dis. 2009;54:248–61.
15. Greenberg JH, Coca S, Parikh CR. Long-term risk of chronic kidney disease and mortality in children after acute kidney injury: a systematic review. BMC Nephrol. 2014;15:184.
16. Shaw NJ, Brocklebank JT, Dickinson DF, Wilson N, Walker DR. Long-term outcome for children with acute renal failure following cardiac surgery. Int J Cardiol. 1991;31:161–5.
17. Scharer K, Krmar R, Querfeld U, Ruder H, Waldherr R, Schaefer F. Clinical outcome of Schonlein-Henoch purpura nephritis in children. Pediatr Nephrol. 1999;13:816–23.
18. Garg AX, Clark WF, Salvadori M, Macnab J, Suri RS, Haynes RB, Matsell D, Walkerton Health Study Investigators. Microalbuminuria three years after recovery from *Escherichia coli* O157 hemolytic uremic syndrome due to municipal water contamination. Kidney Int. 2005;67:1476–82.
19. Morgera S, Kraft AK, Siebert G, Luft FC, Neumayer HH. Long-term outcomes in acute renal failure patients treated with continuous renal replacement therapies. Am J Kidney Dis. 2002;40:275–9.
20. Abitbol CL, Bauer CR, Montane B, Chandar J, Duara S, Zilleruelo G. Long-term follow-up of extremely low birth weight infants with neonatal renal failure. Pediatr Nephrol. 2003;18:887–93.
21. Bucaloiu ID, KirchnerHL NER, Hartle JE, Perkins RM. Increased risk of death and de novo chronic kidney disease following reversible acute kidney injury. Kidney Int. 2012;81:477–85.
22. Askenazi DJ, Feig DI, Graham NM, Hui-Stickle S, Goldstein SL. 3–5 year longitudinal follow-up of pediatric patients after acute renal failure. Kidney Int. 2006;69:184–9.
23. Horne K, Packington R, Monaghan J, et al. Three year outcomes after acute kidney injury: results of a prospective parallel group cohort study. BMJ Open. 2017;7:e015316.
24. Ball EF, Kara T. Epidemiology and outcome of acute kidney injury in New Zealand children. J Paediatr Child Health. 2008;44:642–6.
25. Hui-Stickle S, Brewer ED, Goldstein SL. Pediatric ARF epidemiology at a tertiary care center from 1999 to 2001. Am J Kidney Dis. 2005;45:96–101.
26. Basile DP, Donohoe D, Roethe K, Osborn JL. Renal ischemic injury results in permanent damage to peritubular capillaries and influences long-term function. Am J Physiol Renal Physiol. 2001;281(5):F887–99.
27. Basile DP. Rarefaction of peritubular capillaries following ischemic acute renal failure: a potentialfactor predisposing to progressive nephropathy. Curr Opin Nephrol Hypertens. 2004;13(1):1–7.
28. Burne-Taney MJ, Liu M, Ascon D, Molls RR, Racusen L, Rabb H. Transfer of lymphocytes from mice with renal ischemia can induce albuminuria in naive mice: a possible mechanism linking early injury and progressive renal disease? Am J Physiol Renal Physiol. 2006;291(5):F981–6.
29. Spurgeon-Pechman KR, Donohoe DL, Mattson DL, Lund H, James L, Basile DP. Recovery from acute renal failure predisposes hypertension and secondary renal disease in response to elevated sodium. Am J Physiol Renal Physiol. 2007;293(1):F269–78.
30. Wynn TA. Fibrosis under arrest. Nat Med. 2010;16:523–5.
31. Go AS, et al. Assessment serial evaluation, and subsequent sequelae of acute kidney injury study investigators. The assessment, serial evaluation, and subsequent sequelae of acute kidney injury (ASSESS-AKI) study: design and methods. BMC Nephrol. 2010;11:22.

28 Long-Term Outcome of Acute Kidney Injury in Children: A Practical Approach for Follow-up

Chia Wei Teoh and Michael Zappitelli

28.1 Clinical Case

A previously healthy 3-year-old girl presented with fever, irritability, poor intake, loose stools, cough, and coryza. She was intravascularly depleted, with blood pressure 90/50 mmHg but no respiratory distress. Investigations included leukocytosis, Na^+ 147 mmol/L, blood urea nitrogen (BUN) 20 mmol/L, serum creatinine (SCr) 40 μmol/L, pyuria, proteinuria, and microscopic hematuria. She received a fluid bolus followed by maintenance solution. Over 24 hours, diarrhea and fever (39 °C) continued. She received ibuprofen, acetaminophen, and intravenous ceftriaxone. On day 2, she developed oliguria. Blood pressure (BP) dropped to 70/40 mmHg. SCr was 90 μmol/L. Urine and blood cultures grew *E. coli*. Renal ultrasound was unremarkable. Intravenous gentamicin was added, nephrology was consulted, and she was transferred to the intensive care unit (ICU) for inotropic support. Over 2 days, she stabilized clinically, but SCr peaked at 120 μmol/L. By day 7, SCr decreased to 30 μmol/L with clinical improvement. On day 9, she was discharged from ICU, and SCr was 31 μmol/L. The nephrology service signed off. At hospital discharge from the general ward, she was referred for a voiding cystourethrogram and primary care provider follow-up with a diagnosis of urinary sepsis, possible superimposed viral illness, and instructions to repeat a urine culture and follow imaging results.

Key Points

- AKI may be associated with long-term chronic kidney disease (CKD) and hypertension, which are associated with cardiovascular disease.

C. W. Teoh · M. Zappitelli (✉)
Department of Pediatrics, Division of Nephrology, Hospital for Sick Children, University of Toronto, Toronto, ON, Canada
e-mail: chiawei.teoh@sickkids.ca; michael.zappitelli@sickkids.ca; michele.zappitelli@mcgill.ca

S. K. Sethi et al. (eds.), *Critical Care Pediatric Nephrology and Dialysis: A Practical Handbook*, https://doi.org/10.1007/978-981-13-2276-1_28

- There is currently a lack of evidence-based guidelines and thus poor long-term follow-up, for children who develop AKI.
- Children with high baseline risk for kidney disease, with more severe AKI, and with lack of complete recovery from AKI should be targeted for long-term follow-up of kidney function, proteinuria, and BP.

28.2 Introduction

AKI in children is strongly associated with poor hospital outcomes (mortality, longer stay, and prolonged invasive ventilation) [1, 2]. Hospitalized adults with AKI are also at higher risk for long-term development of CKD, end-stage renal disease (ESRD), hypertension, cardiovascular events, and mortality [3, 4]. The potential importance of AKI as a contributor to poor long-term health in children has only recently been appreciated. As in the clinical case, children develop AKI due to different reasons, described in other chapters. However, few children require acute dialysis. Few healthcare providers would argue that children requiring acute dialysis need follow-up after discharge to ensure that kidney function returns to, and remains, normal. However, a dilemma lies with children who develop non-dialysis-requiring AKI: are they at risk for long-term kidney disease, and if so, how should they be followed and by whom? There are no concrete guidelines on who and how to follow pediatric AKI after hospital discharge; thus, many children with AKI are likely not followed for long-term kidney disease development. Considering systematic follow-up of pediatric AKI must balance potential benefits (early CKD detection/treatment) with burden to families and healthcare systems.

This chapter will briefly summarize the rationale for long-term follow-up of pediatric AKI and review the current evidence on pediatric long-term AKI-outcome associations. In the context of an evolving evidence base, this chapter will provide a practical approach to following up children who develop AKI during hospitalization.

28.3 Rationale for Post-hospital Discharge Follow-Up of Children Who Develop AKI

28.3.1 AKI to Chronic Kidney Injury Pathophysiology

This section briefly summarizes the pathophysiology underlining the relationship between AKI and subsequent CKD (depicted in Fig. 28.1). Several excellent reviews provide more detailed description [3, 5–7].

AKI in most hospitalized patients occurs due to acute renal tubular cell injury (acute tubular necrosis due to hypoxia/ischemia, nephrotoxicity, inflammation, etc.). These events trigger acute cellular responses not only around the injured tubular cells but also within the interstitium and peritubular capillaries (around the tubules). This cellular response causes proliferation of interstitial cells around the

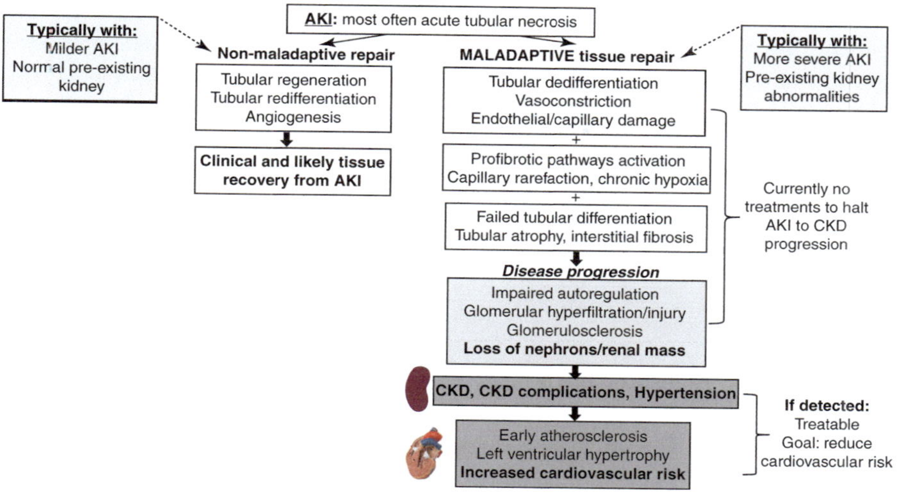

Fig. 28.1 Simplified depiction of progression from acute to chronic kidney injury and later kidney and cardiovascular disease. *Left*: If AKI is mild and the patient has no baseline kidney disease, repair of acute injured kidney tissue will be normal and not lead to long-term chronic kidney disease (CKD). *Right*: In patients with more severe AKI or with baseline kidney conditions, the acute kidney cell injury repair process may be *maladaptive*, leading to fibrosis, abnormalities in renal tubular cells, interstitium and vasculature, and ultimate renal mass loss. This may lead to CKD or hypertension or important, but treatable, cardiovascular risk factors. It is thus worth detecting CKD and hypertension, to prevent cardiovascular disease

tubules and in more severe cases, tubular cell death. With mild AKI, this response is associated with regeneration of renal tubular cells and ultimately, resolution of inflammation/cellular response. Research shows that in some patients, especially with more severe injury, the repair process is "maladaptive"; tubular cell regeneration is incomplete, and cellular responses persist after acute injury. Ongoing inflammation and pro-fibrotic cellular responses ensue (e.g., influx of interstitial myofibroblasts or immune cells), leading to abnormal tubular cell morphology, fewer peritubular capillaries (contributing to chronic hypoxia), and increased interstitial space and cellularity with tubulointerstitial fibrosis. Nephron loss may cause glomerular hyperfiltration in remaining nephrons, potentiating further glomerular injury and, together with chronic hypoxia, glomerulosclerosis. Thus the initial AKI event may propagate initiation and maintenance of fibrosis. Tubulointerstitial fibrosis and glomerulosclerosis ultimately lead to renal function loss over time.

Several factors, including severity of initial AKI insult, contribute to determining whether CKD will occur. Pre-existing CKD and recurrent AKI episodes are important risk factors for CKD development/worsening after AKI in adults [3]. Though pre-existing CKD is rare in children, neonates may present a similar risk for dysregulated response to AKI. Nephrogenesis is only complete at about 34–36 weeks gestational age. Children born prematurely or with intrauterine growth restriction have permanently reduced nephron mass. The neonatal kidney receives increasing proportions of cardiac output in the first weeks of life. Early life hypoxic processes which interfere with normal blood flow rise to the kidney may be detrimental [8]. Neonates, especially premature neonates, should be considered at risk for AKI and also as having a baseline kidney environment which promotes maladaptive repair and subsequent pro-fibrotic processes.

28.3.2 AKI Is Associated with CKD in Adults

Large studies in adults showed that AKI is a strong risk factor for developing *new* CKD, worsening of existing CKD and ESRD [3, 9]. Pre-existing CKD increases likelihood of poorer outcomes after AKI. However, even adults with no pre-existing CKD (often the case for children) who develop AKI have at least double the risk of developing CKD. In normotensive adults, patients with AKI were at 22% adjusted increased risk of developing hypertension [4]. Importantly, AKI in adults is associated with increased risk for overall and cardiovascular mortality [9]. Current recommendations are that adults with AKI should be followed for CKD and other outcome development after hospital discharge [9].

28.3.3 Why Is It Important to Detect Long-Term Kidney Disease in Children?

Most children with AKI will *not* need long-term dialysis. CKD is a disease spectrum, ranging from mildly to severely decreased kidney function, often associated with hypertension. It is well documented that children with dialysis-requiring CKD (ESRD) develop anemia, bone disease, growth/developmental impairment, dyslipidemia, and cardiovascular morbidity and are at $\geq$30 times higher mortality risk than the general pediatric population. How important is it to detect non-dialysis-requiring CKD or hypertension in childhood?—very important.

The association between childhood CKD (even early stages) and early signs of cardiovascular disease is evident. Children with CKD are at risk for hypertension, subclinical atherosclerosis, left ventricle hypertrophy, increased carotid intima-media thickness, and microalbuminuria [10]. Microalbuminuria is one of the strongest CKD progression predictors in several nephropathies. The American Heart Association lists CKD as a "Tier I" cardiovascular risk factor (highest risk) in children [11]. Hypertension is one of the most important childhood cardiovascular risk factors and predicts adult hypertension, cardiovascular morbidity, and mortality [11]. CKD and hypertension are amenable to treatment, e.g., reducing albuminuria, antihypertensives, dyslipidemia screening, and lifestyle modifications. CKD and hypertension-associated cardiovascular disease thus begins in childhood (the beginning of one's lifespan). Measures aimed at preventing long-term kidney disease and promoting cardiovascular health may have important long-lasting effects.

28.4 Evidence Linking Pediatric AKI to CKD or Hypertension Development

It is known that children with AKI caused by primary renal diseases (e.g., hemolytic uremic syndrome) are at risk for long-term kidney outcomes [12]. Few healthcare providers would argue that such patients need long-term kidney follow-up; moreover, many of these patients will have close nephrologist contact in the acute disease course.

There is little published research on the association between AKI and long-term outcomes in children without primary renal diseases. Most studies have included only AKI patients with no non-AKI comparison groups, making it difficult to estimate the risk of late kidney sequelae associated with AKI. However, observational data send a clear message: pediatric AKI survivors have a much higher incidence of CKD and hypertension after hospital discharge, compared to the general pediatric population (Table 28.1 and recently synthesized in reviews) [13–20]. Unfortunately, these studies were of variable quality and follow-up periods. This makes it difficult to understand which patients should be targeted for follow-up and at what frequency. A separate body of literature has shown that children treated for cancer are at high risk for long-term proteinuria, reduced glomerular filtration rate (GFR), and hypertension (Table 28.1). This population is well-known to experience AKI via many mechanisms (including nephrotoxicity, ischemia, and sepsis) [21].

Recently, the pediatric cardiac surgery population has been studied in more detail (Table 28.1). In cardiac transplant recipients, children *without* recovery from AKI before discharge were at higher risk for CKD 1 year later [18]. A large, retrospective study from Denmark found that children with cardiac surgery-associated AKI were 3.8-fold more likely (12% vs. 3% in non-AKI) to develop CKD [22]. However, this study used physician-ordered laboratory data; it is possible that bias by indication (AKI patients more likely to have kidney function followed) favored finding an association of AKI with CKD. A smaller but prospective study found that at 5 years after pediatric cardiac surgery, 13% developed CKD (low GFR or albuminuria) and 17% developed hypertension. However, there was no association of CKD or hypertension with AKI.

Studies to date have not had large enough sample sizes and been mostly performed with lack of non-AKI comparison groups. However, we should be struck by the remarkably high prevalence of CKD or hypertension in children who have had AKI, when considering that the prevalence of both conditions in the pediatric population is <1%. This should be placed in the context that healthcare providers are not currently evaluating renal function in children after AKI development. For example, in the aforementioned prospective cardiac surgery study, only 4% of patients were followed by a nephrologist after discharge [15]. Hessey et al. showed that in >2000 ICU children, less than half of patients had SCr measured before hospital discharge [23]. In addition, 20% of children with Stage 2 AKI (SCr doubling) did not have SCr measured before discharge; yet, of those who did have SCr measured, 30% still fulfilled AKI criteria. Healthcare providers (intensivists, nurses, ward pediatricians, residents) need to begin thinking about long-term AKI morbidity and at least, test for AKI recovery before hospital discharge.

Neonates deserve special mention, for reasons described above. Evidence to date confirms that AKI is very common in neonates and appears to be a risk factor for long-term kidney disease (Table 28.2), at least in part due to the unique neonatal

Table 28.1 Non-exhaustive summary of evidence from pediatric studies with long-term renal sequelae post-AKI

Study	AKI definition	*n*	Follow-up (y)	Prevalence of kidney abnormalities in AKI patients				Additional comments
				Proteinuria	Hypertension	eGFR < 90	eGFR < 60	
Cardiac surgery								
Madsen (2017) [22]	KDIGO	382 (AKI 127)	4.9			12%		AKI had 3.8-fold higher adjusted risk for CKD (12 vs. 3%)
Cooper (2016) [13]	pRIFLE	51 (AKI 33)	7	3.9%	21.2%	14.3%		Past AKI: Higher urine injury biomarker levels at follow-up No AKI vs. non-AKI difference in kidney outcomes
Greenberg (2016) [15]	AKIN	131 (AKI 57)	5.4	6%	11%	0%	0%	Overall cohort prevalence of hypertension and CKD 17% and 18%, respectively No AKI vs. non-AKI difference in kidney outcomes
Hollander (2016) [18]	KDIGO	76 (AKI 54)	1				6%	CKD more common in AKI patients who did not recover function (18%) vs. those who did (0%)
Mel (2014) [14]	Dialysis	25	5.1	0%	0%	4%	0%	No control group
Shaw (1991) [14]	Dialysis	11	3.4	18.2%	0%	18.2%	0%	No control group
Non-cardiac surgery								
Menon (2014) [19] (*nephrotoxic AKI*)	pRIFLE	77	0.5	68.5%	37.7%	23.4%	2.6%	AKI group 3.8-fold greater risk of developing CKD
Mammen (2012) [14] (*ICU cohort*)	AKIN	126	1–3	9.5%	3.2%	38.9%	0.8%	No control group Acute dialysis treatment more common in CKD patients (38 vs. 15%, $p = 0.04$)

Viaud (2012) [14] (*ICU cohort*)	Dialysis	13	16	54%	15%	61.5%	23.1%	No control group
Hoffmeister (2010) [17] (*post-HSCT cohort*)	SCr doubling	689 (AKI 227)	16		18%			AKI 2.5-fold higher hypertension risk vs. non-AKI
Buysse (2008) [14] (*meningococcus*)	SCr doubling	120 (AKI 16)	9.8	18.8%	12.5%	6.3%	0%	No control group
Hingorani (2007) [16] (*post-HSCT cohort*)	SCr doubling	1319 (AKI 332)					32%	AKI 1.6-fold higher CKD risk vs. non-AKI
Askenazi (2006) [14] (*hospital cohort*)	Diagnostic code	29	3–5	27.6%	20.7%	13.8%	6.9%	No control group
Slack (2005) [14] (*meningococcus*)	Dialysis	12	4.2	25%	25%	25%	8.3%	No control group
Georgaki (1989) [14] (*hospital cohort*)	Dialysis	10	7–12			20%		No control group

Reference 14: Is a systematic review which contains the details of the studies for which the Table indicates. *y* year, *eGFR* estimated glomerular filtration rate, *CKD* chronic kidney disease, *KDIGO* Kidney Disease Improving Global Outcomes AKI definition, *pRIFLE* pediatric Risk Injury Failure Loss End-Stage Renal Disease AKI definition, *AKIN* Acute Kidney Injury Network AKI definition, *SCr* serum creatinine, *HSCT* hematopoietic stem cell transplant

Table 28.2 Non-exhaustive summary of some studies in neonates in the last 5 years on long-term renal sequelae post-AKI

Study	AKI definition	*n*	Follow-up (y)	Prevalence of kidney abnormalities in AKI patients				Additional comments
				Proteinuria	Hypertension	eGFR < 90	eGFR < 60	
Harer (2017) [25]	KDIGO	34 (AKI 20) preterm	5	20%	10%	35% (CysC)		AKI (vs. *non-AKI)* 4.5-fold higher risk for renal dysfunction
Maqsood (2017) [26]	KDIGO	222 (AKI 110) preterm	6.6–8.3		6.4%			4% of all ELBW infants had evidence of CKD at ≥2 years. No AKI vs. non-AKI difference
Bruel (2016) [24]	Creatinine > GA-based critical value	74 (AKI 25) preterm	6.6	12%	8%	25%		11% and 23% of the whole cohort had albuminuria and abnormal kidney function, respectively No AKI vs. non-AKI difference
Zwiers (2014) [27]	pRIFLE	169 (AKI 64) term, ECMO	8.2				0%	34% AKI vs. 21% non-AKI had CKD or hypertension at follow-up ($p = 0.004$)

y year, *eGFR* estimated glomerular filtration rate, *KDIGO* Kidney Disease Improving Global Outcomes AKI definition, *CysC* Cystatin C estimated glomerular filtration rate, *CKD* chronic kidney disease, *ELBW* extremely low birth weight, *GA* gestational age, *SCr* serum creatinine, *pRIFLE* pediatric Risk Injury Failure Loss End-Stage Renal Disease AKI definition, *ECMO* extracorporeal membrane oxygenation factors described above [24–27]. This remains an evolving field requiring further evaluation in larger, well-designed studies.

28.5 Translating Current Knowledge into Clinical Practice

International guidelines suggest following patients 3 months after an AKI episode to assess AKI resolution and CKD development or progression [9]. These guidelines were based on evidence in adults that AKI (vs. non-AKI) is independently associated with outcomes. There are no specific pediatric guidelines, because strong evidence for changing how we care for children with AKI after discharge has not been generated. We *do* know that children with AKI are at higher risk for CKD or hypertension than the general pediatric population and that children undergoing cardiac surgery have an overall high long-term CKD and hypertension prevalence. Below, we provide two examples of published approaches to following children with AKI, followed by our proposed approach. Neither has been evaluated for impact on outcomes, should be treated as guides, and considered within the reader's own healthcare context.

28.5.1 A Pediatric AKI Survivor Clinic

An AKI survivor clinic at a US tertiary care pediatric center has been described [28]. Children with Stage 2 AKI or worse (i.e., doubling of SCr) are identified using the institutional electronic health record (EHR) system, which triggers referral. A clinic staff reviews EHR-triggered referrals for eligibility and communicates with medical teams and families. Three-, 6-, and 12-month follow-up visits are scheduled for eligible patients, and the primary care provider is contacted. These clinics include screening and treatment for CKD and hypertension; review of kidney risk for future health events (e.g., surgeries); and healthcare provider and family education surrounding AKI and risk (e.g., nephrotoxins). This clinic is a cutting edge for pediatric AKI follow-up care and an example of an institution-level follow-up program. Such programs require coordination with physicians, institutional support, and an EHR to perform "alerts" of AKI.

28.5.2 A More General Approach to Pediatric AKI Follow-Up

A recent review highlights that current evidence limits developing concrete recommendations on pediatric AKI follow-up; but standardized methods of evaluating late AKI kidney sequelae should be used (modified summary, Table 28.3) [20]. They acknowledge the challenge in many healthcare contexts to systematically follow up all AKI patients. They highlight (a) underlying kidney disease risk (e.g., baseline kidney abnormalities, severe critical illness, conditions known to cause direct kidney damage like severe nephrotoxicity), (b) severe AKI, (c) lack of recovery from

Table 28.3 Suggested definitions for acute kidney injury and kidney health measures

	Definition
AKI	KDIGO criteria for AKI (any AKI = SCr rise from baseline by ≥50% in 7 days or by ≥26.5 μmol/L in 48 h or need for dialysis [SCr criteria]; or urine output <0.5 mL/kg/h × 6 h [urine output criteria]) Severe AKI-KDIGO AKI Stage ≥2
Microalbuminuria	Urine albumin/creatinine ratio > 3 mg/mmol (30 mg/g)
Proteinuria	• Urine protein/creatinine ratio > 20 mg/mmol (0.2 mg/mg) • 24 h urine: – <18 years—protein excretion > 100 mg/m^2/day – >18 years—protein excretion > 150 mg/day
Hypertension	• Systolic or diastolic BP ≥ 95th percentile for age/height/sex • Antihypertensive medication requirement • Confirm high BP with an additional two extra patient visits • Consider using 24 h ambulatory monitoring to confirm
CKD	GFR between 60 and 90 mL/min/1.73 m^2: Grade 2 CKD
	GFR < 60 mL/min/1.73 m^2 for ≥3 months: official CKD definition per guidelines Estimate GFR using SCr-based equations or if available, cystatin C-based equations

KDIGO Kidney Disease Improving Global Outcomes AKI definition, *SCr* serum creatinine, *GFR* glomerular filtration rate, *CKD* chronic kidney disease

AKI before discharge, and (d) recurrent AKI episodes, as potential high-risk AKI factors which should trigger need for long-term kidney follow-up.

28.5.3 A Proposed Guide to Pediatric AKI Follow-Up (Shown in Fig. 28.2)

28.5.3.1 Document the Presence of AKI

Patients at risk for AKI should have SCr measured, especially ICU patients, those receiving nephrotoxins and undergoing stem cell transplant, or patients with deteriorating condition. The KDIGO definition should be used to classify patients by AKI severity (shown in Table 28.3).

28.5.3.2 Estimate Baseline Risk, AKI Severity, and Document Kidney Health Before Hospital Discharge

When preparing a patient who developed AKI for discharge, consider whether the patient has high pre-existing risk for future late kidney sequelae. Ask yourself "is this patient at increased risk for long term kidney or BP issues?". Some risk factors include pre-existing kidney abnormalities, borderline BP, ex-premature, multiple comorbidities, or neonates. Note the AKI severity. Patients with Stage 2 AKI or worse (doubling of SCr from baseline) are more likely to have long-term complications.

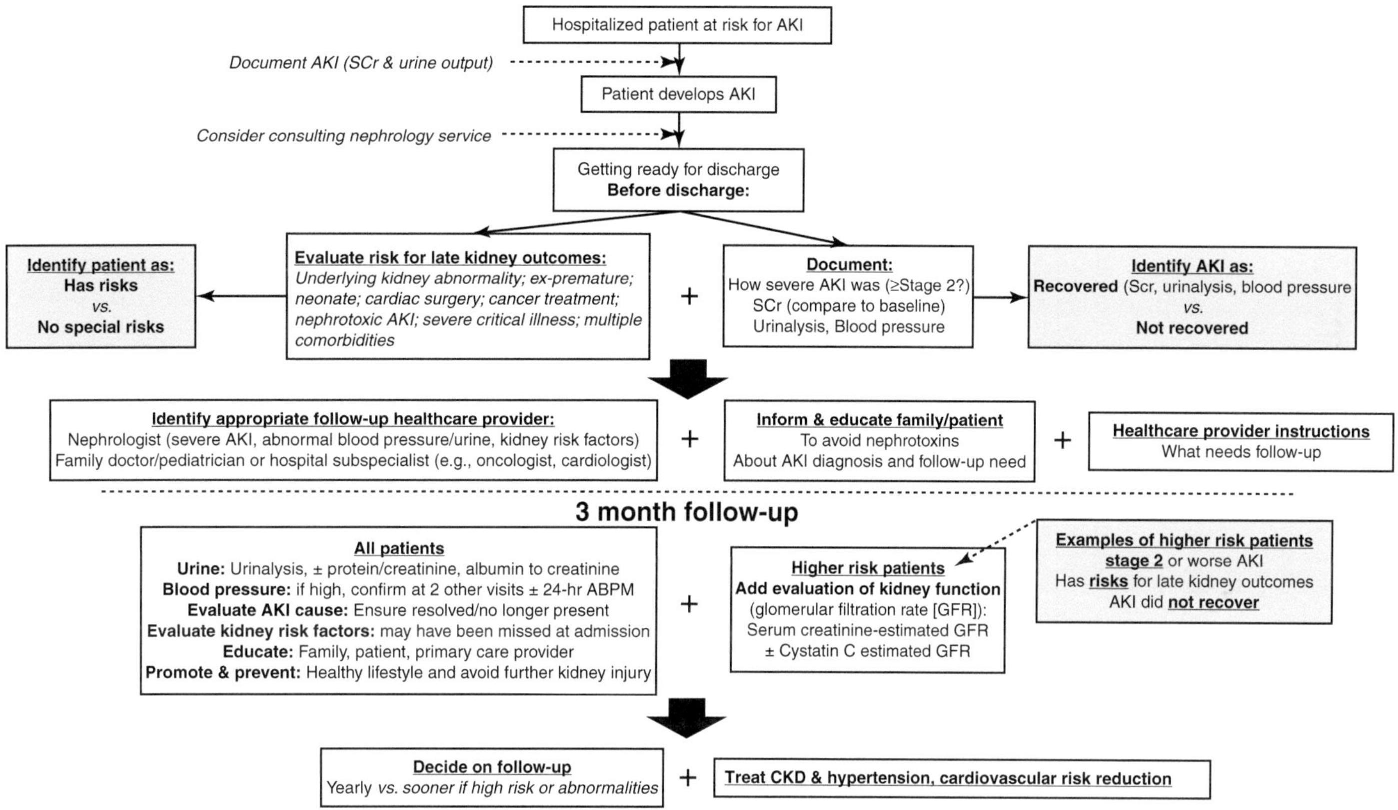

Fig. 28.2 Suggested approach for post-hospital discharge follow-up of children who develop AKI. This panel provides one approach to deciding which AKI patients should be followed after discharge and what measures should be evaluated. *Upper part*: Describes what happens before discharge from a hospitalization with AKI and the decision process in *preparing* for post-discharge follow-up. *Lower part*: Describes a proposed follow-up process, measures, and patient selection for different kidney health measures. *SCr* serum creatinine, *Stage 2* refers to Stage 2 acute kidney injury or at least doubling of SCr from baseline, *ABPM* 24 h ambulatory blood pressure monitoring, the gold standard test for blood pressure evaluation, *CKD* chronic kidney disease

SCr should be measured before hospital discharge to document return of SCr to baseline ("recovery"). Patients discharged with abnormal SCr should be especially targeted for follow-up. Normal urinalysis and BP should also be documented before discharge; if abnormal, they should be targeted for follow-up.

28.5.3.3 Decide Who Should Follow the Patient and When

This can be tricky. In some healthcare contexts, referring all AKI patients to a nephrologist would be an unacceptable burden. Patients with obvious risk for long-term kidney abnormalities, baseline kidney disease, significant kidney dysfunction, or high BP before discharge should ideally be followed by a nephrologist. If unsure, consider discussing with the nephrologist. In patients with milder AKI or no risk factors for poor late outcomes (e.g., no medical history, sepsis or SCr doubling, and SCr normalization before discharge), a reliable non-nephrologist primary care provider can follow BP, urinalysis, and SCr; but instructions must be provided to the physician. Until research is available to guide recommendations, it is reasonable to suggest follow-up in 3 months, as suggested by adult guidelines [9]. Obviously, patients discharged with more severe disease (e.g., high BP, persistent Stage 2 AKI) should be followed sooner.

28.5.3.4 What Should Be Evaluated During Follow-Up?

At the first follow-up visit, the main goals are to determine if the underlying AKI causes have resolved, educate families about AKI (e.g., avoiding nephrotoxins, informing physicians that their child developed AKI), screen for poor kidney health risk factors (e.g., nephrotoxins, obesity), and evaluate the child's kidney health. Kidney health is generally assessed by evaluating GFR (SCr, cystatin C), urinary measures (especially proteinuria), and BP. Urine examination and BP are non-invasive. However, evaluating GFR requires a blood sample. We therefore stratify patients as low and high risk, which helps determine who might require blood testing at follow-up.

28.5.4 Lower-Risk Patients

Previously healthy children, with no risk factors outlined above and with complete AKI resolution before discharge (SCr normalization to pre-AKI baseline, normotensive, no proteinuria), should undergo urine and BP examination at the first follow-up visit. If the patient's history suggests previously unacknowledged kidney disease risk, GFR should be evaluated with SCr (and/or cystatin C) measurement. High BP should be confirmed (two repeat measurements during different visits; 24 h ambulatory BP monitoring). Proteinuria may be evaluated using urinalysis, protein to creatinine ratio, or albumin to creatinine ratio (the latter two being more sensitive). If all parameters are normal, we suggest a reassessment in 1 year; if parameters remain unremarkable, then reassessment every 1 or 2 years is likely reasonable, along with healthy lifestyle promotion. It is unknown how long such children should be followed. However, urine and BP are easy to evaluate during well-child visits. If abnormalities are found, appropriate treatment and referral to a nephrologist should be performed. Moreover, ensuring that kidney imaging (ultrasound) has been performed is important.

28.5.5 Higher-Risk Patients

Children known to or found to have underlying kidney disease should be followed by a nephrologist. Children with other risk factors outlined above, with post-cardiac surgery, or with recurrent and/or severe AKI (≥Stage 2) should be evaluated similarly to low-risk patients but must also have GFR evaluated (SCr and/or Cystatin C) at the first follow-up visit. Though CKD is defined by guidelines as a GFR < 60 mL/min/1.73 m^2, GFR < 90 mL/min/1.73 m^2 should be considered as potentially abnormal and followed up closely. Frequency of follow-up thereafter will be dictated by the severity of abnormalities, but at the very least, re-evaluation in a year, followed by every 1 or 2 years, is strongly recommended.

28.6 Conclusion

Evidence suggests that children with AKI are at higher long-term kidney risk than other children, placing them at increased cardiovascular risk. Future research will increase insight into these associations and provide us with guidance on which patients require specific follow-up. However, AKI follow-up should begin now and be triggered by healthcare providers during hospitalization. If we do not at least document that AKI occurred and *think* about potential negative late AKI outcomes, follow-up will not happen. This is unfortunate because early CKD and hypertension are amenable to intervention. Hopefully, the proposed approach provided by this chapter shows that follow-up need not be onerous and may potentially have a long-lasting positive impact on patient health.

References

1. Alkandari O, Eddington KA, Hyder A, et al. Acute kidney injury is an independent risk factor for pediatric intensive care unit mortality, longer length of stay and prolonged mechanical ventilation in critically ill children: a two-center retrospective cohort study. Crit Care. 2011;15(3):R146.
2. Kaddourah A, Basu RK, Bagshaw SM, Goldstein SL, AWARE Investigators. Epidemiology of acute kidney injury in critically ill children and young adults. N Engl J Med. 2017;376(1):11–20.
3. Chawla LS, Eggers PW, Star RA, Kimmel PL. Acute kidney injury and chronic kidney disease as interconnected syndromes. N Engl J Med. 2014;371(1):58–66.
4. Hsu CY, Hsu RK, Yang J, Ordonez JD, Zheng S, Go AS. Elevated BP after AKI. J Am Soc Nephrol. 2016;27(3):914–23.
5. Venkatachalam M, Weinberg JM, Kriz W, Bidani AK. Failed tubule recovery, AKI-CKD transition, and kidney disease progression. J Am Soc Nephrol. 2015;26(8):1765–76.
6. Kumar S. Cellular and molecular pathways of renal repair after acute kidney injury. Kidney Int. 2018;93(1):27–40.
7. Liu BC, Tang TT, Lv LL, Lan HY. Renal tubule injury: a driving force toward chronic kidney disease. Kidney Int. 2018;93(3):568–79.

8. Zappitelli M, Ambalavanan N, Askenazi DJ, et al. Developing a neonatal acute kidney injury research definition: a report from the NIDDK neonatal AKI workshop. Pediatr Res. 2017;82(4):569–73.
9. KDIGO AKI Work Group. KDIGO clinical practice guideline for acute kidney injury. Kidney Int Suppl. 2012;2(1):1–138.
10. Brady TM, Schneider MF, Flynn JT, et al. Carotid intima-media thickness in children with CKD: results from the CKiD study. Clin J Am Soc Nephrol. 2012;7(12):1930–7.
11. Kavey RE, Allada V, Daniels SR, et al. Cardiovascular risk reduction in high-risk pediatric patients: a scientific statement from the American Heart Association Expert Panel on Population and Prevention Science; the Councils on Cardiovascular Disease in the Young, Epidemiology and Prevention, Nutrition, Physical Activity and Metabolism, High Blood Pressure Research, Cardiovascular Nursing, and the Kidney in Heart Disease; and the Interdisciplinary Working Group on Quality of Care and Outcomes Research: endorsed by the American Academy of Pediatrics. Circulation. 2006;114(24):2710–38.
12. Garg AX, Salvadori M, Okell JM, et al. Albuminuria and estimated GFR 5 years after *Escherichia coli* O157 hemolytic uremic syndrome: an update. Am J Kidney Dis. 2008;51(3):435–44.
13. Cooper DS, Claes D, Goldstein SL, et al. Follow-up renal assessment of injury long-term after acute kidney injury (FRAIL-AKI). Clin J Am Soc Nephrol. 2016;11(1):21–9.
14. Greenberg JH, Coca S, Parikh CR. Long-term risk of chronic kidney disease and mortality in children after acute kidney injury: a systematic review. BMC Nephrol. 2014;15:184.
15. Greenberg JH, Zappitelli M, Devarajan P, et al. Kidney outcomes 5 years after pediatric cardiac surgery: the TRIBE-AKI study. JAMA Pediatr. 2016;170(11):1071–8.
16. Hingorani S, Guthrie KA, Schoch G, Weiss NS, McDonald GB. Chronic kidney disease in long-term survivors of hematopoietic cell transplant. Bone Marrow Transplant. 2007;39(4):223–9.
17. Hoffmeister PA, Hingorani SR, Storer BE, Baker KS, Sanders JE. Hypertension in long-term survivors of pediatric hematopoietic cell transplantation. Biol Blood Marrow Transplant. 2010;16(4):515–24.
18. Hollander SA, Montez-Rath ME, Axelrod DM, et al. Recovery from acute kidney injury and CKD following heart transplantation in children, adolescents, and young adults: a retrospective cohort study. Am J Kidney Dis. 2016;68(2):212–8.
19. Menon S, Kirkendall ES, Nguyen H, Goldstein SL. Acute kidney injury associated with high nephrotoxic medication exposure leads to chronic kidney disease after 6 months. J Pediatr. 2014;165(3):522.e2–7.e2.
20. Sigurjonsdottir VK, Chaturvedi S, Mammen C, Sutherland SM. Pediatric acute kidney injury and the subsequent risk for chronic kidney disease: is there cause for alarm? Pediatr Nephrol. 2018;33(11):2047–55.
21. Knijnenburg SL, Mulder RL, Schouten-Van Meeteren AY, et al. Early and late renal adverse effects after potentially nephrotoxic treatment for childhood cancer. Cochrane Database Syst Rev. 2013;10:CD008944.
22. Madsen NL, Goldstein SL, Froslev T, Christiansen CF, Olsen M. Cardiac surgery in patients with congenital heart disease is associated with acute kidney injury and the risk of chronic kidney disease. Kidney Int. 2017;92(3):751–6.
23. Hessey E, Ali R, Dorais M, et al. Renal function follow-up and renal recovery after acute kidney injury in critically ill children. Pediatr Crit Care Med. 2017;18(8):733–40.
24. Bruel A, Roze JC, Quere MP, et al. Renal outcome in children born preterm with neonatal acute renal failure: IRENEO-a prospective controlled study. Pediatr Nephrol. 2016;31(12):2365–73.
25. Harer MW, Pope CF, Conaway MR, Charlton JR. Follow-up of acute kidney injury in neonates during childhood years (FANCY): a prospective cohort study. Pediatr Nephrol. 2017;32(6):1067–76.

26. Maqsood S, Fung N, Chowdhary V, Raina R, Mhanna MJ. Outcome of extremely low birth weight infants with a history of neonatal acute kidney injury. Pediatr Nephrol. 2017;32(6):1035–43.
27. Zwiers aJM, IJsselstijn H, van Rosmalen J, et al. CKD and hypertension during long-term follow-up in children and adolescents previously treated with extracorporeal membrane oxygenation. Clin J Am Soc Nephrol. 2014;9:2070–8.
28. Silver SA, Goldstein SL, Harel Z, et al. Ambulatory care after acute kidney injury: an opportunity to improve patient outcomes. Can J Kidney Health Dis. 2015;2:36.

Part VI

Advances

Advances in Paediatric Renal Replacement Therapy

29

Malcolm G. Coulthard

29.1 Introduction

Most children who require acute renal replacement therapy (RRT) do not have primary renal diseases, but are managed in paediatric intensive care units (PICUs) for renal impairment that has occurred as a consequence of being critically ill. The primary driver of their acute renal failure (ARF) is usually kidney under-perfusion due to hypotension, which may be caused by intravascular hypovolaemia, or cardiac failure, or vasodilatation associated with sepsis, or combinations of these. Many authors prefer the term acute kidney injury (AKI) to ARF as it emphasises the fact that some children acquire long-term renal damage, but this is not logical because in many cases the kidney dysfunction results from reversible, protective physiological renal responses which do not result in any tissue injury, though acute proximal tubular necrosis (ATN) and more extensive cortical necrosis are frequently seen. The two commonest paediatric indications for RRT today are recent open-heart surgery associated with fluid overload, and multiple-organ dysfunction syndrome (MODS) [1–5]. Sometimes, RRT is used to augment normal kidney function to rapidly remove toxic metabolites, such as ammonia in babies born with rare genetic metabolic conditions [6].

In principle, the factors in children which drive their physicians to undertake RRT, and the indications for selecting one treatment modality over another, are broadly similar to adult practice, but two features make therapy considerably more challenging in the very young. First, their nutritional requirements are proportionately greater, and can only be delivered in relatively large volumes of liquid in babies, which makes fluid restriction more problematic, and intermittent fluid removal less useful. Second, major practical issues of scale are involved in delivering precise fluid and biochemical balance to very small individuals. And, it is

M. G. Coulthard (✉)
Great North Children's Hospital, Newcastle-upon-Tyne, UK

S. K. Sethi et al. (eds.), *Critical Care Pediatric Nephrology and Dialysis: A Practical Handbook*, https://doi.org/10.1007/978-981-13-2276-1_29

disproportionately the smallest children who require RRT. For these reasons, I present an example case of a baby who required RRT in critical care and then discuss her management issues to illustrate advances that have been made in RRT delivery, and ones that are still needed.

29.2 Case

Anne was a 2.9-kg baby girl born at 35-week gestation who had consistently poor peripheral perfusion and hypotension because of her antenatally diagnosed hypoplastic left heart. Her capacity to suck was limited, and she was mostly fed with formula milk via a nasogastric tube. From 2 weeks of age, she developed intermittent abdominal distension and tenderness suggestive of incipient necrotising enterocolitis (NEC), so we changed her from enteral feeding to total parenteral nutrition through a central line. One week later, she became relatively oliguric with an hourly output of just 1.5 mL/kg of concentrated urine (osmolality 600 mOsm/kg), and had developed mild peripheral oedema, though her enzymatically measured plasma creatinine was normal at 27 μmol/L (0.3 mg/dL). We decided to undertake the first of three stages of planned open-heart surgery procedures on her.

The procedure was difficult and prolonged, and post-operatively, she had a distended abdomen and no bowel sounds, her creatinine had risen to 48 μmol/L (0.5 mg/dL), her plasma sodium was slightly elevated at 148 mmol/L, her hourly urine output had fallen to 0.6 mL/kg which was unresponsive to furosemide, and her oedema had increased, so we fluid-restricted her. Her urinary sodium and creatinine concentrations were 58 mmol/L and 4800 μmol/L (54.5 mg/dL), respectively. We delivered all of her intravenous medications in 10% dextrose to maximise her calorie intake, but she went on to develop a metabolic acidosis and hyperkalaemia, with a base excess of −12 mmol/L, and a plasma potassium of 6.2 mmol/L. Her general condition deteriorated, and we commenced RRT.

We did not consider using peritoneal dialysis (PD) because of the state of her abdomen. She had a triple-lumen right-internal-jugular venous line in place for blood sampling, and to allow inotropes and other medications to be infused, but this was too small to allow continuous veno-venous haemofiltration (CVVH) to be performed, so we inserted an additional 6.5-French double-lumen femoral line. We performed CVVH using a paediatric circuit with an extracorporeal volume (ECV) of 60 mL, and primed this with packed red blood cells and plasma, and anticoagulated her with heparin as she was being treated with this post-operatively already. We aimed to remove a net fluid volume (ultrafiltrate, UF) of 30 mL/h over the first 24 h of RRT to reduce her fluid overload by about 300 mL, and to provide a daily 'fluid space' of about 150 mL/kg to administer her intravenous drugs and calories.

She became hypotensive after 15 min of treatment, but responded to a transient increase in inotrope dosage. She became hypotensive again after 18 h, and required a 10-mL/kg saline infusion and a reduction in her prescribed UF rate. Her oedema, acidosis, and electrolyte abnormalities resolved, her creatinine peaked at 109 μmol/L (1.2 mg/dL), and her tissue perfusion improved. After 4 days, her abdominal signs resolved, her urine output increased, her creatinine fell, and we discontinued her CVVH. Within a week, her creatinine had fallen to 23 μmol/L (0.3 mg/dL), she was able to maintain fluid balance, and a urine stick test showed no blood or protein.

29.3 The Decision to Start Renal Replacement Therapy

The diagnosis of ARF is usually made by a combination of a rise in the plasma creatinine and the presence of oliguria, commonly defined either as an hourly urine output of <1 or ≤0.5 mL/kg. It is frequently stated that creatinine is a poor indicator of the onset of ARF because it takes time to rise [7], but this is an inevitable consequence of the first-order elimination kinetics of endogenous markers; substances which rise more promptly are likely to be doing so because they are also markers of inflammation, such as cystatin-C [8]. Enzymatic creatinine concentrations are commonly reported as mg/dL to one-significant-figure, which blunts their sensitivity because the coefficient of variation of the assay is much finer than this, at about ±1 μmol/L, or ±0.012 mg/dL. For instance, Anne's creatinine increase from 27 to 48 μmol/L (0.31–0.54 mg/dL) over a few hours indicates a clinically significant fall in GFR of 78% (68–88%). However, reporting this as 0.3–0.5 mg/dL dumbs the information down; these figures could also represent a change from 0.34 to 0.45 mg/dL, a rise of just 32%.

Unfortunately, none of the existing tubular damage markers for AKI [7] can assist meaningfully in acute decision-making. However, combining Anne's blood and urinary creatinine and sodium concentrations indicates that she is only excreting about 1% of her glomerular filtrate (GFR) as urine, and that her fractional excretion of sodium is even less. This demonstrates physiologically excellent proximal and distal tubular function and excludes extensive ischaemic cellular damage.

The decisions of *if*, *when*, and *how* to initiate RRT in a child are primarily based on clinical imperatives, rather than renal physiology assessments. Severe fluid overload is associated with poorer outcomes, in part because fluid restriction limits our capacity to regulate the babies' biochemical status conservatively (Box 29.1). If we had been able to infuse Anne with sufficient volumes of an intravenous dextrose and sodium bicarbonate formulation, it may have allowed us to provide enough calories and counteract her acidosis and hypernatraemia sufficiently to avoid using RRT.

29.4 Peritoneal Dialysis

Peritoneal dialysis (PD) still has a role in some critically ill children worldwide [9], as it is relatively inexpensive, and it can often deliver gentle chemical control and sufficient UF to provide effective RRT, and it can be scaled down for very small infants. Using bicarbonate-based dialysis fluids avoids the risk of lactic or acetic acidosis in children with compromised or immature liver function, and starting with small cycle volumes (e.g., 10 mL/kg) helps prevent fluid breaching into the pleural spaces, and compromising ventilation with increasing abdominal pressures.

Box 29.1 This shows the ways that ARF may impact on a child's physiology and health. The top section shows the direct effects of fluid overload, and the lower section lists the main chemical disturbances, most of which are difficult to treat if fluid restriction is needed

Fluid overload (directly)	
Limits nutrition	Not typically the prime consideration during a critical care episode, but major nutritional debts may accrue after a series of episodes
Hypertension	Uncommon in most causes of acute renal failure
Systemic oedema	May interfere with wound closure and healing, and impair practical procedures such as siting drips
Pulmonary oedema	May critically limit ventilation efficiency
Biochemical perturbations	
Metabolic acidosis	Common in critically ill children, and can be managed by infusing their sodium as bicarbonate rather than chloride[a]
Hypo-/hypernatremia	Can be avoided or corrected by adjusting the sodium concentration of infusions[a]
Hyperkalaemia	Beta-blockers only produce transient improvement Insulin and glucose therapy is transient[a] Rectal ion-exchange resins can cause local complications
Hyperphosphataemia	May be a clinical problem if there is extensive tissue damage, or following chemotherapy for bulky tumours

[a]These conservative therapies to regulate or prevent biochemical perturbations are typically highly effective so long as sufficient volumes of appropriate fluid can be infused. The need to commence RRT for one of these indications is therefore highly dependent upon the urine output

However, acute PD is contraindicated in a range of conditions, has a high incidence of technical problems, and carries a significant peritonitis risk. In Anne's case, a fluid leak around a PD catheter would be likely as the abdomen was tense with an inelastic oedematous wall, and leaks create a high peritonitis risk. Also, her abdominal signs suggested that she had incipient NEC. Apart from this posing a likely risk of requiring a laparotomy, this implied that her splanchnic blood flow may be reduced, which would limit PD efficiency and UF capacity.

29.5 Haemotherapies

'Haemotherapies' (HT) are increasingly favoured over PD to manage children with ARF. I use this term to include all extracorporeal devices used to remove plasma chemicals and water across a semipermeable membrane, whether the chemicals are cleared by haemofiltration, or haemodialysis, or both.

With *haemofiltration*, replacement fluid added to the blood dilutes the plasma chemical wastes, and then a similar volume is filtered off, taking waste molecules with it by convection. The net fluid loss (UF) is controlled by adjusting these two quantities of water. The nomenclature used for HT devices lacks any system or logic, and hereafter I will use the commonest acronym applied to haemofiltration devices, which is CVVH (C = continuous, even though it may be used intermittently; VV = veno-venous, like all other HT systems; H = haemofiltration). Typically, CVVH has been used continuously in critically ill infants and children in order to deliver smooth regulation of fluid and electrolyte control.

With *haemodialysis* (HD), small molecular-weight waste chemicals in the blood diffuse across the semipermeable membrane down their concentration gradients into the dialysis fluid outside. As with CVVH, UF is achieved by the filtration of plasma water through the membrane (along with its solutes) under a positive transmembrane hydrostatic pressure (TMP). Until now, HD machines have largely been programmed to deliver rapid chemical clearances during short intermittent sessions (e.g., 4 h), which is convenient for well outpatients, but not for unstable critically ill children. However, the mechanism of HD does not in any way dictate this; for example, the Nidus has been designed to deliver continuous dialysis to very small babies [10].

The convective haemofiltration process clears higher molecular-weight solutes through high-flux membranes more efficiently than dialysis, which may confer advantages with long-term use. However, this is irrelevant in paediatric critical care as they clear urea, creatinine, sodium, potassium, phosphate, water, and ammonia equally efficiently. All HT devices which operate with conventional circuits share the same range of challenges and hazards, which are discussed below. The table summarises some of the main points of one widely used HT device, and some emerging alternatives (Table 29.1).

Table 29.1 Features of a haemotherapy device widely used in children, and three recently published systems for treating infants

Feature	Prismaflex	Adapted Aquadex circuit	CARPEDIEM	Nidus
Minimum circuit volume, mL	60	33	27	9
Patient size recommendation	20 kg to adult in USA 8 kg to adult in Europe	<10 kg	2.5–10 kg	0.8–8 kg
Current licensing status	Licensed for use in larger children	Aquadex™ licenced for adult use	Has CE mark (for Europe)	Undergoing UK-wide NHRA-funded trial
Access line sizes (French)	6.5–8 dual-lumen	6–8 dual-lumen *or* two × 5 single-lumens	Only one case: 4 dual-lumen	3.2 to 6.5 single-lumen
UF control precision	±30 mL/h (±300 mL over 24 h of continuous use)	Expressed as % of replacement fluid; range = −9% to 4%	Not reported. Fluid pumps have ±7.5% error	Volumetric syringes give microlitre control
Published experience	Extensive	12 cases (2.7–12.4 kg)	1 case (2.9 kg)	10[a] cases (1.8–7.0 kg)

[a]Another 7 cases have been reported for the pilot versions of Nidus, weighing from 0.6 to 3.8 kg, mean 1.6 kg [21, 22]

29.6 Vascular Access

Conventional CVVH and HD both require two venous access points or a double-lumen cannula that will allow sufficient flow to prevent the circuits from clotting. The physics of liquids flowing through tubing (expressed in Poiseuille's Law) means that most children require 6.5–8 French (2.2–2.8 mm outside diameter) central lines [2, 5, 11–14], which have about a 15% complication rate in small infants, including tearing of blood vessels, external and internal bleeding, and venous thromboses, of which one-fifth require surgical repair. The miniaturised conventional CARPEDIEM device has been designed to treat infants <10 kg, and their one published case only required a 4-French line [15].

The Nidus infant HD device has a novel syringe-driven circuit that only requires a single-lumen patient line [10]. It can dissociate the flow rates of the blood it withdraws from the patient, and the blood it passes across the filter, which means that a small central line does not lead to the circuit clotting. Post-cardiac-surgery babies (similar to Anne) who were treated with the Nidus were mostly dialysed through one 20-gauge lumen of triple-lumen line, while the other lumens were used for fluid and drug delivery, including inotropes. The larger infants on Nidus were managed with 6.5-French surgically placed single-lumen lines.

29.7 Extracorporeal Volumes, and Circuit Priming

Conventional HT circuits need pump-insert segments, pressure-sensor points, an expansion chamber, and a filter, and until recently the smallest available ECV was 60 mL, as used for Anne. When the ECV exceeds 10% of the patient's total blood volume, it may induce clinically important cardiovascular instability. Assuming a total blood volume of 80 mL/kg, this makes conventional circuits unsuitable for infants of <7.5 kg.

As an HT session starts, the circuit fluid mixes rapidly with the patient's blood to produce a single volume, so when that fluid is saline and the patient is small, it promptly dilutes the child's haemoglobin and alters their plasma biochemistry. If we had primed Anne's CVVH device with saline, it would have dropped her haemoglobin from 10.3 to 7.2 g/dL. To prevent this, most units prime HT circuits for children <5 kg with packed red blood cells mixed with saline, plasma, or an albumin solution [4, 6, 12–14, 16, 17], which has extra financial costs and foreign blood exposure risks. The effects of high potassium, phosphate, and citrate concentrations in stored blood, and its low Ph, can be moderated by adding bicarbonate. An alternative is to use a saline prime, and follow it at once with a transfusion of packed cells. The CARPEDIEM circuit is only 27 mL, which avoids blood-priming babies ≥3.4 kg [15], and in the Aquadex circuit adapted for babies it is 33 mL [16]. The Nidus ECV ranges from 9 to 17 mL for babies of 1–8 kg, so blood priming is never needed [10].

29.8 Anticoagulation

All extracorporeal circuits require anticoagulation unless the baby has a coagulopathy. Traditionally, systemic unfractionated heparin infusions have been used, and monitored at the bedside using glass-activated clotting time (ACT) on 0.1 mL of blood, which is typically increased to between 180 and 220 s. Anti-factor-Xa assays may provide an alternative laboratory-based test. The risk of heparin-induced bleeding is minimal in older patients, but this cannot be assumed in immature infants who have an increased risk of intracerebral and pulmonary haemorrhages. An alternative is to anticoagulate just the circuit by infusing citrate into it to chelate the calcium ions, and correcting this with a calcium infusion as the blood is returned to the child. Many children, like Anne, are maintained on systemic heparin after major cardiac surgery, which may simply be continued. Sluggish blood flow and contact with the air-trap promote clotting. Because the Nidus circuit uses much narrower tubing and is air-free, it can operate at lower ACT levels [10].

29.9 Ultrafiltration Control

It is an unfortunate fact that the control systems that regulate the UF in conventional HT circuits are fundamentally imprecise. The concept is simple, with the device making measurements of the UF rate achieved, and then adjusting the TMP to increase or decrease that rate as necessary, by changing the blood and/or fluid flow dynamics. In practice, it is not simple to reliably measure the relatively small volumes of UF that are added to much larger volumes of dialysate and/or replacement fluid. This system generates two types or error, one that the physician is aware of, and one that they can only guess at. First, the machine may report that it has not achieved the 'dialled-in' UF rate, in which case it attempts to go on and correct it to reach its target. Second, the displayed UF may be different from the actual volume removed—a false estimate, and this error is just as likely to occur at zero UF as at high rates. In 2006, the FDA issued a Public Health Notification not to use the Prisma for small children because it identified that its UF inaccuracy of ±60 mL/h had been responsible for several deaths [18]. Hence, there are no HT devices approved for use in children <20 kg in the USA, or <8 kg in Europe.

When devices overestimate UF rates, children may become overloaded, but when they under-report the volume of fluid they remove it may lead to hypovolaemia, sometimes causing hypotension, shock, and rarely death. Most times that these events occur clinically, they are assumed to be due to the child's inherent cardiovascular instability, or ascribed to other specific causes, and treated either with saline infusions or an increase in inotropic dosage. In Anne's case, she was given extra inotropes for an early hypotensive episode, and saline for another 18 h later. As in most clinical situations, we cannot be certain of the exact cause of every individual event, but hypotensive episodes are reported soon after commencing acute HT in between a quarter and a half of infants, helped by providing extra inotropic support [12, 16, 19].

Our unit has demonstrated the size and clinical impact of the UF errors that occur during conventional outpatient HD sessions in infants of about 5 kg [10]. This has changed our management; we now weigh small children at intervals during their treatment where feasible, to identify their true fluid-balance changes, rather than relying on the machine's UF records.

Gambro report that their next-generation CVVH device, the Prismaflex, has an improved UF precision at ±30 mL/h, or up to ±300 mL/day of continuous use [20]. These remain large errors if small babies are treated off-licence. The CARPEDIEM may have better precision, given its smaller ECV and highly accurate weigh balance, but it uses a conventional circuit and algorithms, and its fluid-replacement pumps have an imprecision of ±7.5% [15]. When the Aquadex was adapted for infant use, it used non-occlusive intravenous pumps to control fluid balance, which are known to have back-leakage problems, but its percentage in vitro UF regulation was median (range) −1% (−9 to 4%) [16]. The Nidus is engineered entirely differently from conventional HT devices, and it regulates the UF volume very accurately by the controlled differential movement of two operating syringes within microlitre precision. This method was initially delivered manually to three babies of ≤1.1 kg [21], and then adapted to a pilot automated device [22], before being developed to the Nidus. No episodes of acute hypotension were noted within 2 h of commencing treatment with the Nidus in 350 treatment sessions [10]. Proposals to produce even smaller syringe-driven HT systems have failed to consider the regulation of the UF [23]; a manually operated design would have consistently led to uncontrolled and unmeasured volume fluid depletion [24], and a later automated system to unregulated water retention [25].

Key 'Take Home' Points

1. The available conventional CVVH and HD devices are adequate for treating larger children.
2. There are no established CVVH or HD devices that have sufficiently accurate ultrafiltration (UF) control to be licensed for use in children <20 kg in the USA, or for infants <8 kg in Europe.
3. In addition to poor UF control, established CVVH and HD devices require relatively large double-lumen venous access lines (or two separate lines), and circuit volumes of ≥60 mL, which ideally require blood priming of their circuits in infants <7.5 kg.
4. There are two new options based upon conventional engineering designed for infants of ≤10 kg, with circuits of around 30 mL; the CARPEDIEM which is CE marked for European use and has been reported in one baby, and an adaptation of the Aquadex device which has been tested in 12 babies.
5. A novel system with a circuit of 9–17 mL which requires one single-lumen line has been developed for babies of ≤8 kg, and had precise UF control in ten cases. It is currently undergoing a UK-wide study.
6. Until better devices are readily available, conventional CVVH and HD machines used off-license should be primed with blood in small babies, and UF readings should be viewed with caution, and supplemented with clinical observations of fluid balance and weighing where possible.

References

1. Pichler G, Rödl S, Mache C, Trop M, Ring E, Zobel G. Two decades' experience of renal replacement therapy in paediatric patients with acute renal failure. Eur J Pediatr. 2007;166(2):139–44.
2. Selewski DT, Charlton JR, Jetton JG, Guillet R, Mhanna MJ, Askenazi D, et al. Neonatal acute kidney injury. Pediatrics. 2015;136:e463–73.
3. Jhang WK, Kim YA, Ha EJ, Lee YJ, Lee JH, Park YS, et al. Extrarenal sequential organ failure assessment score as an outcome predictor of critically ill children on continuous renal replacement therapy. Pediatr Nephrol. 2014;29:1089–95.
4. Sutherland SM, Alexander SR. Continuous renal replacement therapy in children. Pediatr Nephrol. 2012;27:2007–16.
5. Santiago MJ, Lopez-Herce J, Urbano J, Solana MJ, del Castillo J, Ballestero Y, et al. Clinical course and mortality risk factors in critically ill children requiring continuous renal replacement therapy. Intensive Care Med. 2010;36:843–9.
6. Westrope C, Morris K, Burford D, Morrison G. Continuous hemofiltration in the control of neonatal hyperammonemia: a 10-year experience. Pediatr Nephrol. 2010;25:1725–30.
7. McCaffrey J, Dhakal AK, Milford DV, Webb NJA, Lennon R. Recent developments in the detection and management of kidney injury. Arch Dis Child. 2017;102(1):91–6.
8. Evangelopoulos AA, Vallianou NG, Bountziouka V, Katsagoni C, Bathrellou E, Vogiatzakis ED, et al. Association between serum cystatin C, monocytes and other inflammatory markers. Intern Med J. 2011;42:517–22.
9. Raina R, Chauvin AM, Bunchman T, Askenazi D, Deep A, Ensley MJ, et al. Treatment of AKI in developing and developed countries: an international survey of pediatric dialysis modalities. PLoS One. 2017;12:e0178233.
10. Coulthard MG, Crosier J, Griffiths C, Smith J, Drinnan M, Whitaker M, et al. Haemodialysing babies weighing <8 kg with the Newcastle infant dialysis and ultrafiltration system (Nidus); comparison with peritoneal and conventional haemodialysis. Pediatr Nephrol. 2014;29:1869–71.
11. Shaheen I, Harvey B, Watson AR. Haemofiltration therapy. Paediatr Child Health. 2008;19:121–6.
12. Sohn YB, Paik KH, Cho HY, Kim SJ, Park SW, Kim ES, et al. Continuous renal replacement therapy in neonates weighing less than 3 kg. Korean J Pediatr. 2012;55:286–92.
13. Liu ID, Ng K-H, Lau PY-W, Yeo WS, Koh P-L, Yap H-K. Use of HF20 membrane in critically ill unstable low-body-weight infants on inotropic support. Pediatr Nephrol. 2013;28:819–22.
14. Askenazi DJ, Goldstein SL, Koralkar R, Fortenberry J, Baum M, Hackbarth RM, et al. Continuous renal replacement therapy for children ≤10 kg: a report from the prospective pediatric continuous renal replacement therapy registry. J Pediatr. 2013;162:587–92.
15. Ronco R, Garzotto F, Brendolan A, Zanella M, Bellettato M, Vedovato S, et al. Continuous renal replacement therapy in neonates and small infants: development and first-in-human use of a miniaturised machine (CARPEDIEM). Lancet. 2014;383:1807–13.
16. Askenazi D, Ingram D, White S, Cramer M, Borasino S, Coghill C, et al. Smaller circuits for smaller patients: improving renal support therapy with Aquadex. Pediatr Nephrol. 2016;31:853–60.
17. Symons JM, Brophy PD, Gregory MJ, McAfee N, Somers MJG, Bunchman TE, et al. Continuous renal replacement therapy in children up to 10 kg. Am J Kid Dis. 2003;41:984–9.
18. FDA Updated public health notification: Gambro Prisma® continuous renal replacement system. 2006. http://www.fda.gov/MedicalDevices/Safety/AlertsandNotices/PublicHealthNotifications/ucm062100.htm.
19. Jander A, Tkaczyk M, Pagowska-Klimek I, Pietrzykowski W, Moll J, Krajewski W, et al. Continuous veno-venous hemodiafiltration in children after cardiac surgery. Eur J Cardiothorac Surg. 2007;31:1022–8.
20. Gambro Lundia AB. The Prismaflex® system. www.gambro.com/PageFiles/6046/Prismaflex-5-System-brochure.pdf.

21. Coulthard MG, Sharp J. Haemodialysis and ultrafiltration in babies weighing under 1000 g. Arch Dis Child Fetal Neonatal Ed. 1995;73:F162–5.
22. Everdell NL, Coulthard MG, Crosier J, Keir MJ. A machine for haemodialysing very small infants. Pediatr Nephrol. 2005;20:636–43.
23. Coulthard MG. Ultra-small neonatal dialysis circuits do not maintain safe fluid balance. Pediatr Nephrol. 2016;31:1033.
24. Nishimi S, Ishikawa K, Oda S, Furukawa H, Takada A, Chida S. In vitro ability of a novel system for neonatal extracorporeal renal replacement therapy with ultra-small volume circuit for removing solutes. J Iwate Med Assoc. 2015;67:215–23.
25. Nishimi S, Ishikawa K, Sasaki M, Furukawa H, Takada A, Chida S. Ability of a novel system for neonatal extracorporeal renal replacement therapy with an ultra-small volume circuit to remove solutes *in vitro*. Pediatr Nephrol. 2016;31:493–500.

MIX
Papier aus verantwortungsvollen Quellen
Paper from responsible sources
FSC® C105338

If you have any concerns about our products,
you can contact us on
ProductSafety@springernature.com

In case Publisher is established outside the EU,
the EU authorized representative is:
Springer Nature Customer Service Center GmbH
Europaplatz 3, 69115 Heidelberg, Germany

Printed by Libri Plureos GmbH
in Hamburg, Germany